Essential Neuropharmacology

The Prescriber's Guide

Essential Neuropharmacology
The Prescriber's Guide

Stephen D. Silberstein

Thomas Jefferson University Hospital, Department of Neurology, Philadelphia

Michael J. Marmura

Thomas Jefferson University Hospital, Department of Neurology, Philadelphia

Consultant Editor

Stephen M. Stahl

University of California, San Diego and University of Cambridge, UK

With illustrations by

Nancy Muntner

Neuroscience Education Institute

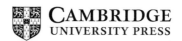
CAMBRIDGE
UNIVERSITY PRESS

CAMBRIDGE UNIVERSITY PRESS
Cambridge, New York, Melbourne, Madrid, Cape Town, Singapore,
São Paulo, Delhi, Dubai, Tokyo

Cambridge University Press
The Edinburgh Building, Cambridge CB2 8RU, UK

Published in the United States of America by Cambridge University Press, New York

www.cambridge.org
Information on this title: www.cambridge.org/9780521136723

First published 2010

Printed in the United Kingdom at the University Press, Cambridge

A catalog record for this publication is available from the British Library

Library of Congress Cataloging in Publication data
Silberstein, Stephen D.
Essential neuropharmacology : the prescriber's guide / Stephen Silberstein, Michael Marmura ; edited
by Stephen M. Stahl ; with illustrations by Nancy Muntner.
    p. ; cm.
Other title: Prescriber's guide
Includes bibliographical references and indexes.
ISBN 978-0-521-13672-3 (pbk.)
1. Neuropharmacology – Handbooks, manuals, etc.   I. Marmura, Michael James.
II. Stahl, S. M.   III. Title.   IV. Title: Prescriber's guide.
[DNLM: 1. Central Nervous System Agents – pharmacology – Handbooks.   2. Central Nervous
System Agents – therapeutic use – Handbooks.   3. Central Nervous System Diseases – drug
therapy – Handbooks.   QV 39 S587e   2010]
RM315.s527   2010
615′.78–dc22

                                                            2010011292

ISBN 978-0-521-13672-3 Paperback

Contents

Introduction   page ix

List of icons   xi

Acknowledgements   xv

1. acetazolamide   1
2. almotriptan   5
3. alteplase   8
4. amantadine   11
5. amitriptyline   14
6. apomorphine   18
7. armodafinil   21
8. aspirin (acetylsalicylic acid)   24
9. azathioprine   28
10. baclofen   32
11. benztropine   36
12. botulinum toxin type A   40
13. botulinum toxin type B   45
14. bromocriptine   48
15. carbamazepine   51
16. carbidopa/levodopa   55
17. carisoprodol   59
18. chlorpromazine   62
19. clonazepam   65
20. clonidine   69
21. clopidogrel   72
22. clozapine   75
23. cyclobenzaprine   78
24. cyclophosphamide   81
25. cyclosporine   84
26. cyproheptadine   87
27. dantrolene   90
28. 3,4-diaminopyridine   93
29. diazepam   96
30. dihydroergotamine   100
31. dipyridamole and aspirin   103
32. donepezil   107

33. droperidol   110
34. duloxetine   113
35. edrophonium   117
36. eletriptan   120
37. entacapone   123
38. ethosuximide   126
39. felbamate   129
40. flunarizine   132
41. fluoxetine   135
42. frovatriptan   139
43. gabapentin   142
44. galantamine   146
45. glatiramer acetate   149
46. guanfacine   152
47. guanidine hydrochloride   155
48. haloperidol   158
49. heparin   161
50. immune globulin intravenous (IGIV)   165
51. indomethacin   169
52. interferon-beta   173
53. lacosamide   177
54. lamotrigine   180
55. levetiracetam   184
56. lithium   187
57. mannitol   191
58. meclizine   194
59. memantine   197
60. metaxalone   200
61. methocarbamol   202
62. methotrexate   205
63. methylergonovine   209
64. methysergide   212
65. metoclopramide   215
66. mexiletine   218
67. mitoxantrone   221
68. modafinil   224
69. mycophenolate mofetil   228
70. naratriptan   231
71. natalizumab   234

72.	nimodipine	237
73.	nortriptyline	240
74.	oxcarbazepine	244
75.	penicillamine	248
76.	phenobarbital	251
77.	phenytoin	255
78.	pizotifen	259
79.	pramipexole	262
80.	prednisone	266
81.	pregabalin	272
82.	primidone	275
83.	prochlorperazine	279
84.	propranolol	282
85.	pyridostigmine	286
86.	quetiapine	289
87.	quinine sulfate	293
88.	rasagiline	296
89.	reserpine	300
90.	riluzole	303
91.	rituximab	306
92.	rivastigmine	309
93.	rizatriptan	312
94.	ropinirole	315
95.	rufinamide	319
96.	selegiline	322
97.	sumatriptan	326
98.	tetrabenazine	329
99.	tiagabine	332
100.	timolol	335
101.	tizanidine	339
102.	topiramate	342
103.	trientine hydrochloride	346
104.	trihexyphenidyl	349
105.	valproic acid	353
106.	venlafaxine	358
107.	verapamil	362
108.	vigabatrin	366
109.	warfarin	369
110.	zolmitriptan	373
111.	zonisamide	376

List of abbreviations   381

Index by drug name   383

Index by use   389

Index by class   401

Introduction

Neurology is the final frontier of medicine, and we are starting to better understand disorders of the central and peripheral nervous system. In the past few decades, we have become increasingly able to diagnose and treat patients with neurologic disorders, resulting in improvements in both their disease and their quality of life. Medication is essential, and understanding its pharmacology is an important part of taking care of patients with neurologic disorders. Despite these advances and our expertise, we still encounter patients who are refractory to the usual therapies. Due to the increasing subspecialization of neurology into fields including epilepsy, stroke, multiple sclerosis, movement disorders, neuromuscular disorders, and headache, physicians require references to guide us in their treatment. This text focuses on the common and less common medications we use in clinical practice and provides useful tips for their use.

Icons

 antiadrenergic

 alpha-2 agonist

 anticonvulsant

 antihistamine

 benzodiazepine

 cholinesterase inhibitor

 antipsychotic

 antiarrhythmic

 lithium

 psychostimulant

 monoamine oxidase inhibitor

 anticholinergic

 anticoagulant

 N-methyl-D-aspartate antagonist

antiemetic

 norepinephrine and dopamine reuptake inhibitor

 antiparkinson agent

 antiplatelet agent

 selective serotonin reuptake inhibitor

 beta-blocker

 serotonin and norepinephrine reuptake inhibitor

 calcium channel blocker

 chelating agent

 cholinergic agonist, potassium channel blocker

 tricyclic/tetracyclic antidepressant

 ergot

 immunomodulator

 neuromuscular drug

neurotoxin

 non-steroidal anti-inflammatory

 osmotic diuretic

 skeletal muscle relaxant

 thrombolytic agent

 triptan

 How the drug works, mechanism of action

 Best augmenting agents to add for partial response or treatment-resistance

 Life-threatening or dangerous adverse effects

 Weight Gain: Degrees of weight gain associated with the drug, with unusual signifying that weight gain is not expected; not unusual signifying that weight gain occurs in a significant minority; common signifying that many experience weight gain and/or it can be significant in amount; and problematic signifying that weight gain occurs frequently, can be significant in amount, and may be a health problem in some patients

 Sedation: Degrees of sedation associated with the drug, with unusual signifying that sedation is not expected; not unusual signifying that sedation occurs in a significant minority; common signifying that many experience sedation and/or it can be significant in amount; and problematic signifying that sedation occurs frequently, can be significant in amount, and may be a health problem in some patients

Tips for dosing based on the clinical expertise of the author

 Drug interactions that may occur

 Warnings and precautions regarding use of the drug

 Dosing and other information specific to children and adolescents

 Information regarding use of the drug during pregnancy

 Clinical pearls of information based on the clinical expertise of the author

 Suggested reading

Acknowledgements

The authors wish to thank Maya Carter MD, Daniel Hexter MD, Daniel Kremens MD, Tso-wei Liang MD, Sangjin Oh MD, and Alex Papangelou MD for their sub-specialty advice and editing. We especially want to thank Lynne Kaiser for her meticulous editing.

Michael Marmura would like to thank his parents, William and Janet, for their boundless love, kindness, and support, which have made me the person I am.

Stephen Silbertstein would like to thank his wife Marsha, children Aaron and Joshua, present and future daughters-in-law Stephanie and Miriam, and his grandson Jake.

ACETAZOLAMIDE

Brands
• Diamox, Azomid, AZM, Dazamide, Novo-Zolamide

Generic?
Yes

Class
• Antiepileptic drug (AED), carbonic anhydrase inhibitor

Commonly Prescribed for
(FDA approved in bold)
• **Adjunctive treatment for centrencephalic epilepsies (petit mal, unlocalized)**
• **Acute mountain sickness**
• **Edema due to congestive heart failure or medication**
• **Glaucoma**
• Idiopathic intracranial hypertension (IIH) (pseudotumor cerebrii)
• Episodic ataxias type 1 and 2
• Hemiplegic migraine
• Marfan syndrome
• Sleep apnea

How the Drug Works
• Blocks the carbonic anhydrase enzyme, which is responsible for converting CO_2 and H_2O to bicarbonate. This increases excretion of sodium, potassium, bicarbonate and water, producing alkaline diuresis. In epilepsy, decreases excessive neuronal discharge in CNS due either to inhibition of carbonic anhydrase or slight degree of acidosis. It also reduces production of CSF and aqueous humor

How Long Until It Works
• Seizures – by 2–3 weeks
• IIH – maximum benefit in 4–6 weeks

If It Works
• Seizures – goal is the remission of seizures. Continue as long as effective and well-tolerated. Consider tapering and slowly stopping after 2 years seizure-free, depending on the type of epilepsy
• IIH – monitor visual fields and papilledema and symptoms such as visual obscurations and headache

If It Doesn't Work
Increase to highest tolerated dose
• Seizures – consider changing to another agent, adding a second agent or referral for epilepsy surgery evaluation. When adding a second agent keep in mind the drug interactions that can occur
• IIH – eliminate symptomatic causes such as drugs or toxins, encourage weight loss if patient is obese, consider loop diuretics or topiramate. Lumbar puncture often provides short-term relief of symptoms. For visual loss, optic nerve defenestration or CSF shunting (lumboperitoneal or ventriculoperitoneal) may be needed

Best Augmenting Combos for Partial Response or Treatment-Resistance
• Epilepsy – acetazolamide itself is usually an augmenting agent. Relatively few interactions with other AEDs. Topiramate and zonisamide have similar mechanisms of action, so acetazolamide is not usually combined with these agents
• IIH – furosemide and topiramate may be helpful. Combine with caution due to risk of kidney stone formation

Tests
• Obtain a CBC when starting drug and during therapy. Check bicarbonate, potassium, and sodium levels if symptoms of metabolic acidosis develop

How Drug Causes AEs
• Related to carbonic anhydrase inhibition, which can cause metabolic acidosis and electrolyte imbalances

Notable AEs
• Paresthesias, tinnitus, anorexia, nausea/vomiting, diarrhea, taste alteration, myopia (transient), renal calculi, and photosensitivity

Life-Threatening or Dangerous AEs
• Blood dyscrasias such as agranulocytosis, hemolytic anemia, leukopenia, thrombocytopenia. Hypokalemia. Rash including Stevens Johnson syndrome

Weight Gain
• Unusual

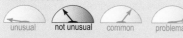

Sedation
• Not unusual

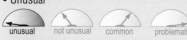

What to Do About AEs
• Lower dose when using for epilepsy or IIH. If AEs are significant, discontinue and change to another agent. Paresthesias may respond to high potassium diets or potassium supplements

Best Augmenting Agents for AEs
• Most AEs cannot be improved by an augmenting agent

DOSING AND USE

Usual Dosage Range
• Epilepsy – 375–1000 mg daily
• IIH – 250–2000 mg daily
• Edema – 250–375 mg qod
• Mountain sickness – 500–1000 mg daily

Dosage Forms
• Tablets: 125, 250 mg. Sustained release 500 mg
• Injection: 500 mg vials

How to Dose
• Epilepsy – Start at 125–250 mg twice daily, with a lower starting dose (250 mg daily) for patients already on other AEDs. Occasionally used at higher doses, but not necessarily more effective
• IIH – Start at 250–500 mg per day in 2 divided doses. Increase as tolerated to 1000 mg/day. Occasionally used at higher doses, depending on tolerability and effect on visual symptoms
• Congestive heart failure – 250–375 mg daily, skipping doses every 2–3 days to maintain effect
• Acute mountain sickness – Start 24–48 hours before ascent and continue for 48 hours or as long as needed to control symptoms. Usual dose 500–1000 mg per day

Dosing Tips
• Citrus juice and fluids may help decrease risk of kidney stone formation. Taking with food can decrease AEs

Overdose
• Ataxia, anorexia, nausea, paresthesias, vomiting, tremor and tinnitus. Induce emesis or gastric lavage. Supplement with bicarbonate or potassium as necessary

Long-Term Use
• Safe for long-term use

Habit Forming
• No

How to Stop
• Taper slowly
• Abrupt withdrawal can lead to seizures in patients with epilepsy
• Papilledema or headaches may recur within days to months of stopping

Pharmacokinetics
• Tablets have peak effect at 1–4 hours, with 8–12 hours duration of action. Sustained release tablets have peak effect at 3–6 hours and duration of 18–24 hours. 70–90% protein bound. Not metabolized and excreted unchanged by kidneys

Drug Interactions
• May decrease levels of primidone
• Increases levels of cyclosporine, possibly leading to nephrotoxicity or neurotoxicity
• Concurrent use with salicyclates can increase AEs of both
• May increase effects of amphetamines

Other Warnings/ Precautions
• Carbonic anhydrase inhibitors are sulfonamides. There may be cross-sensitivity with antibacterial sulfonamides

Do Not Use
• Known hypersensitivity to the drug. Depressed potassium or sodium levels, significant kidney or hepatic disease, hyperchloremic acidosis, adrenocortical insufficiency, and suprarenal gland dysfunction

SPECIAL POPULATIONS

Renal Impairment
- Renal insufficiency can lead to increased toxicity. Use with caution

Hepatic Impairment
- Use with caution. Patients with severe disease have an increased risk of bleeding complications

Cardiac Impairment
- Severe hypokalemia causes cardiac arrhythmias. Chronic metabolic acidosis may lead to hyperventilation and decreases left ventricular function – use with caution in patients on beta-blocker or calcium channel therapy

Elderly
- Use with caution

Children and Adolescents
- Safety and effectiveness in the pediatric population is unknown. Suggested daily dose is 8 to 30 mg/kg

Pregnancy
- Category C. Risks of stopping medication must outweigh risk to fetus for patients with epilepsy. Seizures and potential status epilepticus place the woman and fetus at risk and can cause reduced oxygen and blood supply to the womb
- In IIH, consider lumbar puncture as an alternative to medication, especially in the first few months of pregnancy, and monitor closely for visual changes
- Supplementation with 0.4 mg of folic acid before and during pregnancy is recommended

Breast Feeding
- A small percentage is excreted in breast milk. Monitor infant for sedation, poor feeding or irritability

THE ART OF NEUROPHARMACOLOGY

Potential Advantages
- Inexpensive adjunctive medication for epilepsy and useful in the treatment of IIH and episodic ataxias

Potential Disadvantages
- Not a first-line drug in epilepsy or migraine due to ineffectiveness and AEs

Primary Target Symptoms
- Seizure frequency and severity, headache or papilledema in IIH

 Pearls
- In epilepsy, appears most effective in children with petit mal epilepsy, but may be effective in patients with grand mal, mixed, or myoclonic seizures
- Acetazolamide is occasionally used for treatment of migraine. Large, double-blind, placebo-controlled trials did not indicate effectiveness
- First-line agent for treatment of episodic ataxias at an average dose of 500–750 per day. Type 2 responds better than type 1 in most cases
- Similar to episodic ataxia type 2, familial hemiplegic migraine type 1 is a channelopathy caused by a mutation of the CACNA1A gene. Case reports suggest acetazolamide can be used to treat hemiplegic migraine
- As a diuretic, increased doses do not increase effect. Results are often improved with alternating days of treatment
- The acetazolamide challenge test is used to decide indications for cerebrospinal fluid shunting

Suggested Reading

Celebisoy N, Gökçay F, Sirin H, Akyürekli O. Treatment of idiopathic intracranial hypertension: topiramate vs acetazolamide, an open-label study. Acta Neurol Scand 2007;116(5):322–7.

Kayser B, Hulsebosch R, Bosch F. Low-dose acetylsalicylic acid analog and acetazolamide for prevention of acute mountain sickness. High Alt Med Biol 2008;9(1):15–23.

Kossoff EH, Pyzik PL, Furth SL, Hladky HD, Freeman JM, Vining EP. Kidney stones, carbonic anhydrase inhibitors, and the ketogenic diet. Epilepsia 2002;43(10):1168–71.

Reiss WG, Oles KS. Acetazolamide in the treatment of seizures. Ann Pharmacother 1996;30(5):514–9.

Robbins MS, Lipton RB, Laureta EC, Grosberg BM. CACNA1A nonsense mutation is associated with basilar-type migraine and episodic ataxia type 2. Headache 2009;49 (7):1042–6.

ALMOTRIPTAN

THERAPEUTICS

Brands
- Axert, Almogran

Generic?
No

 Class
- Triptan

Commonly Prescribed for
(FDA approved in bold)
- **Migraine**

 How the Drug Works
- Selective 5-HT1 receptor agonist, working predominantly at the B, D and F receptor subtypes. Effectiveness may be due to blocking the transmission of pain signals from the trigeminal nerve to the trigeminal nucleus caudalis and preventing release of inflammatory neuropeptides rather than just causing vasoconstriction

How Long Until It Works
- 1 hour or less

If It Works
- Continue to take as needed. Patients taking acute treatment more than 2 days/week are at risk for medication overuse headache, especially if they have migraine

If It Doesn't Work
- Treat early in the attack – triptans are less likely to work after the development of cutaneous allodynia, a marker of central sensitization
- For patients with partial response or reoccurrence, add an NSAID
- Change to another agent

 Best Augmenting Combos for Partial Response or Treatment-Resistance
- NSAIDs or neuroleptics are often used to augment response

Tests
- None required

ADVERSE EFFECTS (AEs)

How Drug Causes AEs
- Direct effect on serotonin receptors

Notable AEs
- Tingling, flushing, sensation of burning, vertigo, sensation of pressure, heaviness, nausea

 Life-Threatening or Dangerous AEs
- Rare cardiac events including acute MI, cardiac arrhythmia, and coronary artery vasospasm have been reported with almotriptan

Weight Gain
- Unusual

Sedation
- Unusual

What to Do About AEs
- In most cases, only reassurance is needed. Lower dose, change to another triptan or use an alternative headache treatment

Best Augmenting Agents for AEs
- Treatment of nausea with antiemetics is acceptable. Other AEs improve with time

DOSING AND USE

Usual Dosage Range
- 6.25–12.5 mg

Dosage Forms
- Tablets: 6.25 and 12.5 mg

How to Dose
- Tablets: Most patients respond best at 12.5 mg oral dose. Give 1 pill at the onset of an attack and repeat in 2 hours for a partial response or if headache returns. Maximum 25 mg/day. Limit 10 days per month

Dosing Tips
- Treat early in attack

Overdose
- May cause hypertension, cardiovascular symptoms. Other possible symptoms include seizure, tremor, extremity erythema, cyanosis or ataxia. For patients with angina, perform ECG and monitor for ischemia for at least 20 hours

Long-Term Use
- Monitor for cardiac risk factors with continued use

Habit Forming
- No

How to Stop
- No need to taper. Patients who overuse triptans often experience withdrawal headaches lasting up to several days

Pharmacokinetics
- Half-life about 3 hours. Tmax 2.5 hours. Bioavailability is 80%. Metabolized by MAO A enzyme as well as cytochrome P450 (CYP3A4 and CYP2D6) isozymes. 35% protein binding

 Drug Interactions
- Monoamine oxidase (MAO) inhibitors may make it difficult for drug to be metabolized
- Theoretical interactions with SSRI/SNRI. It is unclear whether triptans pose any risk for the development of serotonin syndrome in clinical practice
- Minimal increase in concentration with CYP-3A4 inhibitors – no need for dose adjustment

Do Not Use
- Within 2 weeks of MAO inhibitors, or 24 hours of ergot-containing medications such as dihydroergotamine
- Patients with proven hypersensitivity to eletriptan, known cardiovascular disease, uncontrolled hypertension, or Prinzmetal's angina
- Almotriptan was not studied in patients with hemiplegic and basilar migraine
- May worsen symptoms in ischemic bowel disease

SPECIAL POPULATIONS

Renal Impairment
- Concentration increases in those with moderate-severe renal impairment (creatinine clearance less than 30 mL/min). May be at increased cardiovascular risk

Hepatic Impairment
- Drug metabolism may be decreased. Do not use with severe hepatic impairment

Cardiac Impairment
- Do not use in patients with known cardiovascular or peripheral vascular disease

Elderly
- May be at increased cardiovascular risk

 Children and Adolescents
- Safety and efficacy have not been established
- Triptan trials in children were negative, due to higher placebo response

 Pregnancy
- Category C. Use only if potential benefit outweighs risk to the fetus. Migraine often improves in pregnancy, and other acute agents (opioids, neuroleptics, prednisone) have more proven safety

Breast Feeding
- Almotriptan is found in breast milk. Use with caution

THE ART OF NEUROPHARMACOLOGY

Potential Advantages
- Effective with good consistency and excellent tolerability, even compared to other oral triptans. Less risk of abuse than opioids or barbiturate-containing treatments

Potential Disadvantages
- Cost, and the potential for medication overuse headache. May not be as effective as other triptans

Primary Target Symptoms

- Headache pain, nausea, photo- and phonophobia

Pearls

- Early treatment of migraine is most effective
- Lower AEs compared to other triptans. Good consistency and pain-free response, making it a good choice for patients with anxiety prone to medication side effects
- May not be effective when taken during the aura, or before headache begins

- In patients with "status migrainosus" (migraine lasting more than 72 hours) neuroleptics and dihydroergotamine are more effective
- Triptans were not originally studied for use in the treatment of basilar or hemiplegic migraine
- Patients taking triptans more than 10 days/ month are at increased risk of medication overuse headache which is less responsive to treatment
- Chest and throat tightness are usually benign and may be related to esophageal spasm rather than cardiac ischemia. These symptoms occur more commonly in patients without cardiac risk factors

Suggested Reading

Diener HC, Gendolla A, Gebert I, Beneke M. Almotriptan in migraine patients who respond poorly to oral sumatriptan: a double-blind, randomized trial. Eur Neurol 2005;53 (Suppl 1):41–8.

Dodick D, Lipton RB, Martin V, Papademetriou V, Rosamond W, MaassenVanDenBrink A, Loutfi H, Welch KM, Goadsby PJ, Hahn S, Hutchinson S, Matchar D, Silberstein S, Smith TR, Purdy RA, Saiers J; Triptan Cardiovascular Safety Expert Panel. Consensus statement: cardiovascular safety profile of triptans (5-HT agonists) in the acute treatment of migraine. Headache 2004;44(5):414–25.

Ferrari MD, Roon KI, Lipton RB, Goadsby PJ. Oral triptans (serotonin 5-HT (1B/1D) agonists) in acute migraine treatment: a meta-analysis of 53 trials. Lancet 2001;358(9294):1668–75.

Gladstone JP, Gawel M. Newer formulations of the triptans: advances in migraine management. Drugs 2003;63(21):2285–305.

Mathew NT, Finlayson G, Smith TR, Cady RK, Adelman J, Mao L, Wright P, Greenberg SJ; AEGIS Investigator Study Group. Early intervention with almotriptan: results of the AEGIS trial (AXERT Early Migraine Intervention Study). Headache 2007;47(2):189–98.

THERAPEUTICS

Brands
• Activase

Generic?
Yes

Class
• Tissue plasminogen activator (TPA), thrombolytic agent

Commonly Prescribed for
(FDA approved in bold)
• **Acute ischemic stroke (AIS)**
• **Acute myocardial infarction (AMI)**
• **Pulmonary embolism (PE)**
• **Restoration of function to central venous access device**

How the Drug Works
• Alteplase is a tissue plasminogen activator. It binds to fibrin in a thrombus and converts the entrapped plasminogen to plasmin, initiating a local fibrinolysis with little systemic effect

How Long Until It Works
• Less than 1 hour, often earlier

If It Works
• After administration, monitor in intensive care – preferably in an acute stroke or cardiac unit

If It Doesn't Work
• Alteplase is not always effective and has risks. After initial monitoring period in intensive care, continue standard AIS, AMI, or PE care

Best Augmenting Combos for Partial Response or Treatment-Resistance
• Not combined with other agents. Use caution with patients already taking anticoagulants or antiplatelet medications

Tests
• Ensure no contraindications are present before administering drug. For all patients with suspected AIS with onset less than 3 hours prior, immediately type and screen, obtain CBC, glucose, coagulation tests, and ensure no intracranial bleeding (usually with head CT)

ADVERSE EFFECTS (AEs)

How Drug Causes AEs
• Activating plasminogen increases bleeding risk

Notable AEs
• Superficial bleeding (i.e., at puncture sites), fever, hypotension, dyspnea, nausea, urticaria, and flushing

Life-Threatening or Dangerous AEs
• Internal bleeding (intracranial, GI, GU, or retroperitoneal), anaphylactic reaction, reperfusion arrhythmias, and thrombocytopenia

Weight Gain
• Unusual

unusual   not unusual   common   problematic

Sedation
• Unusual

unusual   not unusual   common   problematic

What to Do About AEs
• Stop infusion for any serious bleeding. Can use fresh frozen plasma if needed

Best Augmenting Agents for AEs
• Most AEs cannot be improved by an augmenting agent

DOSING AND USE

Usual Dosage Range
• 90 mg or less for AIS, 100 mg or less for AMI or PE

Dosage Forms
• Lyophilized powder for injection: 50 mg in 50 mL or 100 mg in 100 mL

How to Dose

- AIS – Give 0.9 mg/kg (not to exceed 90 mg), with 10% of the dose given in the first 1 minute and the remainder infused over 1 hour
- AMI – Give 15 mg as a bolus for all patients. For patients weighing more than 67 kg, then give another 50 mg over 30 minutes and then 35 mg over the next 60 minutes. For patients less than 67 kg, give 0.75 mg/kg over the 30 minutes after the bolus and then 0.50 mg/kg over the next 60 minutes
- PE – 100 mg over 2 hours and restart heparin once partial thromboplastin or thrombin time is less than twice normal

 Dosing Tips

- Give alteplase as soon after AIS as possible to achieve best functional outcome once it has been determined that there are no contraindications

Overdose

- Bleeding complications are common. Treat, if needed, with fresh frozen plasma. Bradycardia, flushing, dyspnea, or hypotension can occur

Long-Term Use

- May be repeated after weeks of previous use if indicated. Not used for prophylaxis

Habit Forming

- No

How to Stop

- Not applicable

Pharmacokinetics

- Rapid hepatic metabolism by hydrolysis. 80% of drug is cleared within 10 minutes after ending infusion

 Drug Interactions

- Anticoagulants such as heparin, vitamin K antagonists increase bleeding risk
- Antiplatelet agents such as aspirin, dipyridamole, clopidogrel, and abciximab may increase bleeding risk when given prior to or soon after alteplase therapy
- NSAIDs may increase risk of GI bleed

- Nitroglycerin decreases alteplase concentrations. Avoid using
- Valproate may increase concentrations
- Dopamine may reduce activity and cause particulate formation

 Other Warnings/ Precautions

- Cholesterol embolism causing renal failure, pancreatitis, bowel infarction, gangrenous digits, or AMI is a rare complication of thrombolysis

Do Not Use

- Evidence of intracranial hemorrhage or suspected subarachnoid hemorrhage
- Serious head trauma
- History of intracranial bleeding, neoplasm, or arteriovenous malformation
- Active internal bleeding
- Recent intracranial or intraspinal surgery
- Seizure at the onset of stroke
- Bleeding diathesis (current warfarin use, prothrombin time > 15 seconds, heparin use with elevated partial prothrombin time, or platelets count < 100,000 mm^3)
- Uncontrolled hypertension at the time of treatment (greater than 185 systolic or 110 diastolic)

SPECIAL POPULATIONS

Renal Impairment

- No change in dose required

Hepatic Impairment

- Reduce dose and use with caution

Cardiac Impairment

- No known effects

Elderly

- Patients over 75 are more likely to have bleeding complications

 Children and Adolescents

- Not studied in children

Pregnancy

- Category C. Use if potential benefit outweighs risks. Increased risk of hemorrhage when given less than 10 days post-partum

Breast Feeding

- Unknown if present in breast milk, use with caution

THE ART OF NEUROPHARMACOLOGY

Potential Advantages

- Proven treatment for acute stroke

Potential Disadvantages

- Must be used within the acute window. Multiple potential complications

Primary Target Symptoms

- Improving the neurologic disability and reducing disability resulting from ischemic stroke

Pearls

- Effective in improving disability when given in 4.5 hour window. Outcomes are better when treating early. Treat as early as possible after AIS when safe to do so
- In clinical trials use was often followed by anticoagulation with heparin for AMI or AIS
- Control blood pressure and maintain below 185/110 mm Hg during treatment. Blood pressures are often elevated in AIS
- Of 100 patients treated with alteplase for AIS, about 11 of those will recover with minimal or no disability compared with placebo
- Less likely to be effective for larger artery AIS (i.e., carotid occlusion)

Suggested Reading

Albers GW, Bates VE, Clark WM, Bell R, Verro P, Hamilton SA. Intravenous tissue-type plasminogen activator for treatment of acute stroke: the Standard Treatment with Alteplase to Reverse Stroke (STARS) study. JAMA 2000;283 (9):1145–50.

Cumbler E, Glasheen J. Management of blood pressure after acute ischemic stroke: An evidence-based guide for the hospitalist. J Hosp Med 2007;2(4):261–7.

Demchuk AM, Tanne D, Hill MD, Kasner SE, Hanson S, Grond M, Levine SR; Multicentre tPA Stroke Survey Group. Predictors of good outcome after intravenous tPA for acute ischemic stroke. Neurology 2001;57(3):474–80.

Saver JL, Albers GW, Dunn B, Johnston KC, Fisher M; STAIR VI Consortium. Stroke Therapy Academic Industry Roundtable (STAIR) recommendations for extended window acute stroke therapy trials. Stroke 2009;40(7):2594–600.

THERAPEUTICS

Brands
• Symmetrel

Generic?
Yes

Class
• Antiparkinson agent

Commonly Prescribed for
(FDA approved in bold)
• **Parkinson's disease (PD)**
• **Drug-induced extrapyramidal reactions**
• **Influenza-A prophylaxis/treatment**
• Post-encephalitic Parkinsonism
• Vascular Parkinsonism
• Fatigue in multiple sclerosis (MS)
• Enhancing arousal after traumatic brain injury
• Attention deficit hyperactivity disorder
• SSRI-related sexual dysfunction

How the Drug Works
• The mechanism of action in PD is poorly understood but animal studies suggest either that it induces release or decreases reuptake of dopamine. Also is a weak *N*-methyl-D-aspartic acid (NMDA) receptor antagonist which in animals decreases release of acetylcholine from the striatum. Treats and prevents influenza-A by preventing the release of viral nucleic acid into the host cell due to interfering with the function of a viral M2 protein. It may also prevent virus assembly during replication

How Long Until It Works
• PD – 48 hours or less

If It Works
• PD – most patients require dose adjustment over time and most PD patients will need to take other agents, such as levodopa

If It Doesn't Work
• PD – Motor symptoms, such as bradykinesia, gait, and tremor should improve. Reduces extrapyramidal reactions, such as dyskinesias, and can allow reduction of carbidopa-levodopa doses. Non-motor symptoms, including autonomic symptoms such as postural hypotension, depression, and bladder dysfunction, do not improve. If the patient has significantly impaired functioning, add levodopa or a dopamine agonist
• Fatigue – MS-related fatigue may respond to pemoline or modafinil

Best Augmenting Combos for Partial Response or Treatment-Resistance
• For suboptimal effectiveness add carbidopa-levodopa with or without a COMT inhibitor or dopamine agonist depending on disease severity. Monoamine oxidase (MAO)-B inhibitors may also be beneficial
• For younger patOients with bothersome tremor: anticholinergics may help
• For severe motor fluctuations and/or dyskinesias with good "on" time, functional neurosurgery is an option
• Depression is common in PD and may respond to low dose selective serotonin reuptake inhibitors
• Cognitive impairment/dementia is common in mid-late stage PD and may improve with acetylcholinesterase inhibitors
• For patients with late-stage PD experiencing hallucinations or delusions, withdraw amantadine and consider oral atypical neuroleptics (quetiapine, olanzapine, clozapine). Acute psychosis is a medical emergency that may require hospitalization

Tests
• None required

ADVERSE EFFECTS (AEs)

How Drug Causes AEs
• Effects on dopamine concentrations and possible anticholinergic effects

Notable AEs
• Nausea, dizziness, insomnia, and blurry vision most common. Depression, anxiety, confusion, livedo reticularis, dry mouth, constipation, peripheral edema, orthostatic hypotension, nervousness, and headache can occur. Can exacerbate preexisting seizure disorders

Life-Threatening or Dangerous AEs

- Abrupt discontinuation has been associated with the development of neuroleptic malignant syndrome
- Rare suicide attempts or ideation, even in those with no history of psychiatric disorders

Weight Gain

- Unusual

unusual   not unusual   common   problematic

Sedation

- Not unusual

unusual   not unusual   common   problematic

What to Do About AEs

- Titrate slowly to avoid GI side effects. Most AEs require reducing dose or stopping medication

Best Augmenting Agents for AEs

- Most AEs cannot be improved by use of an augmenting agent

DOSING AND USE

Usual Dosage Range

- PD – 100–200 mg in divided doses. Occasionally up to 400 mg/day

Dosage Forms

- Tablets/Capsules: 100 mg
- `Syrup: 50 mg/5ml

How to Dose

- Start at 100 mg daily or 100 mg twice daily in patients on no other PD medications with no other major medical problems. In 1 week or more can increase by 100 mg
- Occasional patients will require doses of 300 mg or 400 mg in divided doses to achieve optimal clinical effect

 Dosing Tips

- Initial sedation may improve with time or dividing doses

Overdose

- Symptoms relate to anticholinergic effects. May include renal, respiratory, or CNS AEs or cardiac effects, including arrhythmia, tachycardia, or hypertension. Deaths have been reported with as little as 1 g

Long-Term Use

- Safe for long-term use. Effectiveness may decrease over time

Habit Forming

- No

How to Stop

- Taper slowly and monitor for parkinsonian crisis. Abrupt withdrawal may also precipitate delirium, hallucinations, agitation, depression, pressured speech, anxiety, stupor, or paranoia

Pharmacokinetics

- Most of the drug is excreted unchanged in the urine. Peak effect is at 1.5–8 hours and half-life an average of 17 hours. Doses over 200 mg may cause greater than proportional increases in levels

 Drug Interactions

- Anticholinergics can increase the mild anticholinergic effects of amantadine
- Quinidine, triamterene, thiazide diuretics, and trimethoprim/sulfamethoxazole impair renal clearance of amantadine and can increase plasma concentrations
- Thioridazine with amantadine can increase PD tremor

 Other Warning Precautions

- May cause mydriasis due to anticholinergic AEs. Do not give to patients with untreated angle closure glaucoma

Do Not Use

- Known hypersensitivity to the drug

SPECIAL POPULATIONS

Renal Impairment
- Decrease dose for impaired function. Creatinine clearance 30–50 mL/min: 200 day 1 then 100 daily. 15–29: 200 day 1 then 100 every other day. <15 or hemodialysis: 200 mg every 7 days

Hepatic Impairment
- May cause elevation of liver enzymes. Use with caution

Cardiac Impairment
- Infrequently causes congestive heart failure or peripheral edema. Use with caution

Elderly
- There is reduced drug clearance, but no dose adjustment needed as the dose used is the lowest that provides clinical improvement

Children and Adolescents
- Use for influenza treatment in children aged 1 or greater. (PD is rare in pediatrics.)

Pregnancy
- Category C. Teratogenic in some animal studies. Risks may include cardiovascular maldevelopment. Use only if benefits of medication outweigh risks

Breast Feeding
- Excreted in breast milk. Do not use

THE ART OF NEUROPHARMACOLOGY

Potential Advantages
- Relief of dyskinesias in PD. Relatively quick-acting and less sedation than other treatments

Potential Disadvantages
- Usually not first-line treatment. No evidence of neuroprotection against PD. Generally less effective than levodopa and risks significant CNS AEs including hallucinations

Primary Target Symptoms
- PD – motor dysfunction and dyskinesias

 Pearls
- Useful for PD patients with dyskinesias
- Can cause anticholinergic AEs (dry mouth, urinary retention) despite no known action on receptors. This and hallucinations may limit treatment
- Used for the treatment of MS-related fatigue at doses of 200–400 mg/day
- May be useful in the treatment of traumatic brain injury, including children, at doses of 200–400 mg/daily

 Suggested Reading

Abdel-Salam OM. Drugs used to treat Parkinson's disease, present status and future directions. CNS Neurol Disord Drug Targets 2008;7(4):321–42.

Chen JJ, Swope DM. Pharmacotherapy for Parkinson's disease. Pharmacotherapy 2007;27(12 Pt 2):161S–173S.

Pucci E, Branãs P, D'Amico R, Giuliani G, Solari A, Taus C. Amantadine for fatigue in multiple sclerosis. Cochrane Database Syst Rev 2007;(1):CD002818.

Sawyer E, Mauro LS, Ohlinger MJ. Amantadine enhancement of arousal and cognition after traumatic brain injury. Ann Pharmacother 2008;42(2):247–52.

AMITRIPTYLINE

THERAPEUTICS

Brands
- Elavil, Triptafen, Tryptanol, Endep, Elatrol, Tryptizol, Trepiline, Laroxyl, Saroten, Triptyl, Redomex

Generic?
Yes

Class
- Tricyclic antidepressant (TCA)

Commonly Prescribed for
(FDA approved in bold)
- **Depression**
- Migraine prophylaxis
- Tension-type headache prophylaxis
- Diabetic neuropathy
- Post-herpetic neuralgia
- Peripheral neuropathy with pain
- Back or neck pain
- Phantom limb pain
- Fibromyalgia
- Bulimia nervosa
- Insomnia
- Anxiety
- Nocturnal enuresis
- Pseudobulbar affect
- Arthritic pain

How the Drug Works
- Blocks serotonin and norepinephrine reuptake pumps increasing their levels within hours, but antidepressant effect takes weeks. Effect is more likely related to adaptive changes in serotonin and norepinephrine receptor systems over time. It also has antihistamine properties which most likely causes the sedation in treating insomnia

How Long Until It Works
- Migraines – effective in as little as 2 weeks, but can take up to 3 months on a stable dose to see full effect
- Neuropathic pain – usually some effect within 4 weeks
- Insomnia, anxiety, depression – may be effective immediately, but effects often delayed 2 to 4 weeks

If It Works
- Migraine – goal is a 50% or greater reduction in migraine frequency or severity. Consider tapering or stopping if headaches remit for more than 6 months or if considering pregnancy
- Neuropathic pain – the goal is to reduce pain intensity and symptoms, but usually does not produce remission
- Insomnia – continue to use if tolerated and encourage good sleep hygiene

If It Doesn't Work
- Increase to highest tolerated dose
- Migraine: address other issues, such as medication-overuse, other coexisting medical disorders, such as anxiety, and consider changing to another agent or adding a second agent
- Chronic pain: either change to another agent or add a second agent
- Insomnia: if no sedation occurs despite adequate dosing, stop and change to another agent

Best Augmenting Combos for Partial Response or Treatment-Resistance
- Migraine: For some patients, low-dose polytherapy with 2 or more drugs may be better tolerated and more effective than high-dose monotherapy. May use in combination with AEDs, antihypertensives, natural products, and non-medication treatments, such as biofeedback, to improve headache control
- Chronic pain: AEDs, such as gabapentin, pregabalin, carbamazepine and capsaicin, mexiletine, are agents used for neuropathic pain. Opioids are appropriate for long-term use in some cases but require careful monitoring

Tests
- Check ECG for QT corrected (QTc) prolongation at baseline and when increasing dose, especially in those with a personal or family history of QTc prolongation, cardiac arrhythmia, heart failure or recent myocardial infarction. If patient is on diuretics, measure potassium and magnesium at baseline and periodically with treatment

ADVERSE EFFECTS (AEs)

How Drug Causes AEs

- Anticholinergic and antihistaminic properties are causes of most common AEs. Blockade of alpha-adrenergic-1 receptor may cause orthostasis and sedation

Notable AEs

- Constipation, dry mouth, blurry vision, increased appetite, nausea, diarrhea, heartburn, weight gain, urinary retention, sexual dysfunction, sweating, itching, rash, fatigue, weakness, sedation, nervousness, restlessness

 ### Life-Threatening and Dangerous AEs

- Orthostatic hypotension, tachycardia, QTc prolongation, and rarely death
- Increased intraocular pressure
- Paralytic ileus, hyperthermia
- Rare activation of mania or suicidal ideation
- Rare worsening of existing seizure disorders

Weight Gain

- Common

Sedation

- Common

What to Do About AEs

- For minor AEs, lower dose or switch to another agent. If tiredness/sedation are bothersome, change to a secondary amine (i.e., nortriptyline). For serious AEs, lower dose and consider stopping

Best Augmenting Agents for AEs

- Try magnesium for constipation. For migraine, consider using with agents that cause weight loss (i.e., topiramate)

DOSING AND USE

Usual Dosage Range

- Migraine/Pain: 10–100 mg/day
- Depression, anxiety: 50–150 mg/day

Dosage Forms

- Tablets: 10, 25, 50, 75, 100 and 150 mg

How to Dose

- Initial dose 10–25 mg/day taken about 1 hour before retiring. Effective range from 10–400 mg but typically 150 mg or less

 ### Dosing Tips

- Start at a low dose, usually 10 mg, and titrate up every few days as tolerated. Low doses are often effective for pain even though they are below the usual effective antidepressant dose

Overdose

- Cardiac arrhythmias and ECG changes; death can occur. CNS depression, convulsions, severe hypotension, and coma are not rare. Patients should be hospitalized. Sodium bicarbonate can treat arrhythmias and hypotension. Treat shock with vasopressors, oxygen, or corticosteroids

Long-Term Use

- Safe for long-term use

Habit Forming

- No

How to Stop

- Taper slowly to avoid withdrawal, including rebound insomnia. Withdrawal usually lasts less than 2 weeks. For patients with well-controlled pain disorders, taper very slowly (over months) and monitor for recurrence of symptoms

Pharmacokinetics

- Metabolized by CYP450 system, especially CYP2D6, 1A2. Half-life 10–28 h and metabolized to nortriptyline

 ### Drug Interactions

- CYP2D6 inhibitors (duloxetine, paroxetine, fluoxetine, bupropion), cimetidine, and valproic acid can increase drug concentration
- Fluvoxamine, a CYP1A2 inhibitor, prevents metabolism to nortriptyline and increases amitriptyline concentrations

- Tramadol increases risk of seizures in patients taking TCAs
- Phenothiazines increase tricyclic levels
- Enzyme inducers, such as rifamycin, smoking, phenobarbital can lower levels
- Use with clonidine has been associated with increases in blood pressure and hypertensive crisis
- May reduce absorption and bioavailability of levodopa
- May alter effects of antihypertensive medications and prolongation of QTc, especially problematic in patients taking drugs that induce bradycardia
- Use together with anticholinergics can increase AEs (i.e., risk of ileus)
- Methylphenidate may inhibit metabolism and increase AEs
- Use within 2 weeks of monoamine oxidase (MAO) inhibitors may risk serotonin syndrome

 Other Warnings/ Precautions

- May increase risk of seizure

Do Not Use
- Proven hypersensitivity to drug or other TCAs
- In acute recovery after myocardial infarction or uncompensated heart failure
- In conjunction with antiarrhythmics that prolong QTc interval
- In conjunction with medications that inhibit CYP2D6

SPECIAL POPULATIONS

Renal Impairment
- Use with caution. May need to lower dose

Hepatic Impairment
- Use with caution. May need to lower dose

Cardiac Impairment
- Do not use in patients with recent myocardial infarction, severe heart failure, history of QTc prolongation, or orthostatic hypotension

Elderly
- More sensitive to AEs, such as sedation, hypotension. Start with lower doses

 Children and Adolescents
- Some data for children over 12 and an appropriate treatment for adolescents with migraine, especially children with insomnia who are not overweight. In children less than 12, most commonly used at low dose for treatment of enuresis

 Pregnancy
- Category C. Crosses the placenta and may cause fetal malformations or withdrawal. Generally not recommended for the treatment of pain or insomnia during pregnancy. For patients with depression or anxiety, selective serotonin reuptake inhibitors (SSRIs) may be safer than TCAs

Breast Feeding
- Some drug is found in breast milk and use while breast feeding is not recommended

THE ART OF NEUROPHARMACOLOGY

Potential Advantages
- Proven effectiveness in multiple pain disorders. Can treat insomnia and depression, which are common in patients with chronic pain

Potential Disadvantages
- AEs are often greater than SSRIs or SNRIs and many AEDs. More anticholinergic AEs than other TCAs. Weight gain and sedation can be problematic

Primary Target Symptoms
- Headache frequency and severity
- Reduction in neuropathic pain

 Pearls
- In patients with chronic pain, offers relief at doses below usual antidepressant doses, and can treat coexisting insomnia
- For patients with significant anxiety or depressive disorders, not as effective as newer drugs with more AEs. Consider treatment of depression or anxiety with

another agent together with a low dose of amitriptyline or other TCA for pain
- TCAs can often precipitate mania in patients with bipolar disorder. Use with caution
- Despite interactions, expert psychiatrists may use with MAO inhibitors for refractory depression
- Many patients do not improve. The number of patients needed to treat for moderate pain relief in neuropathic pain is 2–3
- Increases non-REM sleep time and decreases sleep latency

- Effective for nocturnal enuresis in children. Usual dose is 25 mg for children 6–10 and 50 mg for those 11 and older
- May be used to treat pathologic laughing or crying due to forebrain disease at doses of 30–75 mg per day
- Previously used for ADHD before new treatments became available. May be useful as an adjunct for patients with pain and coexisting ADHD
- TCAs may increase risk of metabolic syndrome

 Suggested Reading

Bryson HM, Wilde MI. Amitriptyline. A review of its pharmacological properties and therapeutic use in chronic pain states. Drugs Aging 1996;8(6):459–76.

Silberstein SD, Goadsby PJ. Migraine: preventive treatment. Cephalalgia 2002;22(7):491–512.

Verdu B, Decosterd I, Buclin T, Stiefel F, Berney A. Antidepressants for the treatment of chronic pain. Drugs 2008;68(18):2611–32.

Zin CS, Nissen LM, Smith MT, O'Callaghan JP, Moore BJ. An update on the pharmacological management of post-herpetic neuralgia and painful diabetic neuropathy. CNS Drugs 2008;22(5):417–42

APOMORPHINE

THERAPEUTICS

Brands
- Apokyn, Apo-go, Uprima

Generic?
No

 ### Class
- Dopamine agonist, non-ergot

Commonly Prescribed for
(FDA approved in bold)
- **Parkinson's disease (PD): acute intermittent treatment of "off" episodes**

 ### How the Drug Works
- Dopamine agonist, with high affinity for the D2 receptor. This action is likely the main reason for effectiveness in PD

How Long Until It Works
- PD – 10–60 minutes

If It Works
- PD – this is an adjunctive medication designed for use with other PD treatments. Continue to adjust other PD treatments to achieve maximum functionality

If It Doesn't Work
- PD – adjust PD medication regimen, determine compliance with medications and reconsider the diagnosis

Best Augmenting Combos for Partial Response or Treatment-Resistance
- Patients requiring frequent injections will need an improved treatment plan to avoid severe "off" periods. Strategies include shortening the interval of levodopa dosing, adding COMT inhibitors, or adding longer-acting dopamine agonists

Tests
- None required

ADVERSE EFFECTS (AEs)

How Drug Causes AEs
- Direct effect on dopamine receptors

Notable AEs
- Injection site reactions, drowsiness, nausea or vomiting, dizziness, postural hypotension, hallucinations, edema. Less common hypersexuality or erections

 ### Life-Threatening or Dangerous AEs
- May cause somnolence or sudden onset sleep. Severe orthostatic hypotension and nausea/vomiting, even when compared to other PD treatments

Weight Gain
- Unusual

unusual | not unusual | common | problematic

Sedation
- Common

unusual | not unusual | common | problematic

What to Do About AEs
- Orthostatic hypotension: the first dose should be given in a monitored setting (such as a physician's office). Check supine and standing blood pressure predose and 20, 40, and 60 minutes after injection. If there is no clinical improvement and no AEs, a dose of 4 mg can be given, no earlier than 2 hours after the initial dose

Best Augmenting Agents for AEs
- Nausea/vomiting: At least 3 days before initiating therapy, start trimethobenzamide 300 mg 3 times a day and continue this for at least 2 months. When given alone, apomorphine causes severe nausea and vomiting. Domperidone, an antidopaminergic drug that does not cross the blood–brain barrier, is an alternative treatment for nausea – typically starting at 10 mg 3–4 times a day

DOSING AND USE

Usual Dosage Range
• PD – 2–6 mg per dose, up to 20 mg per day

Dosage Forms
• SC injection: 10 mg/1 mL in 30 mL cartridges

How to Dose
• PD: Before starting therapy, monitor for orthostatic hypotension
• The usual starting dose for acute "off" episodes is 1 mg less than the tolerated test dose. If the patient tolerates the 4 mg test dose, start at 3 mg. If the patient tolerates 3 mg, start at 2 mg and so on

 Dosing Tips
• Start with low dose and increase as needed and based on response and side effects
• For patients resuming therapy after an interruption of 1 week or more, start at the 2 mg dose. The dose may then be increased by 1 mg every few days as an outpatient to a maximum of 6 mg per dose and total daily dose of 20 mg per day. The average number of daily doses in clinical trials was 3 per patient

Overdose
• Symptoms include severe orthostatic hypotension, nausea and vomiting. Somnolence, agitation, chest and abdominal pain, or dyskinesias can occur

Long-Term Use
• Safe for long-term use

Habit Forming
• No

How to Stop
• Designed for acute use only

Pharmacokinetics
• Peak plasma levels in 10–60 minutes

 Drug Interactions
• Serotonin 5-HT3 antagonists used to treat nausea such as ondansetron, dolasetron can cause profound hypotension and loss of consciousness

• Use with caution with antihypertensives (due to risk of orthostatic hypotension) or QTc prolonging medications
• Dopamine antagonists reduce drug effectiveness

 Other Warnings/ Precautions
• Sodium metabisulfite is a metabolite and can cause reactions in patients allergic to sulfites

Do Not Use
• Hypersensitivity to the drug

SPECIAL POPULATIONS

Renal Impairment
• Mild-moderate impairment: start at 1 mg instead of 2 mg

Hepatic Impairment
• Increased concentrations can occur with mild-moderate impairment. Use with caution

Cardiac Impairment
• No known effects

Elderly
• No dose adjustment needed with normal renal function. The dose used is the lowest that provides clinical improvement

 Children and Adolescents
• Not studied in children (PD is rare in pediatrics)

 Pregnancy
• Category C. Use only if benefits of medication outweigh risks

Breast Feeding
• Unknown if excreted in breast milk

THE ART OF NEUROPHARMACOLOGY

Potential Advantages

- PD: The only drug approved for emergency treatment of "off" episodes in PD. Rapid onset of action

Potential Disadvantages

- Severe nausea. Cost. Advanced PD patients often have difficulty using SC injection during "off" periods and a caregiver may be needed

Primary Target Symptoms

- PD – acute freezing and "off" episodes with markedly impaired motor dysfunction including bradykinesia, hand function, gait and rest tremor

Pearls

- For patients with advanced PD, make sure to ask about "off" periods: how often they occur, severity, and how the patient or caregiver manages them
- In advanced PD, "freezing" becomes more unpredictable over time despite well-designed medication regimens, and apomorphine can be a useful adjunct
- May be particularly helpful for nighttime symptoms, including pain and restless leg syndrome

 Suggested Reading

Gunzler SA. Apomorphine in the treatment of Parkinson disease and other movement disorders. Expert Opin Pharmacother 2009;10(6):1027–38.

Kolls BJ, Stacy M. Apomorphine: a rapid rescue agent for the management of motor fluctuations in advanced Parkinson disease. Clin Neuropharmacol 2006;29(5):292–301.

Kvernmo T, Houben J, Sylte I. Receptor-binding and pharmacokinetic properties of dopaminergic agonists. Curr Top Med Chem 2008;8(12): 1049–67.

Stacy M, Silver D. Apomorphine for the acute treatment of "off" episodes in Parkinson's disease. Parkinsonism Relat Disord 2008; 14(2):85–92.

ARMODAFINIL

THERAPEUTICS

Brands
- Nuvigil

Generic?
No

Class
- Wake-promoting agent

Commonly Prescribed for
(FDA approved in bold)
- **Reducing excessive sleepiness in patients with narcolepsy or shift-work related sleep disorder**
- **Reducing excessive sleepiness in patients with obstructive sleep apnea (OSA)/hypopnea syndrome**

How the Drug Works
- Unlike traditional stimulants which act directly via dopaminergic pathways, it may also act in the hypothalamus by stimulating wake-promoting areas, or inhibiting sleep-promoting areas
- It may also have effects on dopamine transporter pathways similar to other stimulants, hypothetically inhibiting the dopamine transporter
- Increases neuronal activity selectively in the hypothalamus and activates tuberomammillary nucleus neurons that release histamine
- It also activates hypothalamic neurons that release orexin/hypocretin
- Armodafinil is the R-enantiomer of modafinil (a mixture of R- and S-enantiomers)

How Long Until It Works
- Typically 2 hours, although maximal benefit may take days-weeks

If It Works
- Continue to use indefinitely as long as symptoms persist. Complete resolution of symptoms is unusual. Does not cause insomnia when dosed correctly

If It Doesn't Work
- Change to most effective dose or alternative agent. Re-evaluate treatment of underlying cause (i.e., OSA) of fatigue. Consider other causes of fatigue (i.e., anemia, heart disease) as appropriate. Screen for use of CNS depressants that can interfere with sleep, i.e., opioids or alcohol

Best Augmenting Combos for Partial Response or Treatment-Resistance
- In treating OSA, armodafinil is an adjunct to standard treatments such as continuous positive airway pressure (CPAP), weight loss and treatment of obstruction when possible
- In narcolepsy, tricyclic antidepressants or SSRI may be of some help. Sleep hygiene is also important. As a last resort, the CNS depressant sodium oxybate can be used

Tests
- None required

ADVERSE EFFECTS (AEs)

How Drug Causes AEs
- AEs are probably related to drug actions on CNS neurotransmitters

Notable AEs
- Nervousness, insomnia, headache, nausea, anorexia, palpitations, dry mouth, diarrhea, hypertension

Life-Threatening or Dangerous AEs
- Transient ECG changes have been reported in patients with preexisting heart disease. (left ventricular hypertrophy, mitral valve prolapse)
- Rare psychiatric reactions (activation of mania, anxiety)
- Rare severe dermatologic reactions

Weight Gain
- Unusual

unusual | not unusual | common | problematic

Sedation
- Unusual

unusual | not unusual | common | problematic

What to Do About AEs
- Try lowering the dose. If insomnia, do not take later in the day

Best Augmenting Agents for AEs
- Most AEs do not respond to adding other medications

DOSING AND USE

Usual Dosage Range
- 150–250 mg daily

Dosage Forms
- Tablets: 50, 150, 250 mg

How to Dose
- Start at 150 mg in the morning
- Patients with narcolepsy are more likely to require a higher dose. (250 mg)

 Dosing Tips
- Dose requirements can escalate over time due to autoinduction. A drug holiday may restore effectiveness of lower dose
- In patients with shift-work related sleep disorder, take 1 hour prior to beginning a shift

Overdose
- No reported deaths. Insomnia, restlessness, agitation, anxiety, tachycardia, nausea and hypertension have been reported

Long-Term Use
- Although most initial trials were only a few months, appears safe. Periodically re-evaluate need for use

Habit Forming
- Class IV medication, but rarely abused in clinical practice

How to Stop
- Withdrawal is not problematic, unlike traditional stimulants. Symptoms of sleepiness may recur

Pharmacokinetics
- Metabolized by amine hydrolysis and CYP450 system including 3A4/5. Peak concentrations at 2 hours and elimination half-life is 15 hours. Reaches steady state at 7 days. Mild CYP3A4 induction

 Drug Interactions
- Can increase plasma levels and effect of many drugs metabolized by 2C19 or 2D6 including phenytoin, diazepam, propranolol, tricyclic antidepressants, and SSRIs
- Can induce CYP450 3A4 reducing plasma levels of midazolam, triazolam, and many steroidal contraceptives
- May reduce plasma levels of cyclosporine
- CYP3A4/5 inducers (such as carbamazepine, phenobarbital and rifampin) can lower armodafinil plasma levels and inhibitors (ketoconazole, erythromycin, fluvoxamine, and fluoxetine) can increase levels
- Armodafinil can affect warfarin effectiveness requiring closer monitoring of prothrombin times
- May interact with MAO inhibitors

 Other precautions/ warnings
- May adversely affect mood. Can cause activation of psychosis or mania

Do Not Use
- Known hypersensitivity to the drug, severe hypertension or cardiac arrhythmias

SPECIAL POPULATIONS

Renal Impairment
- No known effects. May require lower dose

Hepatic Impairment
- Reduce dose in patients with severe impairment

Cardiac Impairment
- Do not use in patients with ischemic ECG changes, chest pain, left ventricular hypertrophy or recent myocardial infarction

Elderly
- No known effects

 Children and Adolescents
- Not studied in children

Pregnancy
• Category C. Generally not used in pregnancy

Breast Feeding
• Unknown if excreted in breast milk. Do not use

THE ART OF NEUROPHARMACOLOGY

Potential Advantages
• Less risk of addiction, withdrawal and abuse compared to other stimulants. Longer duration of action than modafinil

Potential Disadvantages
• Cost. May be less effective than other stimulants

Primary Target Symptoms
• Sleepiness, fatigue, concentration difficulties

Pearls
• The Epworth sleepiness scale is a reliable way to measure daytime sleepiness and response to treatment. It is a self-administered 8 item questionnaire with scores of 0–24. A score of 10 or greater indicates excessive daytime sleepiness. A reduction of 4 or more points on the Epworth is considered a good response to treatment
• Narcolepsy is characterized by excessive daytime sleepiness, uncontrollable sleep and observed cataplexy. Hypnagogic or hypnopompic hallucinations or sleep paralysis suggest the diagnosis. In sleep studies, a sleep latency of 8 minutes or less and quick onset of REM sleep confirms the diagnosis. The maintenance of wakefulness test can monitor response to treatment or be used to document safety in patients in which wakefulness is important for public safety (e.g., pilots). An increase of 1–2 minutes in maintenance of wakefulness is considered a good response to treatment
• Does not appear to affect sleep architecture
• Technically not a psychostimulant and minimal abuse potential

---

Suggested Reading

Darwish M, Kirby M, Hellriegel ET, Robertson P Jr. Armodafinil and modafinil have substantially different pharmacokinetic profiles despite having the same terminal half-lives: analysis of data from three randomized, single-dose, pharmacokinetic studies. Clin Drug Investig 2009;29(9):613–23.

Lankford DA. Armodafinil: a new treatment for excessive sleepiness. Expert Opin Investig Drugs 2008;17(4):565–73.

Nishino S, Okuro M. Armodafinil for excessive daytime sleepiness. Drugs Today (Barc) 2008;44(6):395–414.

Parmentier R, Anaclet C, Guhennec C, Brousseau E, Bricout D, Giboulot T, Bozyczko-Coyne D, Spiegel K, Ohtsu H, Williams M, Lin JS. The brain H3-receptor as a novel therapeutic target for vigilance and sleep-wake disorders. Biochem Pharmacol 2007;73(8):1157–71.

ASPIRIN
(Acetylsalicylic acid)

THERAPEUTICS

Brands
- Bayer Aspirin, Ecotrin, Halfprin, Heartline, Empirin, Alka-Seltzer, Asprimox, Magnaprin, Bufferin, Ascriptin, Aspergum, ZORprin

Generic?
Yes

Class
- Antiplatelet agent, NSAID, anti-inflammatory

Commonly Prescribed for
(FDA approved in bold)
- **To reduce risk of myocardial infarction (MI), transient ischemic attack (TIA) or ischemic stroke (IS) due to fibrin platelet emboli**
- **Angina (unstable or stable)**
- **Revascularization procedures (coronary artery bypass graft (CABG), angioplasty, and carotid endarterectomy)**
- **Analgesic for mild-moderate pain for relief of headache, muscle aches and pains, toothache, arthritis, menstrual pain**
- **Fever**
- **Rheumatic conditions, such as spondyloarthropathies, rheumatoid arthritis, osteoarthritis, pleurisy associated with systemic lupus erythematosus**
- Reducing risk of stroke in high-risk populations, such as non-valvular atrial fibrillation, when anticoagulants are contraindicated
- Toxemia of pregnancy

How the Drug Works
- By acetylating cyclo-oxygenase-1 (cox-1), aspirin inhibits synthesis of thromboxane A2, a prostaglandin derivative that is a potent vasoconstrictor and inducer of platelet aggregation
- Irreversibly inhibits platelet aggregation even at low doses
- At larger doses, interferes with cox-1 and -2 in arterial walls, interfering with prostaglandin production. Counteracts fever by vasodilation of peripheral vessels, allowing dissipation of excess heat

How Long Until It Works
- A single dose of aspirin inhibits platelet aggregation for the life of the platelet (7–10 days). In pain, effective within 1–2 hours

If It Works
- Continue to use for prevention of MI, IS or TIA, and for pain

If It Doesn't Work
- Only reduces risk of MI or IS. Warfarin is superior for cardiogenic stroke. Control all IS risk factors such as smoking, hyperlipidemia, and hypertension. For acute events, admit patients for treatment and diagnostic testing. Consider screening for aspirin resistance

 ### Best Augmenting Combos for Partial Response or Treatment-Resistance
- In stroke prevention, there is no proven benefit to using clopidogrel in combination with aspirin. In clinical trials, there was no significant difference in IS prevention, and AEs (mostly bleeding) were significantly higher
- Consider changing to dipyridamole-aspirin combination for IS prevention
- Pain: In acute migraine, add caffeine and/or acetaminophen, antiemetics, or triptans

Tests
- None required

ADVERSE EFFECTS (AEs)

How Drug Causes AEs
- Antiplatelet effects increase bleeding risk

Notable AEs
- Stomach pain, heartburn, nausea and vomiting

 ### Life-Threatening or Dangerous AEs
- GI, intracranial or intraocular bleeding. Risk increases with higher doses

Weight Gain
- Unusual

Sedation
- Unusual

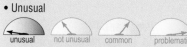

What to Do About AEs
- For significant GI or intracranial bleeding stop drug

Best Augmenting Agents for AEs
- Proton pump inhibitors reduce risk of GI bleeding

DOSING AND USE

Usual Dosage Range
- MI, TIA, or IS prevention: 50–1300 mg/day
- Pain: 325–1000 mg per dose

Dosage Forms
- Chewable Tablets: 81 mg
- Tablets: 325 mg, 500 mg
- Gum Tablets: 227.5 mg
- Enteric-coated: 81 mg, 165 mg, 325 mg, 500 mg, 650 mg
- Extended- or controlled-release: 650 mg, 800 mg
- Suppositories: 120 mg, 200 mg, 300 mg, 600 mg

How to Dose
- Give once daily for prevention of vascular events. For pain, take 325–1000 mg every 4–6 hours as needed up to a maximum of 4000 mg per 24 hours. With extended-release, take 650–1300 mg every 8 hours as needed, maximum 3900 mg/day

 Dosing Tips
- Taking with food decreases absorption and reduces GI AEs

Overdose
- Early: Produces respiratory alkalosis, resulting in hyperpnea and tachypnea. Nausea and vomiting, hypokalemia, tinnitus, dehydration, hyperthermia, thrombocytopenia, and easy bruising
- Late: coma, pulmonary edema, respiratory failure, renal failure, hypoglycemia. Mixed respiratory alkalosis and metabolic acidosis may occur. Treat with emesis or gastric lavage and monitor salicylate levels and electrolytes. In severe cases, hemodialysis is effective

Long-Term Use
- Safe for long-term use

Habit Forming
- No

How to Stop
- No need to taper

Pharmacokinetics
- Aspirin half-life is 20 minutes. > 99% protein binding. Hepatic metabolism and renal excretion

 Drug Interactions
- Alcohol increases risk of GI ulceration and may prolong bleeding time
- Urinary acidifiers (ascorbic acid, methionine) decrease secretion and increase drug effect
- Antacids and urinary alkalinizers may decrease drug effect
- Carbonic anhydrase inhibitors may increase risk of salicylate intoxication, and aspirin may displace acetazolamide from protein binding sites leading to toxicity
- Activated charcoal decreases aspirin absorption and effect
- Corticosteroids may increase clearance and decrease serum levels
- Use with heparin or oral anticoagulants has an additive effect and can increase bleeding risks
- Aspirin may cause unexpected hypotension after treatment with nitroglycerin
- Aspirin use with NSAIDs may decrease NSAID serum levels and increases risk of GI AEs
- May displace valproic acid from binding sites and increase pharmacologic effects
- May blunt effectiveness of beta-blockers and angiotensin-converting enzyme inhibitors
- May decrease effect of loop diuretics and spironolactone
- Increases drug levels of methotrexate

- Reduces the uricosuric effects of probenecid and sulfinpyrazone
- Large doses (> 2 g /day) may produce hypoglycemia when used with insulin or sulfonylurias in diabetics

Other Warnings/ Precautions

- The use of aspirin or other salicylates in children or teens with influenza or chicken pox may be associated with Reye's syndrome. Symptoms include vomiting and lethargy that may progress to delirium or coma
- Tinnitus or dizziness are symptoms of aspirin toxicity
- Aspirin intolerance is not rare, especially in asthmatics. Symptoms include bronchospasm, angioedema, severe rhinitis or shock. It is possible to desensitize patients in a hospital setting, but they will need to maintain daily aspirin to avoid recurrence

Do Not Use

- Known hypersensitivity to salicylates, acute asthma or hay fever, severe anemia or blood coagulation defects, children or teenagers with chicken pox or flu symptoms

Renal Impairment

- Use with caution in chronic renal insufficiency. May temporarily worsen renal function

Hepatic Impairment

- Use with caution in patients with significant disease including those with hypoprothrombinemia or vitamin K deficiency. High doses can cause hepatotoxicity

Cardiac Impairment

- No known effects

Elderly

- No known effects

Children and Adolescents

- Not recommended for prevention of IS or TIA in children younger than age 12

Pregnancy

- Category D. Crosses the placenta and is associated with anemia, ante- or post-partum hemorrhage, prolonged gestation and labor, and constriction of ductus arteriosus. Do not use, especially in 3rd trimester

Breast Feeding

- Excreted in breast milk in low concentrations. Risk to infants and their platelet function is unknown

THE ART OF NEUROPHARMACOLOGY

Potential Advantages

- Effective and inexpensive medication for prevention of both IS and other vascular diseases, such as MI

Potential Disadvantages

- May be less effective in some patients for ischemic stroke prevention. Risk of aspirin resistance

Primary Target Symptoms

- Prevention of the neurological complications that result from ischemic stroke
- Headache or other pain

Pearls

- First-line drug for secondary prevention of IS, along with clopidogrel or extended-release dipyridimole plus aspirin
- May be less effective than clopidogrel for patients with peripheral vascular disease
- Aspirin 325 mg in combination with clopidogrel increased bleeding risk in clinical trials and did not prove superior for IS prevention
- Stop aspirin 1 week before any surgical procedure, given its effect on platelet function

- Standard coagulation tests do not accurately reflect the effect of aspirin. Bleeding times are often unreliable. Multiple assays are now available to measure the effect of a given aspirin on platelet function. These include standard platelet aggregometry and tests measuring the effect on COX-1 by measuring thromboxane metabolites
- Increasing aspirin dose may overcome resistance, but patients may develop aspiring resistance over time on a stable dose
- At this point, there are no guidelines to suggest when to screen for aspirin resistance. It is unclear if aspirin failures should simply increase their dose, change to another agent, or take another agent in combination with aspirin
- Antiplatelets may be equally effective compared to anticoagulants for prevention of recurrent arterial dissection
- When compared to warfarin for the prevention of stroke due to symptomatic intracranial disease (WASID), aspirin 1300 mg was equal to warfarin and associated with lower rates of myocardial infarction or major hemorrhage
- In pain/migraine, combination products containing caffeine and/or acetaminophen may be more effective. Adding antiemetics such as metoclopramide is useful in migraine

Suggested Reading

Bhatt DL, Fox KA, Hacke W, Berger PB, Black HR, Boden WE, Cacoub P, Cohen EA, Creager MA, Easton JD, Flather MD, Haffner SM, Hamm CW, Hankey GJ, Johnston SC, Mak KH, Mas JL, Montalescot G, Pearson TA, Steg PG, Steinhubl SR, Weber MA, Brennan DM, Fabry-Ribaudo L, Booth J, Topol EJ; CHARISMA Investigators. Clopidogrel and aspirin versus aspirin alone for the prevention of atherothrombotic events. N Engl J Med 2006;354(16):1706–17.

Diener HC, Lampl C, Reimnitz P, Voelker M. Aspirin in the treatment of acute migraine attacks. Expert Rev Neurother 2006;6(4):563–73.

Goldstein J, Silberstein SD, Saper JR, Ryan RE Jr, Lipton RB. Acetaminophen, aspirin, and caffeine in combination versus ibuprofen for acute migraine: results from a multicenter, double-blind, randomized, parallel-group, single-dose, placebo-controlled study. Headache 2006;46(3):444–53.

Krasopoulos G, Brister SJ, Beattie WS, Buchanan MR. Aspirin "resistance" and risk of cardiovascular morbidity: systematic review and meta-analysis. BMJ 2008;336(7637):195–8.

Lenz T, Wilson A. Clinical pharmacokinetics of antiplatelet agents used in the secondary prevention of stroke. Clin Pharmacokinet 2003;42(10):909–20.

Serebruany VL, Malinin AI, Sane DC, Jilma B, Takserman A, Atar D, Hennekens CH. Magnitude and time course of platelet inhibition with Aggrenox and Aspirin in patients after ischemic stroke: the AGgrenox versus Aspirin Therapy Evaluation (AGATE) trial. Eur J Pharmacol 2004;499(3):315–24.

AZATHIOPRINE

Brands
• Imuran, Azasan, Azamun, Imurel

Generic?
No

Class
• Immunosuppressive agent, immunomodulator

Commonly Prescribed for
(FDA approved in bold)
• **Prophylaxis of organ rejection in patients with allogenic renal transplants**
• **Rheumatoid arthritis**
• Myasthenia gravis (MG) (monotherapy or adjunctive)
• Inflammatory myopathies: polymyositis (PM) and dermatomyositis (DM)
• Multiple sclerosis (MS)
• Neuromyelitis optica

How the Drug Works
• Azathioprine, a derivative of 6-mercaptopurine, inhibits the synthesis of purine. This interferes with DNA and RNA synthesis, repair and replication cells, predominantly T leukocytes
• The mechanism of action in autoimmune diseases is unclear, but appears to suppress cellular cytotoxicity and blunt hypersensitivity reactions

How Long Until It Works
• At least 3 months

If It Works
• MG: Improves strength and muscle fatigue. Often used as an adjunctive to corticosteroids or acute treatment such as immune globulin or plasma exchange. Taper corticosteroids if clinical symptoms improve
• PM/DM: May allow improvement in strength and discontinuation or reduced dose of corticosteroids. (Corticosteroids are usually tapered first.) Taper slowly over 6 months if clinical remission occurs
• MS: May reduce relapses and new lesions on MRI

If It Doesn't Work
• MG: Effectiveness may not occur until 1 year. For patients with severe disability, consider more rapid-acting treatments, such as IV immune globulin
• DM/PM: Question the diagnosis (inclusion-body myositis, hypothyroidism, muscular dystrophy), rule out corticosteroid-induced myopathy and evaluate for undiagnosed malignancy (especially in DM). Change to methotrexate
• MS: If clearly not helpful, change to another agent

Best Augmenting Combos for Partial Response or Treatment-Resistance
• MG: Usually combined with corticosteroids or other treatments in MG. Most patients also use symptomatic medication, such as pyridostigmine
• DM/PM: Usually used in combination with corticosteroids as a sparing agent
• MS: Occasionally combined with other treatments for the treatment of MS

Tests
• Obtain CBC weekly the first month, then twice monthly months 2–3, then monthly unless dose changes
• Before starting treatment, screen for thiopurine methyltransferase deficiency. Heterozygous patients often need a lower dose and closer monitoring. Homozygous patients are at risk for severe bone marrow toxicity

---

ADVERSE EFFECTS (AEs)

How Drug Causes AEs
• Inhibits purine synthesis of DNA and RNA

Notable AEs
• Anorexia, nausea, or vomiting
• Skin rash, alopecia, arthralgias
• Idiosyncratic reaction (fever, myalgia, malaise) in about 10% – usually but not always within days of first dose

Life-Threatening or Dangerous AEs

- Bone marrow suppression: Severe leukopenia, macrocytic anemia, thrombocytopenia, or pancytopenia. Dose-dependent and can occur at any time during treatment
- Pancreatitis, liver toxicity
- Serious infection

Weight Gain

- Unusual

Sedation

- Not unusual

What to Do About AEs

- Reducing dose or temporary withdrawal allows reversal of bone marrow toxicity. Check serum amylase for symptoms of pancreatitis and discontinue if elevated

Best Augmenting Agents for AEs

- H2 blockers may relieve GI symptoms

DOSING AND USE

Usual Dosage Range

- MG – 150–200 mg/day
- DM/PM – 50–200 mg/day
- MS – 100–200 mg/day

Dosage Forms

- Tablets: 50 mg, 75 mg, 100 mg
- Injection: 100 mg per vial

How to Dose

- Start at 50 mg daily. Increase every 2–4 weeks to maintenance dose of 2–3 mg/kg/day

 Dosing Tips

- For patients with significant GI AEs, divide doses

Overdose

- Nausea and vomiting, diarrhea, leukopenia, and liver function abnormalities have been reported. Very large doses can cause severe bleeding, infection, or death

Long-Term Use

- Safe with appropriate monitoring

Habit Forming

- No

How to Stop

- In patients with clinical remission, taper by about 25 mg every 4 weeks and monitor for recurrence

Pharmacokinetics

- Azathioprine is cleaved to mercaptopurine. Drug is cleared by oxidation by xanthine oxidase and thiol methylation, by thiopurine methyltransferase. Peak levels of drug and metabolites in 1–2 hours and half-life 5 hours

 Drug Interactions

- Concurrent use with ACE inhibitors may induce severe leukopenia
- Allopurinol (a purine analog) may increase effects
- Methotrexate increases plasma levels of metabolite
- May decrease action of anticoagulants, such as warfarin
- Decreases cyclosporine levels
- May reverse actions of neuromuscular blockers

 Other Warnings/Precautions

- May increase risk of malignancy

Do Not Use

- Known hypersensitivity, previous treatment with alkalating agents such as cyclophosphamide (due to risk of neoplasia)

Renal Impairment

- Unclear to what extent renal disease predicts effectiveness or toxicity. Consider reducing dose

Hepatic Impairment

- Hepatotoxicity is an uncommon AE. Use with caution and monitor closely

Cardiac Impairment

- No known effects

Elderly

- No known effects

Children and Adolescents

- Effectiveness and safety unknown

Pregnancy

- Category D. Multiple fetal abnormalities have been reported. Generally not used except in renal transplant patients

Breast Feeding

- Do not breast feed while on drug

THE ART OF NEUROPHARMACOLOGY

Potential Advantages

- Generally well tolerated first-line treatment in MG. Useful corticosteroid-sparing agent in PM/DM

Potential Disadvantages

- Very slow onset of action. Effectiveness in MG may be less than other drugs

Primary Target Symptoms

- Preventive treatment of complications from diseases, such as MG, PM, DM or MS

Pearls

- Slow onset of action in MG limits effectiveness. Not proven effective in 1 year in small clinical trials, but did show significant effect in 2 and 3 years. The average patient was able to discontinue prednisone treatment in 3 years
- In patients with contraindications to corticosteroids and less severe disability, may be used as monotherapy. Its effectiveness as monotherapy is unclear
- In DM or PM, azathioprine is an effective corticosteroid-sparing agent. Generally a first-line treatment, especially in those with interstitial lung or liver disease
- Improvement in muscle strength is a better predictor of improvement in PM or DM than a decrease in creatine kinase
- Anti-Jo-1 antibodies are predictive of worsening response in PM and DM
- PM in general is less likely to respond to corticosteroids (about 50%) than DM (over 80%), but DM patients may have a more difficult time tapering corticosteroids
- Small clinical trials demonstrate decrease in number of new MRI lesions in relapsing-remitting MS at doses up to 3 mg/kg/day. Larger trials are needed to conclusively demonstrate effectiveness
- Therapeutic effects may correlate with increasing mean corpuscular volume in CBC. Start to consider tapering corticosteroids after this increase

Suggested Reading

Casetta I, Iuliano G, Filippini G. Azathioprine for multiple sclerosis. J Neurol Neurosurg Psychiatry 2009;80(2):131–2.

Hart IK, Sathasivam S, Sharshar T. Immunosuppressive agents for myasthenia gravis. Cochrane Database Syst Rev 2007;(4): CD005224.

Havrdova E, Zivadinov R, Krasensky J, Dwyer MG, Novakova I, Dolezal O, Ticha V, Dusek L, Houzvickova E, Cox JL, Bergsland N, Hussein S, Svobodnik A, Seidl Z, Vaneckova M, Horakova D. Randomized study of interferon beta-1a, low-dose azathioprine, and low-dose corticosteroids in multiple sclerosis. Mult Scler 2009;15(8):965–76.

Hengstman GJ, van den Hoogen FH, van Engelen BG. Treatment of the inflammatory myopathies: update and practical recommendations. Expert Opin Pharmacother 2009;10(7):1183–90.

Massacesi L, Parigi A, Barilaro A, Repice AM, Pellicanò G, Konze A, Siracusa G, Taiuti R, Amaducci L. Efficacy of azathioprine on multiple sclerosis new brain lesions evaluated using magnetic resonance imaging. Arch Neurol 2005;62(12):1843–7.

Palace J, Newsom-Davis J, Lecky B. A randomized double-blind trial of prednisolone alone or with azathioprine in myasthenia gravis. Myasthenia Gravis Study Group. Neurology 1998;50(6):1778–83.

BACLOFEN

THERAPEUTICS

Brands
• Lioresal, Kernstro

Generic?
Yes

Class
• Skeletal muscle relaxant, centrally acting

Commonly Prescribed for
(FDA approved in bold)
• **Spasticity and pain related to disorders such as multiple sclerosis or spinal cord diseases**
• Trigeminal neuralgia
• Tourette syndrome
• Tardive dyskinesias
• Chorea in Huntington's disease
• Acquired peduncular nystagmus
• Migraine prophylaxis
• Neuropathic pain
• Alcohol dependence

How the Drug Works
• Baclofen is an analog of $GABA_B$, an inhibitory neurotransmitter. However, the exact mechanism of action is unknown but presumably is related to hyperpolarization of afferent terminals inhibiting monosynaptic and polysynaptic reflexes at the spinal level. Has CNS depressant properties

How Long Until It Works
• Pain – hours-weeks

If It Works
• Slowly titrate to most effective dose as tolerated. Many patients will need gradual titration to maintain response and limit sedation

If It Doesn't Work
• Make sure to increase to highest tolerated dose – as high as 200 mg/day. If ineffective, slowly taper and consider alternative treatments for pain. In general, baclofen is more effective for spasticity related to MS or spinal cord disease than other causes of spasticity

Best Augmenting Combos for Partial Response or Treatment-Resistance
• For focal spasticity, i.e., post-stroke spasticity, botulinum toxin is often more effective and is better tolerated
• Use other centrally acting muscle relaxants with caution due to potential synergistic CNS depressant effect
• Baclofen is usually used in combination with neuroleptics for the treatment of tardive dyskinesias or chorea
• Trigeminal neuralgia often responds to anticonvulsants. Pimozide is another option. For truly refractory patients, surgical interventions may be required

Tests
• None required

ADVERSE EFFECTS (AEs)

How Drug Causes AEs
• Most AEs are related to CNS depression

Notable AEs
• Drowsiness, dizziness, weakness, fatigue are most common. Nausea, constipation, hypotension, and confusion

Life-Threatening or Dangerous AEs
• Worsening of seizure control. The most dangerous AEs occur with rapid baclofen withdrawal including high fever, confusion, hallucinations, rebound spasticity, muscle rigidity and, in severe cases, rhabdomyolysis, multi-system organ failure, and death

Weight Gain
• Unusual

Sedation
• Problematic

What to Do About AEs
• Lower the dose and titrate more slowly

Best Augmenting Agents for AEs

- Most AEs cannot be improved by an augmenting agent. MS-related fatigue can respond to CNS stimulants, such as modafinil, but in most cases it is easier to temporarily lower the baclofen dose until tolerance develops

DOSING AND USE

Usual Dosage Range

Spasticity
Oral: 40–80 mg/day in divided doses.
Intrathecal: 300 mcg – 800 mcg/day, rarely more than 1000 mcg/day.

Dosage Forms

- Tablets: 10, 20 mg
- Orally disintegrating tablets: 10, 20 mg
- Intrathecal: 0.05 mg/mL, 10 mg/20 mL and 10 mg/5 mL I in single-use amps

How to Dose

- Oral: start at 15 mg daily in 3 divided doses. Increase by 15 mg every 3 days as tolerated to 60 mg per day in 3 divided doses or until desired clinical effect. Patients may further benefit from increasing dose to 80 mg per day. Doses above 80 mg per day are usually not recommended but doses up to 200 mg/day have been used in patients that tolerate the medication well
- Intrathecal: Patients must demonstrate a positive clinical response to treatment. A dose of 50 mcg is given on day 1 over greater than 1 minute. Observe 4–8 hours for a clinical response. If the response is inadequate, can repeat with dose of 75 mcg 24 hours later and again observe 4–8 hours for improvement. If no response, inject 100 mcg on day 3. Patients who do not respond to a dose of 100 mcg are not candidates for intrathecal treatment
- If the positive effect of the test dose lasts less than 8 hours, the starting dose should be doubled with the bolus dose given over 24 hours. If the response lasts over 8 hours, use the bolus dose as the original daily dose. In patients with spasticity of spinal cord origin, increase the daily dose by 10–30% after 24 hours and then every 24 hours until the desired clinical effect is achieved. In patients with spasticity related to cerebral origin and in children increase the dose more slowly – about 5–15% each increase per 24 hours until desired effect reached
- When to consider intrathecal baclofen: For treatment of spasticity related to a stable, irreversible neurologic disease or trauma that disables the patient or causes severe pain. The patient must have failed at least 3–4 oral medications or experience intolerable side effects at effective doses. The patient or the caregiver must understand the risks and benefits of the pump and the required follow-up care

 Dosing Tips

- About 5% of patients will become refractory to increasing doses of intrathecal baclofen. In those patients, consider careful withdrawal and treatment with other anti-spasticity agents for 2–4 weeks, then restart at the initial continuous infusion dose

Overdose

- Vomiting, hypotonia, drowsiness, coma, respiratory depression, and seizures. In an alert patient induce emesis and lavage. In obtunded patients, intubation is often required

Long-Term Use

- Safe for long-term use. Effectiveness may decrease over time and tolerance to clinical effects occurs in about 5%

Habit Forming

- No

How to Stop

- To avoid withdrawal symptoms, taper slowly over a week or more depending on the dose and time on drug

Pharmacokinetics

- Orally: Rapidly absorbed with excretion half-life 3–4 h. Intrathecal: bolus lasts 4–8 hours, with initial onset 0.5–1 hour after bolus. Continuous infusion lasts 6–8 hours. The peak action is 4 hours after a bolus and 24–48 hours after starting continuous infusion. Excreted unchanged in the kidney

Drug Interactions

- Use with other CNS depressants will exacerbate sedation. No hepatic metabolism, therefore no major drug interactions to consider

 Other Warnings/ Precautions

- Decreased spasticity can be problematic for some patients who require tone to maintain upright posture, balance, and ambulate
- May cause an increase in ovarian cysts
- May worsen symptoms of psychiatric disorders, such as schizophrenia or confusional states
- May worsen control of epilepsy

Do Not Use

- Known hypersensitivity. Never start intrathecal baclofen in patients with an active infection

SPECIAL POPULATIONS

Renal Impairment

- Since baclofen is renally excreted, lower the dose with significant renal dysfunction

Hepatic Impairment

- No known effects

Cardiac Impairment

- No known effects

Elderly

- Titrate carefully but no contraindications

 Children and Adolescents

- Children over age 12 have similar dose requirements as adults. Children under 12 usually have a lower dose requirement for intrathecal baclofen – on average 274 mcg/day. For small children, start with a test dose of 25 mcg

 Pregnancy

- Category C. Use only if benefits of medication outweigh risks

Breast Feeding

- Oral baclofen is excreted in breast milk. Do not use

THE ART OF NEUROPHARMACOLOGY

Potential Advantages

- First-line treatment for spasticity in MS and spinal cord injury patients. Effect is maintained with extended use

Potential Disadvantages

- Poor effectiveness and tolerability in patients with spasticity unrelated to MS or spinal cord injuries. Severe withdrawal AEs. Sedation often limits use

Primary Target Symptoms

- Spasticity, pain

 Pearls

- Effective and important adjunctive medication for MS and spinal cord injury spasticity and pain. With slow titration, baclofen is usually well tolerated
- Baclofen is generally NOT effective for spasticity related to Parkinson's disease, stroke, and traumatic brain injury, although it occasionally is used in severe cases. In general these patients are much more susceptible to AEs
- Do not attempt to use intrathecal baclofen before 1 year after traumatic brain injury
- Intrathecal baclofen should be administered in centers that commonly treat MS and spinal cord diseases
- For patients on intrathecal baclofen with rapidly escalating dose requirements or new onset depression, fever, or confusion, consider the possibility of a shunt catheter malfunction
- Some spasticity can be helpful for patients with MS or spinal cord injuries to support circulatory function, prevent deep vein thrombosis, and optimize activities of daily living
- A second-line treatment for trigeminal neuralgia, usually at doses of 60 mg/day or less
- Baclofen has been used off-label for many other conditions such as chorea, migraine, and neuropathic pain. These studies have been mostly negative

Suggested Reading

Coffey RJ, Edgar TS, Francisco GE, Graziani V, Meythaler JM, Ridgely PM, Sadiq SA, Turner MS. Abrupt withdrawal from intrathecal baclofen: recognition and management of a potentially life-threatening syndrome. Arch Phys Med Rehabil 2002;83(6):735–41.

Green MW, Selman JE. Review article: the medical management of trigeminal neuralgia. Headache 1991;31(9):588–92.

Metz L. Multiple sclerosis: symptomatic therapies. Semin Neurol 1998;18(3): 389–95.

Nielsen JF, Hansen HJ, Sunde N, Christensen JJ. Evidence of tolerance to baclofen in treatment of severe spasticity with intrathecal baclofen. Clin Neurol Neurosurg 2002;104(2):142–5.

Taricco M, Pagliacci MC, Telaro E, Adone R. Pharmacological interventions for spasticity following spinal cord injury: results of a Cochrane systematic review. Eura Medicophys 2006;42(1):5–15.

Vender JR, Hughes M, Hughes BD, Hester S, Holsenback S, Rosson B. Intrathecal baclofen therapy and multiple sclerosis: outcomes and patient satisfaction. Neurosurg Focus 2006;21(2):e6.

THERAPEUTICS

THERAPEUTICS

Brands
- Cogentin

Generic?
Yes

Class
- Antiparkinson agent, anticholinergic

Commonly Prescribed for
(FDA approved in bold)
- **Extrapyramidal disorders**
- **Parkinsonism**
- Acute dystonic reactions
- Idiopathic generalized dystonia
- Focal dystonias
- Dopa-responsive dystonia

How the Drug Works
- In PD, there is a relative excess of cholinergic input. Benztropine is a synthetic anticholinergic with relatively greater CNS activity than most other anticholinergics. May also inhibit the reuptake and storage of dopamine at central dopamine receptors, prolonging dopamine action

How Long Until It Works
- PD/extrapyramidal disorders – minutes-hours

If It Works
- PD – do not abruptly discontinue or change doses of other PD treatments. Usually most effective in combination with other medications

If It Doesn't Work
- PD – Generally benztropine is an adjunctive medication for common PD symptoms, such as tremor, rigidity, and drooling. Other cardinal PD symptoms, such as bradykinesia and gait difficulties, are most likely to improve with other PD treatments, such as levodopa, dopamine agonists, amantadine, or MAO-B inhibitors
- Acute dystonic reactions – diphenhydramine is another option, if not effective consider benzodiazepines. If possible, discontinue the agent that precipitated the extrapyramidal AE

Best Augmenting Combos for Partial Response or Treatment-Resistance
- For bradykinesia or gait disturbances causing significant functional disturbance, levodopa is most effective. For idiopathic PD patients, especially younger patients with normal cognition and milder disability, dopamine agonists are a good first choice. Amantadine and MAO-B inhibitors may also be useful
- Depression is common in PD and may respond to low dose SSRIs

Tests
- None

ADVERSE EFFECTS (AEs)

How Drug Causes AEs
- Prevents the action of acetylcholine on muscarinic receptors

Notable AEs
- Dry mouth, tachycardia, palpitations, hypotension, disorientation, confusion, hallucinations, constipation, nausea/vomiting, dilation of colon, rash, blurred vision, diplopia, urinary retention, elevated temperature, decreased sweating, erectile dysfunction

Life-Threatening or Dangerous AEs
- May precipitate narrow-angle glaucoma. Risk of heat stroke, especially in elderly patients. Can cause tachycardia, cardiac arrhythmias and hypotension in susceptible patients. May cause urinary retention in patients with prostate hypertrophy

Weight Gain
- Unusual

unusual | not unusual | common | problematic

Sedation
- Common

unusual | not unusual | common | problematic

What to Do About AEs

- Confusion, hallucinations – stop benztropine and any other anticholinergics
- Sedation – can take entire dose at night or lower dose
- Dry mouth – chewing gum or water can help
- Urinary retention: if drug cannot be discontinued, obtain urological evaluation

Best Augmenting Agents for AEs

- Most AEs cannot be improved with the use of an augmenting agent

DOSING AND USE

Usual Dosage Range

- PD – 0.5–6 mg/daily
- Extrapyramidal reactions: 2–8 mg/daily

Dosage Forms

- Tablets: 0.5, 1 and 2 mg
- Injection: 1 mg/mL

How to Dose

- PD: use oral tablets. Start at 0.5 mg once daily and increase by 0.5 mg at 5–6 day intervals until reaching best tolerated and effective dose. Patients may take either once daily at night to improve sleep and allow for easier rising in the morning, or divide doses 2–4 times per day
- Drug-induced extrapyramidal disorders: 1 to 4 mg once or twice a day orally or parenterally. If the reaction occurs soon after the initiation of neuroleptic drugs (i.e., phenothiazines) they are likely to be transient. Attempt to withdraw benztropine after 1–2 weeks to determine if still needed. Disorders that develop after prolonged neuroleptic use may not respond to treatment
- Acute dystonic reactions: 1–2 mg injection (IV or IM) and tablets 1–2 mg twice per day prevent recurrence

 Dosing Tips

- Taking with meals can reduce AEs. IM and IV dosing are equally effective and fast acting

Overdose

- Complications may include circulatory collapse, cardiac arrest, respiratory depression or arrest, CNS depression or stimulation, psychosis, shock, coma, seizures, ataxia, combativeness, anhidrosis and hyperthermia, fever, dysphagia, decreased bowel sounds, and sluggish pupils. Induce emesis, use gastric lavage or activated charcoal. Oxygen or intubation may be needed for respiratory depression. Catheterize for urinary retention. Treat hyperthermia appropriately with cooling devices, local miotics for mydriasis/cycloplegia. Use physostigmine to reverse cardiac effects and use fluids and vasopressors if needed

Long-Term Use

- Safe for long-term use. Effectiveness may decrease over time (years) in PD and AEs such as sedation and cognitive impairment can worsen

Habit Forming

- No

How to Stop

- No need to taper

Pharmacokinetics

- Half-life is 36 hours, but the greatest effect lasts about 6–8 hours. Mostly urinary excretion. Bioavailability and metabolism not well understood

 Drug Interactions

- Use with amantadine may increase AEs
- Benztropine and all other anticholinergics may increase serum levels and effects of digoxin
- Can lower concentration of haloperidol and other phenothiazines, causing worsening of schizophrenia symptoms. Phenothiazines tend to increase anticholinergic AEs with concurrent use
- Can decrease gastric motility, resulting in increased gastric deactivation of levodopa and reduction in efficacy

 Other Warning Precautions

- Use with caution in hot weather – may increase susceptibility to heat stroke
- Anticholinergics have additive effects when used with drugs of abuse such as cannabinoids, barbiturates, opioids, and alcohol

Do Not Use

- Patients with known hypersensitivity to the drug, glaucoma (especially angle-closure type), pyloric or duodenal obstruction, stenosing peptic ulcers, prostate hypertrophy or bladder neck obstructions, achalasia, or megacolon

SPECIAL POPULATIONS

Renal Impairment

- Use with caution but no known effects

Hepatic Impairment

- Use with caution but no known effects

Cardiac Impairment

- Use with caution in patients with known arrhythmias, especially tachycardia

Elderly

- Use with caution. More susceptible to AEs

Children and Adolescents

- Do not use in ages 3 or less. Generalized dystonias may respond to anticholinergic treatment and young patients usually tolerate the medication better than the elderly. Typical dose 0.05 mg/kg once or twice daily

Pregnancy

- Category C. Use only if benefit of medication outweighs risks

Breast Feeding

- Concentration in breast milk unknown. May inhibit lactation. Use only if benefits outweigh risk

THE ART OF NEUROPHARMACOLOGY

Potential Advantages

- Useful adjunctive agent for some PD patients, especially post-encephalitic. Long duration of action. First-line agent for extrapyramidal disorders related to neuroleptics, especially in acute setting

Potential Disadvantages

- Multiple dose-dependent AEs associated with muscarinic effects limit use. Not effective for most idiopathic PD patients. Patients with long-standing extrapyramidal disorders may not respond to treatment. Less established as treatment for generalized dystonias than trihexyphenidyl

Primary Target Symptoms

- Tremor, akinesia, rigidity, drooling

 Pearls

- Useful adjunct in younger PD patients with tremor, but trihexiphenidyl is more commonly used
- Useful in the treatment of post-encephalitic PD and for extrapyramidal reactions, other than tardive dyskinesias
- Sedation limits use, especially in older patients. Patients with mental impairment do poorly
- Post-encephalitic PD patients usually tolerate higher doses better than idiopathic PD patients
- Generalized dystonias are more likely to benefit from anticholinergic therapy than focal dystonias. Trihexyphenidyl is used more commonly than benztropine

Suggested Reading

Brocks DR. Anticholinergic drugs used in Parkinson's disease: An overlooked class of drugs from a pharmacokinetic perspective. J Pharm Pharm Sci 1999;2(2):39–46.

Colosimo C, Gori MC, Inghilleri M. Post-encephalitic tremor and delayed-onset parkinsonism. Parkinsonism Relat Disord 1999;5(3):123–4.

Costa J, Espírito-Santo C, Borges A, Ferreira JJ, Coelho M, Sampaio C. Botulinum toxin type A versus anticholinergics for cervical dystonia. Cochrane Database Syst Rev 2005;(1):CD004312.

Hai NT, Kim J, Park ES, Chi SC. Formulation and biopharmaceutical evaluation of transdermal patch containing benztropine. Int J Pharm 2008;357(1–2):55–60.

BOTULINUM TOXIN TYPE A
(Onabotulinumtoxin A/Abobotulinumtoxin A)

Brands
• Botox, Botox cosmetic, Dysport, Xeomin, Vistabel, Neuronox

Generic?
No

 Class
• Neurotoxin

Commonly Prescribed for
(FDA approved in bold)
• **Cervical dystonia (CD)**
• **Glabellar lines**
• **Axillary hyperhidrosis (Onabotulinum toxin A only)**
• **Strabismus and blepharospasm associated with dystonia (Onabotulinum toxin A only)**
• **Upper limb spasticity in adults**
• Hemifacial spasm
• Spasmodic torticollis
• Spasmodic dysphonia (laryngeal dystonia)
• Writer's cramp and other task-specific dystonias
• Spasticity associated with stroke
• Dynamic muscle contracture in cerebral palsy
• Acquired nystagmus
• Oscillopsia
• Sialorrhea (drooling)
• Headache
• Temporomandibular joint dysfunction
• Diabetic neuropathic pain
• Myofascial pain
• Detrusor sphincter dyssynergia
• Palmar hyperhidrosis
• Tics
• Cosmesis
• Incontinence due to overactive or neurogenic bladder
• Achalasia (esophageal motility disorder)

 How the Drug Works
• Blocks neuromuscular transmission by cleaving SNAP-25 protein, which inhibits the vesicular release of acetylcholine from nerve terminals
• In CD and other dystonias, produces partial denervation of muscle and localized reduction in muscle activity. In hyperhidrosis, produces chemical denervation of sweat gland
• Also appears to inhibit release of neurotransmitters involved in pain transmission (including glutamate, calcitonin gene-related peptide, and substance P) and may enter CNS via retrograde axonal transport

How Long Until It Works
• Usually 2–3 days, with peak effect beginning at 2–3 weeks. Effect is quicker in blepharospasm compared to CD

If It Works
• Continue to use as long as effective, but monitor for clinical effects

If It Doesn't Work
• Increase dose or change injection technique. Some pain disorders may respond better to oral medications
• Patients can develop neutralizing antibodies from prior exposure. Response to a test dose of 15 units (u) in the frontalis muscle indicates a physiologic response. Antibody formulation has not been reported with newer type-A formulations

 Best Augmenting Combos for Partial Response or Treatment-Resistance
• Increase dose, number of injections or change site of location

Tests
• None

How Drug Causes AEs
• Most AEs are related to muscle weakness adjacent to the site of injection. Serious systemic AEs are rare, but injectors should use the lowest dose and be familiar with injection technique to minimize AEs

Notable AEs
• Injection site pain and hemorrhage, infection, fever, headache, pruritus, and myalgia. Most AEs depend on site of injection
• CD – dysphagia, neck weakness, upper respiratory infection

- Blepharospasm/strabismus – ptosis, diplopia, dry or watery eyes, keratitis (from reduced blinking)
- Spasmodic dysphonia – hypophonia ("breathy" voice)
- Writer's cramp – hand weakness

 Life-Threatening or Dangerous AEs

- Rarely patients may experience severe dysphagia requiring a feeding tube or leading to aspiration pneumonia
- Use with caution in patients with motor neuropathies or neuromuscular junctional disorders. These patients may be at greater risk for systemic weakness or respiratory problems

Weight Gain
- Unusual

Sedation
- Unusual

What to Do About AEs
- Most AEs will improve with time (weeks)

Best Augmenting Agents for AEs
- Most AEs cannot be improved with an augmenting agent

DOSING AND USE

Usual Dosage Range
- The following units are for Botox formulation. The appropriate conversion from Botox to Dysport is unknown, but studies of CD suggest a ratio of 1:3 or less (100 u Botox less than or equal to 300 u Dysport). Xeomin has a similar strength to Botox
- CD – Botox mean dose 236 u (usually 150–300). Per muscle: sternocleidomastoid 12.5–70 u, trapezius 25–100 u, levator scapulae 25–60 u, splenius 20–100 u, scalenus 15–50 u
- Dysport – typical dose 250–1000 u
- **Blepharospasm** – 1.25–5 u at each site (15–100 u total)

- **Oromandibular dystonia** – Masseter 10–75 u, temporalis 5–50 u, medial and lateral pterygoids 5–40 u each
- **Spasmodic dysphonia** – 2.5–5 u
- **Sialorrhea** – 7.5–40 u
- **Limb dystonia** – Intrinsic hand muscles 2.5–12.5 u, arm 5–45 u, intrinsic hand muscles 35–85 u, leg muscles 50–200 u
- **Primary axillary hyperhidrosis** – 50 u per axilla
- **Headache** – 50–200 u
- **Upper limb spasticity** – 75–360 u

Dosage Forms
- Powder for injection: 100 u, 50 u

How to Dose
- Administer every 3 months using the lowest effective dose
- The following units are for Botox formulation
- **CD** – start at a low dose and adjust as needed. Limiting the dose injected into the sternocleidomastoid muscles to 100 u or less may decrease incidence of dysphagia
- **Blepharospasm** – use 1.25–2.5 u per injection initially. Injecting more than 5 u per site does not produce added benefit. Inject the medial and lateral pretarsal orbicularis oculi of the upper lid and lateral pretarsal orbicularis oculi of the lower lid
- **Oromandibular dystonia** – For jaw-closing inject the masseter at 2–3 sites, and for jaw-opening inject the submentalis complex
- **Spasmodic dysphonia** – for more common adductor type inject 1–2.5 u into each side of the thyroarytenoid muscles, for abductor type inject the posterior cricoarytenoid
- **Sialorrhea** – inject 5–20 u into each parotid gland initially. The mandibular or sublingual glands may also be injected
- **Limb dystonia** – Inject using EMG guidance and dose based on muscle size and severity. Large shoulder and lower limb muscles may require hundreds of units for clinical benefit
- **Primary axillary hyperhidrosis** – perform 10–15 injections approximately 1–2 cm apart
- **Headache** – common sites include procerus (2.5–5 u), corregators (2.5–5 u each side), frontalis (10–25 u, 2.5 u per site), temporalis (5–20 u), occipitalis (2.5–10 u each side), and splenius capitus (5–15 u each side)

• **Upper limb spasticity** – common sites include biceps brachii (100–200 u total), flexor carpi radialis/ulnaris (12.5–50 u), and flexor digitorum profundis (25–50 u)

 Dosing Tips

• Physicians should be familiar with the anatomy of the injection site and the specific disorders
• Inject using a needle or hollow electrode
• EMG recording helps to identify muscle involved in complex dystonias
• Reconstitute with 0.9% sodium chloride. Rotate gently to mix with the saline. Administer within 4 hours
• Dilute with 1, 2, 4 or 8 mL depending on the type of injections to be performed. Dilute more when injecting smaller muscles (such as ocular muscles) that require fewer units
• When injecting for blepharospasm, avoid the levator palpebrae superioris to reduce incidence of ptosis

Overdose

• Signs and symptoms of overdose may be delayed for several weeks. If accidental overdose occurs, monitor for signs of systemic weakness or paralysis

Long-Term Use

• Safe for long-term use

Habit Forming

• No

How to Stop

• No need to taper

Pharmacokinetics

• Does not reach peripheral blood after injection with recommended doses. There may be changes in clinical electromyography in muscles distant to the injection site. The cause of this spread (circulation, axonal transport) is unclear

 Drug Interactions

• Use with caution in patients taking medications, such as aminoglycosides or curae-like compounds, that can interfere with neuromuscular transmission

 Other Warning Precautions

• Contains albumin, a blood derivative that can theoretically carry risk of viral infection of Creutzfeldt-Jacob disease
• Hypersensitivity reactions such as anaphylaxis, urticaria, and soft tissue edema have been reported

Do Not Use

• Patients with known hypersensitivity to the drug or any of its components; infection at the proposed injection sites

Renal Impairment

• No known effects

Hepatic Impairment

• No known effects

Cardiac Impairment

• There are rare reports of cardiac events including myocardial infarction following administration of Botulinum toxin type A. The relationship of the events to the injections is unclear and some of these patients had risk factors for heart disease

Elderly

• No known effects

 Children and Adolescents

• Studied in children 12 and older for strabismus and blepharospasm, 16 and older for CD, and 18 and over for hyperhidrosis. Used for treatment of sialorrhea in cerebral palsy

 Pregnancy

• Category C. Use only if benefit of medication outweighs risks

Breast Feeding

• Concentration in breast milk unknown. Use only if benefits outweigh risk

THE ART OF NEUROPHARMACOLOGY

Potential Advantages

- Effective in multiple refractory conditions, including pain, with very few AEs or drug interactions

Potential Disadvantages

- Cost and need for frequent injections to maintain effect. Dose requirement increases with muscle size

Primary Target Symptoms

- Dystonia, spasticity, pain, drooling, or sweating (depending on indication)

 Pearls

- Botulinum toxin is most effective in focal dystonias. Generalized dystonias can be treated with anticholinergic therapy, especially in younger, cognitively normal patients
- It often takes a series of injections to determine the optimal dose for a given patient
- Anterocollis (forward neck flexion) is often associated with neuroleptic exposure and Parkinsonism and is the most difficult cervical dystonia to treat. Injections of sternocleidomastoid and anterior scalene muscles are standard but fluoroscopic injections of deep cervical flexors may reduce clinical failures
- In oromandibular dystonia, Botulinum toxin appears more effective in jaw-closing dystonias than jaw-opening or mixed dystonias
- Meige syndrome is a combination of dystonias, including blepharospasm plus oromandibular dystonia. Symptoms may also include tongue protrusion, light sensitivity, muddled speech, contraction of the platysma muscle, and laryngeal dystonia. In addition to the usual sites for blepharospasm and oromandibular dystonia, consider injections of zygomaticus (usually 2.5–7.5 u) and risorius (2.5–10 u)
- Some studies report benefit in patients with chronic migraine at a dose of 50–250 u. Patients with allodynia, ocular headache and "imploding" pain may be more likely to benefit. Patients with episodic migraine and chronic tension-type headache did not do better than with placebo injections
- Consider as an alternative for patients with focal "nummular" (coin-shaped) headache and trigeminal neuralgia
- A recent double-blind trial found the Botulinum toxin type A was effective in some patients for reducing pain associated with diabetic neuropathy. This suggests the toxin has an effect on nerve rather than muscle alone
- Studies of CD suggest the appropriate conversion factor between Botox and Dysport units is less than 3 (100 units of Botox equal or less potent than 300 units of Dysport). Compared to Botox, Dysport appears to disperse to a greater area. It is unknown if this might cause problems when doing injections for CD, strabismus, or blepharospasm
- The most effective agent for post-stroke spasticity due to its focal action and lack of system side effects. Use to improve specific functions such as dressing, eating, etc. Higher doses may be needed
- Recently Botulinum toxin type A was renamed Onabotulinumtoxin A (for Botox and Botox cosmetic) and Abobotulinumtoxin A (Dysport)

Suggested Reading

Ashkenazi A, Silberstein S. Is botulinum toxin useful in treating headache? Yes. Curr Treat Options Neurol 2009;11(1):18–23.

Klein AW, Carruthers A, Fagien S, Lowe NJ. Comparisons among botulinum toxins: an evidence-based review. Plast Reconstr Surg 2008;121(6):413e–422e.

Lennerstrand G, Nordbø OA, Tian S, Eriksson-Derouet B, Ali T. Treatment of strabismus and nystagmus with botulinum toxin type A. An evaluation of effects and complications. Acta Ophthalmol Scand 1998;76(1):27–7.

Mathew NT, Jaffri SF. A double-blind comparison of onabotulinumtoxina (BOTOX) and topiramate (TOPAMAX) for the prophylactic treatment of chronic migraine: a pilot study. Headache 2009;49(10):1466–78.

Maurri S, Brogelli S, Alfieri G, Barontini F. Use of botulinum toxin in Meige's disease. Riv Neurol 1988;58(6):245–8.

Pappert EJ, Germanson T; Myobloc/Neurobloc European Cervical Dystonia Study Group. Botulinum toxin type B vs. type A in toxin-naïve patients with cervical dystonia: Randomized, double-blind, noninferiority trial. Mov Disord 2008;23(4):510–7.

Petri S, Tölle T, Straube A, Pfaffenrath V, Stefenelli U, Ceballos-Baumann A; Dysport Migraine Study Group. Botulinum toxin as preventive treatment for migraine: a randomized double-blind study. Eur Neurol 2009;62(4):204–11.

Zesiewicz TA, Stamey W, Sullivan KL, Hauser RA. Botulinum toxin A for the treatment of cervical dystonia. Expert Opin Pharmacother 2004; 5(9):2017–24.

BOTULINUM TOXIN TYPE B
(Rimabotulinum toxin B)

Brands
• Myobloc, Neurobloc

Generic?
No

 Class
• Neurotoxin

Commonly Prescribed for
(FDA approved in bold)
• **Cervical Dystonia (CD)**
• Glabellar lines
• Axillary hyperhidrosis
• Strabismus and blepharospasm associated with dystonia
• Hemifacial spasm
• Spasmodic torticollis
• Spasmodic dysphonia (laryngeal dystonia)
• Writer's cramp and other task-specific dystonias
• Spasticity associated with stroke
• Dynamic muscle contracture in cerebral palsy
• Sialorrhea (drooling)
• Headache
• Myofascial pain

 How the Drug Works
• Blocks neuromuscular transmission by cleaving the vesicle-associated membrane protein synaptobrevin, which inhibits the vesicular release of acetylcholine from nerve terminals
• In CD and other dystonias, produces partial denervation of muscle and localized reduction in muscle activity.
In hyperhidrosis, produces chemical denervation of sweat glands
• Also appears to inhibit release of neurotransmitters involved in pain transmission (including glutamate, calcitonin gene-related peptide, and substance P) and may enter CNS via retrograde axonal transport

How Long Until It Works
• Usually 1–3 days with peak effect beginning at 2 weeks

If It Works
• Continue to use as long as effective, but monitor for clinical effects

If It Doesn't Work
• Increase dose or change injection technique. Some pain disorders may respond better to oral medications

 Best Augmenting Combos for Partial Response or Treatment-Resistance
• Increase dose, number of injections or change site of location

Tests
• None

How Drug Causes AEs
• Most AEs are related to muscle weakness adjacent to the site of injection. Serious systemic AEs are rare, but injectors should use the lowest dose and be familiar with injection technique to minimize AEs

Notable AEs
• Injection site pain and hemorrhage, dry mouth, infection, fever, headache, pruritus, and myalgia. Most AEs depend on site of injection
• CD – dysphagia, neck weakness, upper respiratory infection
• Spasmodic dysphonia – hypophonia ("breathy" voice)

 Life-Threatening or Dangerous AEs
• Rarely patients may experience severe dysphagia requiring a feeding tube or leading to aspiration pneumonia
• Use with caution in patients with motor neuropathies or neuromuscular junctional disorders. These patients may be at greater risk for systemic weakness or respiratory problems

Weight Gain
• Unusual

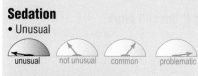

Sedation
• Unusual

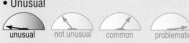

What to Do About AEs
• Most AEs will improve with time (weeks)

Best Augmenting Agents for AEs
• Most AEs cannot be improved with an augmenting agent

DOSING AND USE

Usual Dosage Range
• **CD** – Total dose 5000–10,000 units (u)
• **Hemifacial spasm** – Total dose 200–800 u
• **Spasmodic dysphonia** – 50–250 u
• **Sialorrhea** – 1000 u each side, up to 2500 bilaterally

Dosage Forms
• Solution for injection: 5000 u/mL

How to Dose
• Administer every 3 months using the lowest effective dose
• **CD** – start at a low dose and adjust as needed. Limiting the dose injected into the sternocleidomastoid muscles to 2000 u or less may decrease incidence of dysphagia
• **Spasmodic dysphonia** – for more common adductor type inject 50–100 u into each side of the thyroarytenoid muscles, for abductor type inject the posterior cricoarytenoid
• **Sialorrhea** – inject 500–1000 u into each parotid gland and 250 u into each submandibular gland. The mandibular glands may also be injected

 Dosing Tips
• Physicians should be familiar with the anatomy of the injection site and the specific disorders
• Inject using a needle or hollow electrode

• EMG recording helps to identify muscle involved in complex dystonias
• May dilute with saline but administer within 4 hours as product does not contain a preservative

Overdose
• Signs and symptoms of overdose may be delayed for several weeks. If accidental overdose occurs, monitor for signs of systemic weakness or paralysis

Long-Term Use
• Safe for long-term use

Habit Forming
• No

How to Stop
• No need to taper

Pharmacokinetics
• Does not reach peripheral blood after injection with recommended doses

 Drug Interactions
• Use with caution in patients taking medications, such as aminoglycosides or curae-like compounds, that can interfere with neuromuscular transmission

 Other Warning Precautions
• Contains albumin, a blood derivative that can theoretically carry risk of viral infection of Creutzfeldt-Jacob disease

Do Not Use
• Hypersensitivity to the drug or any of its components; infection at the proposed injection sites

SPECIAL POPULATIONS

Renal Impairment
• No known effects

Hepatic Impairment
• No known effects

Cardiac Impairment
• No known effects

Elderly
• No known effects

Children and Adolescents
• Safety and effectiveness unknown

Pregnancy
• Category C. Use only if benefit of medication outweighs risks

Breast Feeding
• Concentration in breast milk unknown. Use only if benefits outweigh risk

---

THE ART OF NEUROPHARMACOLOGY

Potential Advantages
• Effective in CD and most likely other pain disorders, with very few AEs or drug interactions. Compared to type A may have faster onset of action

Potential Disadvantages
• Cost and need for frequent injections to maintain effect. Dose requirement increases with muscle size. Effect may wear off sooner than with type A formulations

Primary Target Symptoms
• Dystonia, spasticity, pain, drooling, or sweating (depending on indication)

Pearls
• Botulinum toxin is most effective in focal dystonias. Generalized dystonias can be treated with anticholinergic therapy, especially in younger, cognitively normal patients
• It often takes a series of injections to determine the optimal dose for a given patient
• Botulinum toxin has not been extensively studied for the treatment of headache, neuropathic pain, or blepharospasm
• Some studies indicate that type B starts working earlier than A, but that the duration of effect might be less. This could be due to the inability to convert doses, making it difficult to compare different formulations
• Type B may disperse from injection sites to a greater extent than type A toxin
• To date, there does not appear to be antibody production against type B toxin

---

 Suggested Reading

Brashear A, McAfee AL, Kuhn ER, Fyffe J. Botulinum toxin type B in upper-limb poststroke spasticity: a double-blind, placebo-controlled trial. Arch Phys Med Rehabil 2004;85(5):705–9.

Colosimo C, Chianese M, Giovannelli M, Contarino MF, Bentivoglio AR. Botulinum toxin type B in blepharospasm and hemifacial spasm. J Neurol Neurosurg Psychiatry 2003; 74(5):687.

Costa J, Espírito-Santo C, Borges A, Ferreira JJ, Coelho M, Moore P, Sampaio C. Botulinum toxin type B for cervical dystonia. Cochrane Database Syst Rev 2005;(1):CD004315.

Klein AW, Carruthers A, Fagien S, Lowe NJ. Comparisons among botulinum toxins: an evidence-based review. Plast Reconstr Surg 2008;121(6):413e–422e.

Pappert EJ, Germanson T; Myobloc/Neurobloc European Cervical Dystonia Study Group. Botulinum toxin type B vs. type A in toxin-naïve patients with cervical dystonia: Randomized, double-blind, noninferiority trial. Mov Disord 2008;23(4):510–7.

Winner P. Botulinum toxins in the treatment of migraine and tension-type headaches. Phys Med Rehabil Clin N Am 2003;14(4):885–99.

BROMOCRIPTINE

THERAPEUTICS

Brands
• Parlodel, Serocryptin

Generic?
Yes

Class
• Dopamine agonist, ergot

Commonly Prescribed for
(FDA approved in bold)
• **Parkinson's disease (PD)**
• **Acromegaly**
• **Hyperprolactinemia**

How the drug works
• Dopamine agonist, with high affinity for the D2 receptor. This action is the reason for effectiveness. Also has weak alpha-agonist activity. In the treatment of hormone-secreting pituitary adenomas, bromocriptine works as a dopamine agonist, which inhibits prolactin-secreting cells in the anterior pituitary, reducing tumor size

How Long Until It Works
• PD – weeks

If It Works
• PD – may require dose adjustments over time or augmentation with other agents. Most PD patients will eventually require levodopa-carbidopa to manage their symptoms

If It Doesn't Work
• PD – Bradykinesia, gait and tremor should improve. Non-motor symptoms including autonomic symptoms such as postural hypotension, depression, and bladder dysfunction do not improve. If the patient has significantly impaired functioning, add or replace with levodopa

Best Augmenting Combos for Partial Response or Treatment-Resistance
• For suboptimal effectiveness add carbidopa-levodopa with or without a COMT inhibitor. MAO-B may also be beneficial
• For younger patients with bothersome tremor: anticholinergics may help

• For severe motor fluctuations and/or dyskinesias with good "on" time, functional neurosurgery (deep brain stimulation) is an option
• Depression is common in PD and may respond to low dose SSRIs
• Cognitive impairment/dementia is common in mid-late stage PD and may improve with acetylcholinesterase inhibitors
• For patients with late-stage PD experiencing hallucinations or delusions, withdraw bromocriptine and consider oral atypical neuroleptics (quetiapine, olanzapine, clozapine). Acute psychosis is a medical emergency that may require hospitalization for stabilization

Tests
• None required

ADVERSE EFFECTS (AEs)

How Drug Causes AEs
• Direct effect on dopamine receptors

Notable AEs
• Nausea/vomiting, constipation, orthostatic hypotension/syncope, confusion, dyskinesias, hallucinations, nervousness, drowsiness, and anorexia
• Signs of ergotism such as digital vasospasm, tingling in the fingertips, Raynaud phenomenon, cold feet and muscle cramps are uncommon, especially at lower doses

Life-Threatening or Dangerous AEs
• May cause somnolence or sudden onset sleep, often without warning
• Rare pulmonary or retroperitoneal fibrosis, pleural or pericardial effusions
• High doses are associated with confusion, mental disturbances and hallucinations
• Rare but significant increases in blood pressure can occur, often delayed until a week after initiating therapy. Seizures or stroke have occurred rarely, often preceded by severe progressive headache or visual disturbances. Less commonly myocardial infarction has occurred

Weight Gain
• Unusual

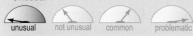

Sedation
• Common

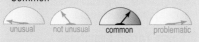

What to Do About AEs
• Nausea can be problematic when starting – titrate slowly
• Hallucinations or delusions may require stopping the medication
• Warn patients about the risk of excessive sleepiness while driving

Best Augmenting Agents for AEs
• Amantadine may help suppress dyskinesias
• Orthostatic hypotension: adjust dose or stop antihypertensives, add dietary salt, and consider fludrocortisone or midodrine
• Urinary incontinence: reducing PM fluids, voiding schedules, oxybutynin, desmopressin nasal spray, hyoscyamine sulfate, urological evaluation

---

DOSING AND USE

Usual Dosage Range
• PD – 5–40 mg daily, divided into 2 daily doses
• Hyperprolactinemia – 2.5–15 mg daily
• Acromegaly – 20–60 mg daily

Dosage Forms
• Tablets: 2.5 and 5 mg

How to Dose
• Start at 1.25 or 2.5 mg at bedtime to increase tolerance, then dose twice daily. Increase the daily dose by 1.25 or 2.5 mg every 1–2 weeks

 Dosing Tips
• Slow titration will minimize nausea and dizziness

Overdose
• Symptoms may include nausea/vomiting, constipation, diaphoresis, dizziness, severe hypotension, lethargy, malaise, and hallucinations. Treatment of hypotension with vasopressors may be required in severe cases

Long-Term Use
• Retroperitoneal fibrosis has been reported with patients using more than 2 years at high doses (30 mg or more). Effectiveness may decrease over time in PD

Habit Forming
• No

How to Stop
• Discontinue over a period of 1 week. PD symptoms may worsen, but serious AEs from discontinuation are rare. In patients using for pituitary disorders, tumor regrowth can occur

Pharmacokinetics
• About 28% of drug is absorbed. Elimination half-life 2–8 hours. Highly protein-bound

 Drug Interactions
• Increases the effect of levodopa
• Erythromycin increases levels
• Dopamine antagonists such as phenothiazines, metoclopramide diminish effectiveness
• Use with caution in patients on antihypertensive medications due to orthostatic hypotension
• Sympathomimetics such as isometheptene, phenylpropanolamine can increase AEs and case reports of ventricular tachycardia and cardiac dysfunction exist

Do Not Use
• Known hypersensitivity to the drug or other ergots. Uncontrolled hypertension. Patients with eclampsia, preeclampsia or pregnancy-induced hypertension, or post-partum patients with coronary artery disease or other severe cardiovascular condition

---

SPECIAL POPULATIONS

Renal Impairment
• No known effects

Hepatic Impairment
• No known effects

Cardiac Impairment
- Infrequently causes cardiac arrhythmias, rarely ventricular tachycardia. Use with caution

Elderly
- No known effects

 Children and Adolescents
- Use in PD is not studied in children (PD is rare) but does appear effective for the treatment of prolactin-secreting tumors in ages 16 and up. Has been used in children as young as 11

 Pregnancy
- Category B. Safety has not been established. For PD, use only if benefits of medication outweigh risks. In patients with prolactin-secreting adenomas, do a pregnancy test every 4 weeks as long as no menses occur. If pregnancy is established, discontinue bromocriptine and monitor closely for signs of tumor regrowth

Breast Feeding
- Inhibits prolactin secretion. Do not use

THE ART OF NEUROPHARMACOLOGY

Potential Advantages
- In PD, may delay need for levodopa and decreases risk of motor dyskinesias. Less likely to cause sleep disturbances than non-ergot agonists

Potential Disadvantages
- Generally less effective than levodopa and more AEs such as hallucinations, somnolence, and orthostatic hypotension. Risk of serious complications (retroperitoneal fibrosis) with long-term use

Primary Target Symptoms
- PD – motor dysfunction including bradykinesia, hand coordination, gait and rest tremor

 Pearls
- More serious AEs than some of the newer dopamine agonists which limits use
- For patients with mildly symptomatic disease, dopamine agonists are also appropriate for initial therapy, but for patients with significant disability, use levodopa early. Patients with poor response to levodopa will not benefit from bromocriptine
- Bromocriptine has minimal effect on the secretion of other pituitary hormones other than prolactin and growth hormone. About 75% of patients with galactorrhea respond to therapy, usually within 12 weeks. Menses are usually reinitiated prior to complete cessation of galactorrhea, on average in 6 to 8 weeks

 Suggested Reading

Brocks DR. Anticholinergic drugs used in Parkinson's disease: an overlooked class of drugs from a pharmacokinetic perspective. J Pharm Pharm Sci 1999; 2(2):39–46.

Costa J, Espírito-Santo C, Borges A, Ferreira JJ, Coelho M, Sampaio C. Botulinum toxin type A versus anticholinergics for cervical dystonia. Cochrane Database Syst Rev 2005;(1): CD004312.

Mizuno Y, Yanagisawa N, Kuno S, Yamamoto M, Hasegawa K, Origasa H, Kowa H; Japanese Pramipexole Study Group. Randomized, double-blind study of pramipexole with placebo and bromocriptine in advanced Parkinson's disease. Mov Disord 2003;18(10):1149–56.

van Hilten JJ, Ramaker CC, Stowe R, Ives NJ. Bromocriptine versus levodopa in early Parkinson's disease. Cochrane Database Syst Rev 2007;(4):CD002258.

CARBAMAZEPINE

Brands
- Tegretol, Carbatrol, Tegretol XR, Equetro, Teril, Timonil, Carbagen, Arbil, Epimaz, Mazepine, Novo-Carbamaz

Generic?
Yes

Class
- Antiepileptic drug (AED)

Commonly Prescribed for
(FDA approved in bold)
- **Complex partial seizures with or without secondary generalization (adults and children, monotherapy and adjunctive)**
- **Generalized tonic-clonic seizures**
- **Mixed seizure patterns**
- **Trigeminal neuralgia**
- Glossopharyngeal neuralgia
- Lennox-Gastaut syndrome
- Temporal lobe epilepsy (children and adults)
- Neuropathic pain
- Alcohol withdrawal
- Restless legs syndrome
- Bipolar I Disorder (acute manic and mixed episodes)
- Psychosis/Schizophrenia (adjunctive)

How the Drug Works
- Blocks voltage-dependent sodium channels
- Modulates sodium and calcium channels and GABA and glutamate transmission

How Long Until It Works
- Seizures – 2 weeks or less
- Trigeminal neuralgia or neuropathic pain – hours to weeks
- Mania – weeks

If It Works
- Seizures – goal is the remission of seizures. Continue as long as effective and well-tolerated. Consider tapering and slowly stopping after 2 years without seizures, depending on the type of epilepsy
- Trigeminal neuralgia – should dramatically reduce or eliminate attacks, pain may recur. Periodically attempt to reduce to lowest effective dose or discontinue

If It Doesn't Work
- Increase to highest tolerated dose. Subject to autoinduction, meaning that dose requirements can change over time
- Epilepsy: consider changing to another agent, adding a second agent or referral for epilepsy surgery evaluation. Check level if compliance is in question. When adding a second agent, keep drug interactions in mind
- Trigeminal neuralgia: Try an alternative agent. For truly refractory patients referral to tertiary headache center, consider surgical or other procedures

Best Augmenting Combos for Partial Response or Treatment-Resistance
- Epilepsy: drug interactions can complicate multi-drug therapy
- Pain: Can combine with other AEDs (gabapentin or pregabalin) or tricyclic antidepressants

Tests
- Baseline CBC, liver, kidney, and thyroid tests
- Check CBC biweekly for 2 months then every 3 months
- Liver, kidney, and thyroid tests every 6–12 months
- Check sodium levels for symptoms of hyponatremia

How Drug Causes AEs
- CNS AEs are probably caused by sodium channel blockade effects
- Mild anticholinergic side effects

Notable AEs
- Sedation, dizziness, ataxia, headache, nystagmus
- Nausea, vomiting, abdominal pain, constipation, pancreatitis, loss of sex drive
- Aching joints and leg cramps
- Elevated liver enzymes
- Benign leukopenia (transient; in up to 10%)

Life-Threatening or Dangerous AEs
- Rare blood dyscrasias: aplastic anemia, agranulocytosis

- Dermatologic reactions including toxic epidermal necrolysis and Stevens-Johnson syndrome. (More common in Asian patients.) Can aggravate rash of lupus
- Can reduce thyroid function
- Hyponatremia/SIADH (syndrome of inappropriate antidiuretic hormone secretion)
- May increase seizure frequency in patients with generalized seizure disorders

Weight Gain
- Not unusual

Sedation
- Problematic

- May limit use

What to Do About AEs
- Take with food, split dose, and take higher dose at night to improve tolerability
- Extended-release form may be better tolerated
- Rashes are common but usually not severe. Usually resolves with time or decreased dose. If severe stop drug. Do HLA typing prior to use in Asian patients
- Elevated liver enzymes usually resolve spontaneously

Best Augmenting Agents for AEs
- Topical steroids or antihistamines for rash

DOSING AND USE

Usual Dosage Range
- Epilepsy: 800–2000 mg/day
- Pain: Often a low dose is effective for trigeminal neuralgia. Usually 1200 mg/day or less
- Bipolar disorder: 400–1600 mg/day

Dosage Forms
Trade (Tegretol/Equ): Chewable tablets: 100 mg; tablets: 200 mg; oral solution: 100 mg/5 mL; extended-release tablets: 100 mg, 200 mg, 400 mg; extended-release capsules 200 mg, 300 mg

Generic: 200 mg tablets, 100 mg or 200 mg chewable tablets, 100 mg/5 mL suspension

How to Dose
- Epilepsy: Start at 400 mg/day. Give in 2 divided doses for ER and 3–4 doses/day with short-acting. Increase every 1–3 weeks to goal dose
- Trigeminal neuralgia/pain: Start at 200 mg/day and increase by 200 mg/week to goal dose
- Do not check levels in the first few weeks due to autoinduction
- Adjust dose as needed when using with AEDs or other drugs that affect levels

 Dosing Tips
- Take with food to avoid GI side effects
- Slow titration will help avoid blood dyscrasias and other AEs
- Carbamazepine induces its own metabolism (autoinduction), meaning the dose can decrease with time
- Oral suspension has higher peak levels than other formulations. Start at a lower dose and titrate more slowly

Overdose
- Coma, ataxia, nystagmus, cerebellar signs, dizziness. Less commonly urinary retention, chorea or seizures. Intraventicular conduction delay

Long-Term Use
- Safe for long-term use. Monitor blood counts, sodium, liver, kidney, and thyroid function

Habit Forming
- No

How to Stop
- Taper slowly
- Abrupt withdrawal can lead to seizures in patients with epilepsy

Pharmacokinetics
- Hepatic metabolism via CYP450 system, CYP3A4. Inducer of CYP3A4 metabolism
- Highly protein bound, renally excreted
- Bioavailability is 75–85%

- Peak levels at 4–8 h, plasma half-life 18–55 h initially, decreasing to 5–26 after autoinduction

Drug Interactions

- Carbamazepine decreases levels of many AEDs (Valproate, clonazepam, topiramate, zonisamide, tiagabine, and ethosuximide) and also warfarin, doxicycline, acetaminophen, haloperidol, nortriptyline, nifedipine, trazodone, alprazolam, among many
- Carbamazepine increases levels of flunarizine, digitalis, lithium, furosemide, isoniazide, and MAO inhibitors
- Variable effect on phenytoin and phenobarbital
- AEDs lamotrigine, phenytoin, primidone, phenobarbital, felbamate and many CYP450 3A4 inducers (including carbamazepine itself) decrease levels
- Acetazolamide, caffeine, verapamil, fluoxetine, desipramine, and many other CYP450 3A4 inhibitors increase levels
- Valproate and Clonazepam have a variable effect on levels

Other Warnings/ Precautions

- CNS AEs increase when used with other CNS depressants
- Rare systemic disorders: dermatomyositis, diabetes insipidus
- Rare worsening of acute angle-closure glaucoma
- Long-term treatment may affect bone metabolism
- May cause alterations in sex hormone levels and impair effectiveness of oral contraceptives
- Decrease of sex drive or fertility
- May worsen absence or mixed absence epilepsy syndromes
- Asian patients have a greater risk of rash

Do Not Use

- Patients with a proven allergy to carbamazepine

Renal Impairment

- Highly protein bound, makes easier to use. Patients with severe renal insufficiency may need lower dose

Hepatic Impairment

- Use with caution in patients with moderate-severe disease and monitor for AEs with regular hepatic function panels. Stop if any worsening

Cardiac Impairment

- Can produce arrhythmias in patients with cardiac disease or conduction disease. Use with caution and obtain baseline ECG

Elderly

- May need lower dose. More likely to experience AEs except rash. Increased risk of aplastic anemia

Children and Adolescents

- Ages 6–12: Start at 200 mg/day in divided doses. Increase by 100 mg/day every 1–2 weeks to goal dose, usually less than 1000 mg/day
- Age 5 or less: 5–10 mg/kg/day in divided doses, increase by 5–10 mg/kg/day every week until goal dose, usually 35 mg/kg/day or less
- Children have less risk of rash

Pregnancy

- Risk category D. Teratogenicity includes increased rate of neural tube defects with use in 1st trimester
- Drug does cross placenta
- Plasma levels and effectiveness may change during pregnancy – monitor serum levels
- Supplementation with 0.4 mg of folic acid before and during pregnancy is recommended
- Patients taking for headache, pain, or bipolar disorder should generally stop before considering pregnancy

Breast Feeding

- Some drug is found in mother's breast milk
- Generally recommendations are to discontinue drug or bottle feed
- Monitor infant for sedation, poor feeding or irritability

THE ART OF NEUROPHARMACOLOGY

Potential Advantages
- Proven effectiveness as monotherapy for partial seizures
- Effective for trigeminal neuralgia

Potential Disadvantages
- Ineffective for many primary generalized epilepsies
- Multiple interactions with other AEDs and other drugs and potential AEs
- Need for blood monitoring. Oxcarbazepine is often better tolerated

Primary Target Symptoms
- Seizure frequency and severity
- Pain

Pearls
- Effective for partial epilepsies but may worsen absence, atonic, or myoclonic seizures
- May worsen or improve generalized tonic-clonic seizure control
- Autoinduction means dose requirements can increase after initial titration
- First-line drug for trigeminal neuralgia, effective in about 80% of patients, often in hours or days. Benefit may not be sustained
- Second-line treatment for SUNCT (Short-lasting unilateral neuralgiform headache with conjunctival injection and tearing)
- Little evidence for use in migraine
- Useful in mania and mixed bipolar states, not necessarily depression

Suggested Reading

Ettinger AB, Argoff CE. Use of antiepileptic drugs for nonepileptic conditions: psychiatric disorders and chronic pain. Neurotherapeutics 2007;4(1):75–83.

Harden CL, Pennell PB, Koppel BS, Hovinga CA, Gidal B, Meador KJ, Hopp J, Ting TY, Hauser WA, Thurman D, Kaplan PW, Robinson JN, French JA, Wiebe S, Wilner AN, Vazquez B, Holmes L, Krumholz A, Finnell R, Shafer PO, Le Guen C; American Academy of Neurology; American Epilepsy Society. Practice parameter update: management issues for women with epilepsy–focus on pregnancy (an evidence-based review): vitamin K, folic acid, blood levels, and breastfeeding: report of the Quality Standards Subcommittee and Therapeutics and Technology Assessment Subcommittee of the American Academy of Neurology and American Epilepsy Society. Neurology 2009;73(2):142–9.

Tomson T. Clinical pharmacokinetics of carbamazepine. Cephalalgia 1987;7(4):219–23.

Wiffen PJ, McQuay HJ, Moore RA. Carbamazepine for acute and chronic pain. Cochrane Database Syst Rev 2005;(3): CD005451.

CARBIDOPA/LEVODOPA

Brands
- Sinemet, Sinemet CR, Parcopa, Laradopa (levodopa), Lodosyn (carbidopa), Atamet, Caramet, Co-careldopa

Generic?
Yes

 Class
- Antiparkinson agent

Commonly Prescribed for
(FDA approved in bold)
- **Parkinson's disease (PD)** including idiopathic PD, post-encephalitic parkinsonism, symptomatic parkinsonism
- Dopa-responsive dystonia (DRD)
- Restless legs syndrome (RLS)

 How the Drug Works
- In PD, there is a loss of dopaminergic neurons in the substantia nigra and relative excess of cholinergic input. In DRD, there is a deficiency of tetrahydrobiopterin, a co-factor for tyrosine hydroxylase, the rate-limiting enzyme in dopamine synthesis
- Levodopa crosses the blood-brain barrier and is converted to dopamine in the brain
- Carbidopa is a peripheral decarboxylase inhibitor that prevents levodopa from being metabolized in the gut, increasing CNS dopamine

How Long Until It Works
- PD – hours, but may take 4–8 weeks to receive maximal benefit from a particular dose level when starting
- DRD – usually improves within days or weeks
- RLS – days to weeks

If It Works
- PD – may require dose adjustments over time or augmentation with other agents
- DRD – effective at low doses

If It Doesn't Work
- PD – Bradykinesia, gait, and tremor should improve. Non-motor symptoms, including autonomic symptoms such as postural hypotension, depression, and bladder dysfunction, do not improve with carbidopa/levodopa. If the response is poor, reconsider the diagnosis of idiopathic PD. Drug-induced parkinsonism or atypical parkinsonism syndromes are possibilities
- RLS – Rule out peripheral neuropathy, iron deficiency, thyroid disease. Change to dopamine agonist or another drug

 Best Augmenting Combos for Partial Response or Treatment-Resistance
- For end-of-dose failure (wearing-off), early morning or nocturnal akinesia, and end-of-dose dystonia: increase frequency and decrease amount of each dose of medication, add a dopamine agonist with a longer half-life, add an MAO-B or COMT inhibitor
- For younger patients with bothersome tremor: anticholinergics may help
- For severe motor fluctuations and/or dyskinesias with good "on" time, functional neurosurgery is an option
- Amantadine may help suppress dyskinesias, although benefit is often short-lived
- Depression is common in PD and may respond to low dose SSRIs
- Cognitive impairment/dementia is common in mid-late stage PD and may improve with acetylcholinesterase inhibitors
- For patients with late-stage PD experiencing hallucinations or delusions, withdraw dopamine agonists and consider oral atypical neuroleptics (quetiapine, olanzapine, clozapine). Acute psychosis is a medical emergency that may require hospitalization
- For patients with DRD, anticholinergic drugs are also helpful
- For RLS, can add or change to dopamine agonist or anticonvulsant, such as clonazepam or gabapentin

Tests
- May cause elevation of liver enzymes or anemia. Regular blood work may be needed

How Drug Causes AEs
- Direct effect of levodopa systemically and dopamine in CNS. Carbidopa – does not

have AEs but can reduce systemic AE (nausea) and increase CNS AE (hallucinations)

Notable AEs

- Nausea/vomiting, orthostatic hypotension, urinary retention, psychosis, depression, dry mouth, dysphagia, nightmares, edema, change in urine color, muscle twitching, and blepharospasm. Rare GI bleeding, hypertension, and hemolytic anemia

 Life-Threatening or Dangerous AEs

- May cause somnolence or sudden-onset sleep, often without warning

Weight Gain

- Unusual

unusual   not unusual   common   problematic

Sedation

- Not Unusual

unusual   not unusual   common   problematic

What to Do About AEs

- Nausea can be problematic when starting. Taking after meals will reduce the peak dose and AEs, but delays effect and reduces effectiveness
- For severe peak-dose dyskinesias, use extended-release form, use a dopamine agonist, lower the amount of each levodopa dose, and shorten the dosing interval

Best Augmenting Agents for AEs

- For nausea, increase dose of carbidopa relative to levodopa
- Amantadine may help suppress dyskinesias, although benefit is often short-lived
- Dopamine agonists are less likely to cause dyskinesias
- Orthostatic hypotension: adjust dose or stop antihypertensives, add dietary salt, and consider fludrocortisone or midodrine
- Urinary incontinence: reduce PM fluids, voiding schedules, oxybutynin, desmopressin nasal spray, hyoscyamine sulfate, urological evaluation

Usual Dosage Range

- PD – 300–800 mg levodopa with at least 75 mg carbidopa per day
- Dopa-responsive dystonia – lower doses may be effective. 50–200 mg levodopa per day, max 400 mg/day

Dosage Forms

- Levodopa tablets: 100, 250 and 500 mg
- Carbidopa/levodopa tablets: 25/100 mg, 10/100 mg, 25/250 mg
- Carbidopa/levodopa controlled release (CR): 25/100 mg, 50/200 mg
- Orally disintegrating tablets (Parcopa) 10/100 mg, 25/100 mg, 25/250 mg
- Carbidopa tablets: 25 mg

How to Dose

- Immediate release: Start either 10/100 or 25/100 3–4 times per day. Dosage may be increased by 1 tablet every other day up to a dosage of 8 tablets
- Extended release: 1 50/200 tablet twice a day, increase by ½ to 1 tablet every other day, up a dosage of 8 tablets
- Give extra carbidopa for patients with AEs such as nausea or orthostatic hypotension. This will increase CNS dopamine and may require lowering levodopa dose. Watch for worsening hallucinations and dyskinesias
- For RLS: take extended-release form before bedtime

 Dosing Tips

- Take before meals for best effect. Distributing protein throughout the day may help avoid fluctuations. Low protein meals may reduce "wearing-off."

Overdose

- Monitor for cardiac arrhythmias. Gastric lavage and intravenous fluids. Pyridoxine may help

Long-Term Use

- Safe for long-term use. Effectiveness may decrease over time in PD (years) and RLS (months)

Habit Forming

- No

How to Stop

- Stopping abruptly will worsen symptoms of PD and lead to confusion, rigidity, and hyperpyrexia similar to neuroleptics malignant syndrome

Pharmacokinetics

- Dopamine is metabolized to dopamine and homovanillic acid in the brain. The peak effect is at 0.5 hours for the immediate-release tablets. Levodopa has a half-life of 50 minutes alone but 90 minutes when taken with carbidopa. The extended-release form has decreased systemic bioavailability (70–75%), decreased maximum concentration, and longer half-life, with peak effect at 2 hours. Absorbed by large neutral amino acid transporter in large intestine and blood-brain barrier absorption through gut and across blood-brain barrier can be affected by protein loads

 Drug Interactions

- Pyridoxine (Vitamin B6), benzodiazepines, phenytoin, methionine, papaverine can impair effectiveness of levodopa
- Anticholinergics and tricyclic antidepressants may decrease bioavailability and absorption
- Non-selective MAO inhibitors can cause hypertensive crisis
- Antacids increase bioavailability
- Levodopa may decrease effectiveness of metoclopramide
- Use levodopa with caution in patients on antihypertensive medications due to orthostatic hypotension
- Dopamine receptor antagonists may reduce therapeutic response

 Other Warning Precautions

- May worsen intraocular pressure in patients with chronic wide-angle glaucoma
- Leukopenia, increased incidence of melanoma in PD with or without levodopa treatment has been reported
- May worsen existing peptic ulcers

Do Not Use

- Patients on non-selective MAO inhibitors, narrow-angle closure glaucoma or known hypersensitivity to the drug

Renal Impairment

- Use with caution but no known effects

Hepatic Impairment

- Use with caution but no known effects

Cardiac Impairment

- Use with caution in patients with known arrhythmias,

Elderly

- Safe for use

 Children and Adolescents

- Not studied in children (PD is rare in pediatrics)
- Children with dopa-responsive dystonia usually tolerate well, and dyskinesias are rare

 Pregnancy

- Category C. Teratogenic in some animal studies. Benefit of medication may outweigh risks in some patients

Breast Feeding

- Concentration in breast milk unknown. Breast feeding is not recommended.

Potential Advantages

- The most effective symptomatic treatment for PD. Less postural hypotension and fewer hallucinations than dopamine agonists

Potential Disadvantages

- Risk for motor complications, dyskinesias, and response fluctuations after 3–5 years of therapy. Not indicated for restless legs syndrome. Need for frequent dosing, especially in late-stage PD

Primary Target Symptoms

- PD – bradykinesia, hand function, gait and rest tremor
- RLS – pain, insomnia

CARBIDOPA/LEVODOPA (continued)

Pearls

- Levodopa, when given alone, causes severe anorexia and nausea. In clinical practice it is almost always used with carbidopa. Carbidopa alone has no therapeutic benefit without levodopa
- For patients with mildly symptomatic disease, dopamine agonists are also appropriate for initial therapy, but for patients with significant disability, use carbidopa/levodopa early
- Both immediate-release and CR levodopa are effective, although some measures suggest CR is more likely to improve quality of life. Motor complications and dyskinesias can occur with either form
- Changing from immediate to CR does not require changing the daily dose
- For RLS, carbidopa/levodopa is usually effective but often patients develop tolerance or rebound symptoms in the morning. This phenomenon, called "augmentation," is why dopamine agonists are generally preferred for RLS

Suggested Reading

Koller WC, Hutton JT, Tolosa E, Capilldeo R. Immediate-release and controlled-release carbidopa/levodopa in PD: a 5-year randomized multicenter study. Carbidopa/Levodopa Study Group. Neurology 1999;53(5):1012–19.

Lang AE. When and how should treatment be started in Parkinson disease? Neurology 2009; 72(7 Suppl):S39–43.

Manyam BV, Hare TA, Robbs R, Cubberley VB. Evaluation of equivalent efficacy of sinemet and sinemet CR in patients with Parkinson's disease applying levodopa dosage conversion formula. Clin Neuropharmacol 1999;22(1):33–9.

Olanow CW, Stern MB, Sethi K. The scientific and clinical basis for the treatment of Parkinson disease. Neurology 2009;72(21 Suppl 4): S1–136.

Robottom BJ, Weiner WJ. Dementia in Parkinson's disease. Int Rev Neurobiol 2009;84:229–44.

Trenkwalder C, Hening WA, Montagna P, Oertel WH, Allen RP, Walters AS, Costa J, Stiasny-Kolster K, Sampaio C. Treatment of restless legs syndrome: an evidence-based review and implications for clinical practice. Mov Disord 2008;23(16):2267–302.

CARISOPRODOL

THERAPEUTICS

Brands
• Soma, Sanoma, Carisoma

Generic?
Yes

 Class
• Skeletal muscle relaxant, centrally acting

Commonly Prescribed for
(FDA approved in bold)
• **Acute painful musculoskeletal conditions**
• Muscle spasm
• Insomnia

 How the Drug Works
• Sedative, may block interneuronal activity in the descending reticular formation and spinal cord

How Long Until It Works
• Pain – as little as 30 minutes

If It Works
• Titrate to most effective tolerated dose

If It Doesn't Work
• Increase dose. If ineffective, consider alternative medications

 Best Augmenting Combos for Partial Response or Treatment-Resistance
• Botulinum toxin is effective, especially as an adjunct for focal spasticity, i.e., post-stroke or head injury affecting the upper limbs
• Use other centrally acting muscle relaxants with caution due to potential additive CNS depressant effect

Tests
• None required

ADVERSE EFFECTS (AEs)

How Drug Causes AEs
• Most are related to sedative effects

Notable AEs
• Drowsiness, dizziness, vertigo, ataxia, depression, nausea/vomiting, tachycardia, postural hypotension, facial flushing

 Life-Threatening or Dangerous AEs
• Hypersensitivity reactions rarely occur after the first dose. Symptoms include extreme weakness, ataxia, vision loss, dysarthria, and euphoria. Serious allergic reactions, such as erythema multiforme, eosinophilia, asthmatic episodes, fever, angioedema, and anaphylactoid shock have been reported

Weight Gain
• Unusual

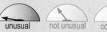

Sedation
• Common

What to Do About AEs
• Reduce dosing frequency for mild AEs and discontinue for serious AEs

Best Augmenting Agents for AEs
• Most AEs cannot be improved by an augmenting agent

DOSING AND USE

Usual Dosage Range
• 1 tablet 3–4 times daily

Dosage Forms
• Tablets: 250, 350 mg

How to Dose
• Give 1 tablet 3 times a day and at bedtime

 Dosing Tips
• May start by dosing at night; 250 mg may be better tolerated

Overdose
• Can produce stupor, coma, shock, respiratory depression, and rarely death.

Additive effects when using with other CNS depressants. Use respiratory assistance and pressors if needed. Dialysis or diuresis may be helpful in some cases

Long-Term Use
• Not well studied

Habit Forming
• Potentially yes

How to Stop
• Patients on low doses do not need to taper. Withdrawal can occur in patients on higher doses. This may include anxiety, tremor, insomnia, hallucinations, and confusion

Pharmacokinetics
• Onset of action in about 30 minutes, with effects lasting 2–6 hours and half-life 8 hours. Hepatic metabolism via CYP2C19 into active metabolite meprobamate and renal excretion

 Drug Interactions
• Use with CNS depressants or psychotropic drugs may be additive

Do Not Use
• Hypersensitivity to the drug. Use with caution in addiction-prone individuals

SPECIAL POPULATIONS

Renal Impairment
• Use with caution, as decreased drug clearance may increase toxicity

Hepatic Impairment
• Use with caution, as decreased drug metabolism may increase toxicity

Cardiac Impairment
• No known effects

Elderly
• May be more prone to AEs

 Children and Adolescents
• Not studied in children

 Pregnancy
• Category C. Use only if there is a clear need

Breast Feeding
• Drug is excreted in breast milk and can cause sedation. Do not use

THE ART OF NEUROPHARMACOLOGY

Potential Advantages
• Quick onset of action

Potential Disadvantages
• Risk of abuse and dependence. Sedation and potential for overdose

Primary Target Symptoms
• Pain, muscle spasm

 Pearls
• Usage in clinical practice has decreased compared to other agents for muscle spasm due to risk of addiction, sedation, and risk of serious hypersensitivity reactions
• Misused by opioid-addicted patients to increase the effect of smaller opioid doses. It particularly affects codeine-derived semi-synthetics, such as codeine, oxycodone, and hydrocodone

Suggested Reading

Chou R, Peterson K, Helfand M. Comparative efficacy and safety of skeletal muscle relaxants for spasticity and musculoskeletal conditions: a systematic review. J Pain Symptom Manage 2004;28(2):140–75.

Littrell RA, Hayes LR, Stillner V. Carisoprodol (Soma): a new and cautious perspective on an old agent. South Med J 1993;86(7):753–6.

Reeves RR, Beddingfield JJ, Mack JE. Carisoprodol withdrawal syndrome. Pharmacotherapy 2004;24(12):1804–6.

CHLORPROMAZINE

THERAPEUTICS

Brands
- Thorazine, Largactil

Generic?
Yes

 ### Class
- Antiemetic, antipsychotic

Commonly Prescribed for
(FDA approved in bold)
- **Antiemetic**
- **Intractable hiccups**
- **Psychosis, schizophrenia**
- Mania in bipolar disorder
- **Acute intermittent porphyria**
- **Tetanus**
- **Restlessness and apprehension before surgery**
- Hyperactivity and behavioral problems (children)
- Migraine (acute)

 ### How the Drug Works
- Dopamine receptor antagonist with greatest action at D2 receptors. Also has antihistamine, anticholinergic effects, and blocks alpha-adrenergic receptors

How Long Until It Works
- Migraine – 1 hour (oral) or less than 30 minutes (IV)

If It Works
- Use at lowest required dose
- Monitor QT corrected (QTc) interval

If It Doesn't Work
- Change to another agent

 ### Best Augmenting Combos for Partial Response or Treatment-Resistance
- For migraine, can be used with dihydroergotamine or NSAIDs

Tests
- Obtain blood pressure and pulse before initial IV and monitor QTc with ECG

ADVERSE EFFECTS (AEs)

How Drug Causes AEs
- Anticholinergic effects produce most AEs (sedation, blurred vision, dry mouth). Hypotension and dizziness are related to alpha-adrenergic blockade, and motor AEs are related to dopamine blocking effects

Notable AEs
- Akathisia, extrapyramidal symptoms, parkinsonism
- Dizziness, sedation, orthostatic hypotension, tachycardia, urinary retention, depression
- Long-term use: weight gain, glucose intolerance, sexual dysfunction, hyperprolactinemia

 ### Life-Threatening or Dangerous AEs
- Tardive dyskinesias
- Neuroleptic malignant syndrome (rare)
- Jaundice, agranulocytosis (rare)

Weight Gain
- Common (with chronic use)

 unusual   not unusual   common   problematic

Sedation
- Problematic

 unusual   not unusual   common   problematic

What to Do About AEs
- Lowering dose or changing to another antiemetic improves most AEs
- Rarely causes ECG changes. Use with caution in patients if QTc is above 450 (females) or 440 (males) and do not administer with QTc greater than 500
- If excessive sedation, use only as a rescue agent for intractable migraine in hospitalized patients or when patients can lie down or sleep

Best Augmenting Agents for AEs
- Give fluids to avoid hypotension, tachycardia, and dizziness
- Give anticholinergics (diphenhydramine or benztropine) or benzodiazepines for extrapyramidal reactions
- Amantadine may improve motor AEs

DOSING AND USE

Usual Dosage Range
- Migraine: up to 200 mg/day IV, IM, or oral in divided doses

Dosage Forms
- Tablets: 10 mg, 25 mg, 50 mg, 100 mg, 200 mg
- Injection: 25 mg/mL
- Liquid: 25 mg/5 mL, 100 mg/5 mL
- Suppository: 25 mg, 100 mg

How to Dose
- Oral: Give 10–25 mg and repeat as needed every 4–6 hours. Patients with previous exposure and few significant AEs may increase dose and use up to 200 mg/day in divided doses
- IV/IM: Give 12.5–50 mg every 4–8 hours up to 200 mg/day

Dosing Tips
- In hospitalized patients, start with lower dose to ensure drug is tolerated and increase as needed to effective dose
- Warn patients not to drive
- Check ECG daily while patients are treated and monitor blood pressure

Overdose
- CNS depression, hypotension, or extrapyramidal reactions are most common. Tachycardia, restlessness, convulsions, and respiratory depression may occur

Long-Term Use
- Safe for long-term use with appropriate monitoring. Tardive dyskinesias may be irreversible

Habit Forming
- No

How to Stop
- No need to taper

Pharmacokinetics
- Metabolized by CYP2D6. Tmax 1–4 hours and half-life 8–33 hours

Drug Interactions
- Use with CNS depressants (barbiturates, opiates, general anesthetics) potentiates CNS AEs
- May enhance effects of antihypertensives
- Use with alcohol or diuretics may increase hypotension
- May decrease effectiveness of dopaminergic agents
- Reduces effectiveness of anticoagulants
- May increase phenytoin levels
- The combination of lithium and neuroleptics has been reported to produce an encephalopathy similar to neuroleptic malignant syndrome

Other Warnings/ Precautions
- Neuroleptic malignant syndrome is characterized by fever, rigidity, confusion, and autonomic instability, and is most common with IV typical neuroleptics such as chlorpromazine

Do Not Use
- Hypersensitivity to drug, CNS depression or QTc greater than 500

SPECIAL POPULATIONS

Renal Impairment
- No known effects

Hepatic Impairment
- No known effects

Cardiac Impairment
- May worsen orthostatic hypotension

Elderly
- More sensitive to CNS AEs, use lower doses

Children and Adolescents
- Appears safe in children over age 1, but mostly used for behavioral problems. Not a first-line agent in pediatric migraine

Pregnancy
- Category C. Use only if benefit outweighs risks

Breast Feeding
- Some drug is found in breast milk and may cause sedation or movement problems in infants. Do not use for migraine

THE ART OF NEUROPHARMACOLOGY

Potential Advantages
- Effective drug for severe migraine. Sedation may be helpful for some patients and akathisia may be less common than with other antiemetics

Potential Disadvantages
- Significant AEs including extrapyramidal reactions, sedation, and hypotension.

Children and elderly patients may tolerate poorly

Primary Target Symptoms
- Headache, nausea

 Pearls
- Effective in refractory migraine and status migrainosus. Often combined with dihydroergotamine, given about 30 minutes after chlorpromazine
- Pretreat or combine with diphenydramine, 25–50 mg, to reduce rate of akathisia and dystonic reactions
- Generally used as a "rescue" treatment in severe migraine when first-line medications (triptans, dihydroergotamine, NSAIDs) have failed

 Suggested Reading

Evans RW, Young WB. Droperidol and other neuroleptics/antiemetics for the management of migraine. Headache 2003;43(7):811–3.

Leucht S, Wahlbeck K, Hamann J, Kissling W. New generation antipsychotics versus low-potency conventional antipsychotics: a systematic review and meta-analysis. Lancet 2003;361:1581–9.

Brands
- Klonopin, Rivotril

Generic?
Yes

Class
- Benzodiazepine, antiepileptic drug (AED)

Commonly Prescribed for
(FDA approved in bold)
- **Seizure disorders. Used as monotherapy or adjunctive for the treatment of Lennox-Gastaut syndrome, akinetic, myoclonic or absence seizures**
- **Panic disorder, with or without agoraphobia**
- Periodic leg movements disorder (PLMD)
- Restless legs syndrome (RLS)
- Tic disorders
- Parkinsonian (hypokinetic) dysarthria
- Muscle relaxation
- Insomnia
- Burning mouth syndrome
- Generalized anxiety disorder
- Schizophrenia (adjunctive)
- Acute mania in bipolar disorder

How the Drug Works
- Benzodiazepines bind to and potentiate the effect of GABA-A receptors, boosting chloride conductance through GABA-regulated channels, and other inhibitory neurotransmitters. There are at least 2 benzodiazepine receptors, 1 of which is associated with sleep mechanisms, the other with memory, sensory and cognitive functions. They act at spinal cord, brainstem, cerebellum, limbic and cortical areas
- In petit mal seizures clonazepam suppresses spike and wave discharges, and in motor seizures decreases the frequency, amplitude, duration and spread of discharge

How Long Until It Works
- There is often an immediate effect in treatment of epilepsy, PLMD, RLS, insomnia and panic disorders, but usually weeks are required for optimal dose adjustments and maximal therapeutic benefit

If It Works
- Seizures – goal is the remission of seizures. Continue as long as effective and well-tolerated. Consider tapering and slowly stopping after 2 years seizure-free, depending on the type of epilepsy
- PLMD, RLS, tic disorders – continue to adjust dose to find the lowest dose that produces relief of symptoms with fewest AEs
- Anxiety – often used only on a short-term basis. Consider adding an SSRI or SNRI for long-term treatment

If It Doesn't Work
- Epilepsy: consider changing to another agent, adding a second agent or referral for epilepsy surgery evaluation
- PLMD, RLS: change to or use combination with a dopamine agonist or an AED such as gabapentin or carbamazepine. Rule out iron-deficiency; if obese, weight loss may be helpful

Best Augmenting Combos for Partial Response or Treatment-Resistance
- Epilepsy: often used in combination with other AEDs for optimal control but sedation can increase
- PLMD, RLS: dopamine agonists or gabapentin
- Anxiety: SSRI or SNRIs. In most cases it is best to avoid combining with other benzodiazepines
- Insomnia: may be combined with low-dose tricylic antidepressants (amitriptyline), or tetracyclics (trazodone, mirtazapine)

Tests
- None required

How Drug Causes AEs
- Actions on benzodiazepine receptors including augmentation of inhibitory neurotransmitter effects

Notable AEs
- Most common: sedation, fatigue, depression, weakness, ataxia, nystagmus, confusion, and psychomotor retardation

- Less common: bradycardia, anorexia, hypotonia, and anterograde amnesia

 Life-Threatening or Dangerous AEs

- CNS depression and decreased respiratory drive, especially in combination with opiates, barbiturates, or alcohol
- Rare blood dyscrasias or liver function abnormalities

Weight Gain
- Unusual

Sedation
- Not unusual

What to Do About AEs
- May decrease or remit in time as tolerance develops
- Lower the total dose and take more at bedtime
- For severe, life-threatening AEs, administer flumazenil to reverse effects

Best Augmenting Agents for AEs
- Most AEs cannot be improved by adding an augmenting agent

DOSING AND USE

Usual Dosage Range
- Epilepsy: up to 20 mg/day in adults in divided doses
- PLMD, RLS: 0.5–2 mg/night
- Panic/anxiety disorders: usually best dose in panic disorder is 1 mg per day in divided doses. Maximum is generally 4 mg/day

Dosage Forms
- Tablets: 0.5, 1 and 2 mg
- Orally disintegrating (wafer): 0.125, 0.25, 0.5, 1, and 2 mg

How to Dose
- Epilepsy: Start at 0.5 mg twice or 3 times daily. Increase dose in increments of 0.5 mg to 1 mg every 3 days until seizures are adequately controlled or AEs develop. Use

the largest dose at bedtime. Tolerance to drug occasionally requires increasing dose to a maximum of 20 mg/day in divided doses 2–3 times daily
- RLS: Start at 0.5 mg at bedtime. Increase by 0.5 mg every few nights until symptoms improve to maximum of 2 mg at night
- Panic disorder: Start at 0.25 mg twice daily and increase to either 0.5 twice daily or 1 mg at night in 3 days

 Dosing Tips

- Dose in epilepsy often requires adjustment over time due to tolerance. Tolerance and dependence are less common in doses used to treat RLS or anxiety
- Assess need to continue treatment in all disorders
- Use disintegrating tablets for patients with swallowing difficulties

Overdose
- Confusion, drowsiness, decreased reflexes, incoordination, and lethargy are common. Ataxia, hypotension, coma, and death are rare. Coma, respiratory or circulatory depression are rare when used alone. Use with other CNS depressants such as alcohol, narcotics, or barbiturates place patients at greater risk. Induce vomiting and use supportive measures along with gastric lavage or ipecac and in severe cases forced diuresis
- Flumazenil reverses effect of clonazepam but provokes seizures in patients with epilepsy

Long-Term Use
- Safe for long-term use with appropriate monitoring

Habit Forming
- Schedule IV drug with risk of tolerance and dependence. Dependence is most common with use after 6 weeks or more. Patients with a history of drug or alcohol abuse have an increased risk of dependency

How to Stop
- Taper slowly, as abrupt withdrawal can cause seizures, even in patients without epilepsy. The seizures often occur over a week after stopping drug due to long half-life
- Taper by 0.25 mg/day every 3 days to reduce risk of withdrawal. Once at a lower dose

(1.5 mg per day or less) decrease speed of taper to as little as 0.125 mg/week or less. Slow tapers are especially recommended for patients on clonazepam for many months or years
- Monitor for re-emergence of disease symptoms (seizures, RLS or anxiety)

Pharmacokinetics
- Peak plasma level at 1–2 hours but long elimination half-life compared to other benzodiazepines (18–50 hours). 97% protein bound and bioavailability over 80%. Mostly metabolized by CYP3A4 isoenzyme

 Drug Interactions
- Alcohol and CNS depressants (barbiturates, narcotics) increase CNS AEs
- CYP3A4 inhibitors such as nefazodone, fluoxetine, fluvoxamine, ketoconazole, clarithromycin, and many antivirals decrease clearance of drug but dose adjustment is rarely needed
- Antacids may alter the rate of absorption
- May increase serum concentrations of digoxin and phenytoin, leading to toxicity

⚠️ **Other Warnings/ Precautions**
- May increase salivation. Use with caution in patients with chronic respiratory disease
- May cause drowsiness and impair ability to drive or perform tasks that require alertness

Do Not Use
- Patients with a proven allergy to clonazepam or any benzodiazepine. Significant liver disease or narrow angle-closure glaucoma

SPECIAL POPULATIONS

Renal Impairment
- Metabolites are renally excreted. Reduce dose

Hepatic Impairment
- Do not use in patients with significant disease

Cardiac Impairment
- No known effects

Elderly
- May clear drug more slowly and have lower dose requirement. Due to slower drug clearance, elderly patients may better tolerate benzodiazepines with a shorter half-life, such as diazepam

 Children and Adolescents
- In infants and children under 10 or under 30 kg body weight, initial dose should be between 0.01–0.03 mg/kg/day in 2 or 3 divided doses and maximal dose no more than 0.05 mg/kg/day. Increase dose by 0.25 or 0.5 mg every 3 days to a maximum maintenance dose of 0.1–0.2 mg/kg/day
- Not studied for use in anxiety/panic disorders

 Pregnancy
- Risk category D. Drug crosses placenta and accumulates in fetal circulation. May increase risk of fetal malformations. Use during labor can cause "floppy infant" syndrome with hypotonia, lethargy, and sucking difficulties
- In epilepsy, use with caution due to risk of seizures in pregnancy or change to another agent. Do not use for treatment of anxiety or RLS

Breast Feeding
- Drug is found in mother's breast milk and may cause accumulation of drug and metabolites. Do not breast feed on drug

THE ART OF NEUROPHARMACOLOGY

Potential Advantages
- Rapid onset of action in epilepsy, RLS, and anxiety disorders, with longer duration of action compared to other benzodiazepines. Useful in even intractable seizures disorders and can be used in children. Most commonly used medication for PLMD

Potential Disadvantages
- Not a first-line agent in most patients with epilepsy. Development of tolerance and CNS depression can be problematic. Potential for abuse. Not as effective as diazepam or

lorazepam for seizure emergencies (status epilepticus)

Primary Target Symptoms

- Seizure frequency and severity
- Pain in PLMD, RLS
- Anxiety or panic attacks

Pearls

- The most commonly used benzodiazepine for the treatment of epilepsy
- The use of clonazepam with divalproate may exacerbate absence seizures

- In patients with multiple types of seizures, may increase the incidence or precipitate generalized tonic-clonic (grand mal) seizures
- In PLMD, proven to reduce the number of limb movements as shown in sleep studies and is the first-line treatment. Usually used in RLS only if dopamine agonists ineffective or poorly tolerated
- In most patients with anxiety, used as an adjunctive medication with an SSRI or SNRI. Longer half-life makes it easier to taper and may have less abuse potential than other benzodiazepines

 Suggested Reading

Biary N, Pimental PA, Langenberg PW. A double-blind trial of clonazepam in the treatment of parkinsonian dysarthria. Neurology 1988; 38(2):255–8.

DeVane CL, Ware MR, Lydiard RB. Pharmacokinetics, pharmacodynamics, and treatment issues of benzodiazepines: alprazolam, adinazolam, and clonazepam. Psychopharmacol Bull 1991;27:463–73.

Isojärvi JI, Tokola RA. Benzodiazepines in the treatment of epilepsy in people with intellectual disability. J Intellect Disabil Res 1998;42 (Suppl 1):80–92.

Karatas M. Restless legs syndrome and periodic limb movements during sleep: diagnosis and treatment. Neurologist 2007;13(5):294–301.

Zakrzewska JM, Forssell H, Glenny AM. Interventions for the treatment of burning mouth syndrome. Cochrane Database Syst Rev 2005; (1):CD002779.

CLONIDINE

THERAPEUTICS

Brands
- Catapres, Dixarit, Clorpres, Duraclon (injection only)

Generic?
Yes

Class
- Antiadrenergic, alpha-2 agonist

Commonly Prescribed for
(FDA approved in bold)
- **Hypertension**
- Gilles de la Tourette syndrome (GTS)
- Tics
- Attention deficit hyperactivity disorder (ADHD)
- Restless legs syndrome (RLS)
- Neuropathic pain
- Opioid detoxification
- Alcohol withdrawal
- Atrial fibrillation
- Growth delay
- Ulcerative colitis
- Hypertensive "urgency"
- Menopausal symptoms such as hot flashes
- Insomnia
- Hyperhidrosis
- Anesthesia

How the Drug Works
- Alpha-2 adrenergic agonist at 2A/B/C receptors Reduces sympathetic output from CNS, which decreases cardiac output, peripheral vascular resistance, and blood pressure. Specifically targets alpha-2 receptors in the brainstem vasomotor center, decreasing presynaptic calcium levels and the release of norepinephrine. May also reduce plasma renin activity and catecholamine excretion
- Its effect in GTS and ADHD may be due to actions at the level of the prefrontal cortex

How Long Until It Works
- Hypertension, withdrawal – less than 2 hours
- GTS – weeks to months
- RLS – days

If It Works
- In neurologic conditions such as tics, continue to assess effect of the medication and if it is still needed

If It Doesn't Work
- GTS/Tics – Neuroleptics are often effective, but their use should be reserved for patients with significant social isolation or embarrassment
- RLS – Generally used as an adjunctive agent. Dopamine agonists are more effective

 ### Best Augmenting Combos for Partial Response or Treatment-Resistance
- In hypertension, combine with treatments less likely to affect heart rate or cause orthostasis (angiotensin-converting enzyme inhibitors, diuretics)
- Tics and GTS symptoms may change over time. Many patients improve with age. Behavioral and psychological therapies are useful, and education and reassurance are all that is needed in mild cases
- Identify and treat comorbid conditions such as ADHD or obsessive compulsive disorder

Tests
- Monitor blood pressure and pulse at office visits

ADVERSE EFFECTS (AEs)

How Drug Causes AEs
- Related to alpha-2 agonist effect – hypotension and sedation

Notable AEs
- Dry mouth, hypotension/syncope, weakness, fatigue, sedation, dizziness, impotence, vivid dreams/nightmares, rash or pruritus, nausea, and depression

 ### Life-Threatening or Dangerous AEs
- Bradycardia, AV block, and prolongation of QTc interval may occur with higher doses. Rapid withdrawal can cause rebound hypertension

Weight Gain
- Unusual

unusual   not unusual   common   problematic

Sedation
• Common

unusual   not unusual   common   problematic

What to Do About AEs
• Lower the dose and take the highest dose in the evening. Many AEs improve with time

Best Augmenting Agents for AEs
• Most AEs cannot be improved by an augmenting agent

DOSING AND USE

Usual Dosage Range
• 0.1–0.8 mg/day in 2 divided doses

Dosage Forms
• Tablets: 0.1, 0.2, 0.3 mg
• Transdermal patches: 0.1/24 h, 0.2/24 h, 0.3/24 h
• Injection: 100 or 200 mg/mL

How to Dose
• Hypertension: start 0.05 or 0.1 mg twice daily, and increase by 0.1 mg/day weekly with tablets or start with 0.1 mg patch and increase by 0.1 mg/week as tolerated
• GTS/Tics: start at 0.05 mg twice daily and increase weekly by 0.05 or 0.1 mg/day as tolerated with tablets. Can take a larger dose in evening if sedation is problematic. The patch is rarely used in neurological disorders: if used titrate more slowly

 Dosing Tips
• Take the final dose before bedtime
• Rebound hypertension usually occurs 2–4 days after discontinuation

Overdose
• Hypertension may occur first, followed by severe hypotension, bradycardia, respiratory depression, hypothermia, drowsiness, decreased reflexes, weakness, or coma. Consider gastric lavage or activated charcoal for large ingestions

Long-Term Use
• Safe, but tolerance to antihypertensive effects is common

Habit Forming
• There are reports of abuse in opioid-dependent patients

How to Stop
• Taper slowly to avoid rebound tachycardia and hypertension. Other withdrawal symptoms may include nervousness, tremor, agitation, and headache

Pharmacokinetics
• Half-life is 12 hours in most, but sometimes longer. The peak effect is at 2–4 hours. Bioavailability is 75–95%, with about half of the drug metabolized into inactive metabolites and the other half excreted unchanged in urine

 Drug Interactions
• Clonidine may reduce effectiveness of levodopa
• Prazosin and tricyclic antidepressants may block the antihypertensive effects of clonidine
• Use with beta-blockers, digitalis, or verapamil can have a synergistic effect, possibly causing AV block
• Use with other CNS depressants increases sedation

 Other Warnings/ Precautions
• Do not discontinue therapy perioperatively and monitor blood pressure closely
• Therapeutic blood levels do not occur until about 2–3 days of starting transdermal patch
• In animal studies, corneal lesions (with concurrent amitriptyline) and retinal degeneration occurred

Do Not Use
• Known hypersensitivity to the drug

SPECIAL POPULATIONS

Renal Impairment
• Clearance is reduced in patients with severe renal insufficiency. Consider reducing dose

Hepatic Impairment
• No known effects

Cardiac Impairment

- Avoid using in patients with known coronary artery disease, conduction disturbances, recent myocardial infarction, or cerebrovascular events. Concurrent beta-blocker or digitalis use may exacerbate AEs

Elderly

- No known effects

 Children and Adolescents

- Children may be more sensitive to CNS AEs than adults. Doses for GTS and tics are similar to adults but titrate more slowly. Consider giving the entire oral dose at night

 Pregnancy

- Category C. Use only if there is a clear need

Breast Feeding

- Excreted in breast milk. Do not use

THE ART OF NEUROPHARMACOLOGY

Potential Advantages

- Fewer AEs than neuroleptics in the treatment of GTS and tic disorders. Useful agent for multiple neurologic conditions, including ADHD

Potential Disadvantages

- Less effective than neuroleptics for GTS or tics. Hypotension, sedation, and rebound hypertension may limit use

Primary Target Symptoms

- Tics, attention-deficit, hyperactivity, pain, sweating, and hot flashes

 Pearls

- The first clinical decision in the treatment of GTS or tics is to decide if pharmacologic treatment is indicated. If the patient is not severely disabled, then reassure the patient and family that symptoms may improve and the prognosis is good. For patients with significant disability, clonidine is a good initial choice due to lack of long-term AEs, especially in patients with coexisting ADHD
- In patients with severe ADHD, stimulants are generally more effective
- Useful in anxiety disorders and opioid withdrawal due to blocking of autonomic symptoms, such as sweating or palpitations
- Chemically similar to another alpha-2 adrenergic agonist, tizanidine, but much more effective for lowering blood pressure. Because the treatment of spasticity related to spinal cord injury often requires high doses, clonidine is not used in these patients
- Guanfacine is a similar alpha-2 adrenergic agonist occasionally used for GTS or tics. It is not as well-studied as clonidine

---

 Suggested Reading

Jiménez-Jiménez FJ, García-Ruiz PJ. Pharmacological options for the treatment of Tourette's disorder. Drugs 2001; 61(15):2207–20.

Sandor P. Pharmacological management of tics in patients with TS. J Psychosom Res 2003; 55(1):41–8.

Smith H, Elliott J. Alpha(2) receptors and agonists in pain management. Curr Opin Anaesthesiol 2001;14(5):513–8.

Webster J, Koch HF. Aspects of tolerability of centrally acting antihypertensive drugs. J Cardiovasc Pharmacol 1996;27 (Suppl 3): S49–54.

CLOPIDOGREL

Brands
• Plavix

Generic?
No

Class
• Antiplatelet agent

Commonly Prescribed for
(FDA approved in bold)
• **Recent myocardial infarction (MI), recent ischemic stroke, or established peripheral arterial disease as secondary prevention**
• **Acute coronary syndrome**
• Prevention of cardiac events as loading dose in patients receiving coronary stent implantation

How the Drug Works
• Inhibitor of platelet aggregation. Clopidogrel works by irreversibly modifying the platelet adenosine diphosphate (ADP) receptor and inhibits the activation of the GPIIb/IIIa complex

How Long Until It Works
• Inhibition of platelet aggregation begins as soon as 2 hours after a single oral dose of clopidogrel. Reaches steady state between days 3–7

If It Works
• Continue to use for MI or stroke prevention

If It Doesn't Work
• Patients can still have MI or stroke despite treatment. Warfarin is superior for cardiogenic stroke. Control all stroke risk factors such as smoking, hyperlipidemia, and hypertension. For acute events, admit patients for treatment and diagnostic testing

Best Augmenting Combos for Partial Response or Treatment-Resistance
• In stroke prevention, there is no proven benefit to using clopidogrel in combination with aspirin. In clinical trials there was no significant difference in stroke prevention, and AEs (mostly bleeding) were significantly higher

Tests
• None required

How Drug Causes AEs
• Antiplatelet effect increases bleeding risk

Notable AEs
• Nausea, vomiting, rash, diarrhea

Life-Threatening or Dangerous AEs
• GI hemorrhage occurred in about 2% of stroke patients in clinical trials (with 0.7% requiring hospitalization), intracranial hemorrhage (0.4%), or intraocular bleeding leading to vision loss

Weight Gain
• Unusual

unusual   not unusual   common   problematic

Sedation
• Unusual

unusual   not unusual   common   problematic

What to Do About AEs
• For significant GI or intracranial bleeding, stop drug

Best Augmenting Agents for AEs
• Most AEs cannot be improved by an augmenting agent

Usual Dosage Range
• 75 mg daily

Dosage Forms
• Tablets: 75 mg

How to Dose

- Give once daily. Occasionally used off-label as a loading dose of 300 mg after coronary or intracranial stenting, followed by daily use at 75 mg

 Dosing Tips

- Food does not affect absorption

Overdose

- Unknown but if occurs consider platelet transfusion for any bleeding

Long-Term Use

- Safe for long-term use

Habit Forming

- No

How to Stop

- No need to taper

Pharmacokinetics

- Metabolized in liver to its carboxylic acid derivative. Onset of action in 2 hours with half-life of 8 hours. Peak action at 3–7 days and duration of action at least 5 days

 Drug Interactions

- Increases GI bleeding or bleeding time when used with NSAIDs, other antiplatelets, or anticoagulants

⚠️ **Other Warnings/ Precautions**

- Thrombotic thrombocytopenic purpura is a rare complication that can occur in as little as 2 weeks and is characterized by thrombocytopenia, hemolytic anemia, neurological dysfunction, renal dysfunction, and fever
- Neutropenia/agranulocytosis is a common AE (0.8%) of ticlopidine, a chemically similar drug to clopidogrel. The risk of myelotoxicity with clopidogrel is quite low

Do Not Use

- Known hypersensitivity to the drug or active pathological bleeding, such as a peptic ulcer or intracranial hemorrhage

Renal Impairment

- No known effects

Hepatic Impairment

- Use with caution. Patients with severe disease have an increased risk of bleeding complications

Cardiac Impairment

- No known effects

Elderly

- No known effects

 Children and Adolescents

- Not studied in children

 Pregnancy

- Category B but not studied. Only use in pregnancy if clearly needed

Breast Feeding

- Excreted in breast milk. Do not use

THE ART OF NEUROPHARMACOLOGY

Potential Advantages

- Avoids issue of aspirin resistance. AEs similar to aspirin. Useful for prevention of both stroke and MI. May be especially useful in patients with coronary artery stenting or peripheral vascular disease

Potential Disadvantages

- There are fewer trials that suggest clopidogrel is superior to aspirin compared to dipyridimole plus aspirin. Cost

Primary Target Symptoms

- Prevention of the neurological complications that result from ischemic stroke

 Pearls

- First-line drug for secondary prevention of ischemic stroke along with aspirin or extended-release dipyridimole plus aspirin

- In the CAPRIE trial comparing aspirin 325 mg/day and clopidogrel 75 mg/day, there was a relative risk reduction with clopidogrel but no statistically significant difference between the 2 groups for stroke prevention. The risk reduction in the clopidogrel group was greatest in patients with peripheral artery disease
- The MATCH trial compared clopidogrel to clopidogrel plus aspirin 325 mg. The CHARISMA trial compared aspirin 75–162 mg to aspirin 75–162 mg plus clopidogrel. In both trials there was no significant difference in stroke prevention between the 2 groups, but bleeding complications were higher in the combination groups
- Stop clopidogrel at least 5 days before any surgical procedure
- In patients with coronary artery disease, stenting or peripheral vascular disease, clopidogrel may be superior to aspirin for the secondary prevention of vascular disease

Suggested Reading

Bhatt DL, Fox KA, Hacke W, Berger PB, Black HR, Boden WE, Cacoub P, Cohen EA, Creager MA, Easton JD, Flather MD, Haffner SM, Hamm CW, Hankey GJ, Johnston SC, Mak KH, Mas JL, Montalescot G, Pearson TA, Steg PG, Steinhubl SR, Weber MA, Brennan DM, Fabry-Ribaudo L, Booth J, Topol EJ; CHARISMA Investigators. Clopidogrel and aspirin versus aspirin alone for the prevention of atherothrombotic events. N Engl J Med 2006;354(16):1706–17.

Biller J. The role of antiplatelet therapy in the management of ischemic stroke: implementation of guidelines in current practice. Neurol Res 2008;30(7):669–77.

Diener HC, Sacco RL, Yusuf S, Cotton D, Ounpuu S, Lawton WA, Palesch Y, Martin RH, Albers GW, Bath P, Bornstein N, Chan BP, Chen ST, Cunha L, Dahlöf B, De Keyser J, Donnan GA, Estol C, Gorelick P, Gu V, Hermansson K, Hilbrich L, Kaste M, Lu C, Machnig T, Pais P, Roberts R, Skvortsova V, Teal P, Toni D, VanderMaelen C, Voigt T, Weber M, Yoon BW; Prevention Regimen for Effectively Avoiding Second Strokes (PRoFESS) study group. Effects of aspirin plus extended-release dipyridamole versus clopidogrel and telmisartan on disability and cognitive function after recurrent stroke in patients with ischaemic stroke in the Prevention Regimen for Effectively Avoiding Second Strokes (PRoFESS) trial: a double-blind, active and placebo-controlled study. Lancet Neurol 2008;7(10):875–84.

Lenz T, Wilson A. Clinical pharmacokinetics of antiplatelet agents used in the secondary prevention of stroke. Clin Pharmacokinet 2003;42(10):909–20.

Sacco RL, Diener HC, Yusuf S, Cotton D, Ounpuu S, Lawton WA, Palesch Y, Martin RH, Albers GW, Bath P, Bornstein N, Chan BP, Chen ST, Cunha L, Dahlöf B, De Keyser J, Donnan GA, Estol C, Gorelick P, Gu V, Hermansson K, Hilbrich L, Kaste M, Lu C, Machnig T, Pais P, Roberts R, Skvortsova V, Teal P, Toni D, Vandermaelen C, Voigt T, Weber M, Yoon BW; PRoFESS Study Group. Aspirin and extended-release dipyridamole versus clopidogrel for recurrent stroke. N Engl J Med 2008;359(12): 1238–51.

Usman MH, Notaro LA, Nagarakanti R, Brahin E, Dessain S, Gracely E, Ezekowitz MD. Combination antiplatelet therapy for secondary stroke prevention: enhanced efficacy or double trouble? Am J Cardiol 2009;103(8):1107–12.

CLOZAPINE

THERAPEUTICS

Brands
- Clozaril, Clopine, Denzapine, Zaponex, Leponex

Generic?
Yes

Class
- Antipsychotic

Commonly Prescribed for
(FDA approved in bold)
- **Schizophrenia**
- **Recent suicidal behavior in patients with schizophrenia or schizoaffective disorder**
- Psychosis in patients with Parkinson's disease (PD) or dementia with Lewy bodies (DLB)
- Bipolar disorder (treatment resistant)
- Severe psychosis

How the Drug Works
- Blocks D2 receptors similar to other antipsychotics, but also blocks serotonin 2A receptors, which improves motor side effects and perhaps depression and cognitive problems. Also blocks alpha adrenergic receptors, and has anticholinergic and antihistamine effects. May stimulate serotonin 1A receptors

How Long Until It Works
- Psychosis – may be effective in days, more commonly takes weeks or months to determine best dose and achieve best clinical effect

If It Works
- Continue to use at lowest required dose with appropriate monitoring. Patients with PD and DLB may improve more than patients with schizophrenia

If It Doesn't Work
- Increase dose
- In psychosis related to PD or DLB, eliminate or reduce dose of offending medications, such as dopamine agonists or amantadine

Best Augmenting Combos for Partial Response or Treatment-Resistance
- PD and DLB: cholinesterase inhibitors may improve symptoms (particularly in DLB)

Tests
- Obligatory. Prior to starting treatment, obtain CBC, including white count and absolute neutrophil count. Repeat CBC weekly for the first 6 months of treatment, then biweekly for months 6–12 and every 4 weeks thereafter

ADVERSE EFFECTS (AEs)

How Drug Causes AEs
- Motor AEs – blocking of D2 receptors
- Sedation, weight gain – blocking of histamine 1 receptors
- Hypotension – blocking of alpha-1 adrenergic receptors
- Dry mouth, constipation – blocking of muscarinic receptors

Notable AEs
- Most common: Constipation, dry mouth, increased salivation, weight gain, nausea, tachycardia, tremor, urinary retention, sweating. May increase risk of metabolic syndrome

Life-Threatening or Dangerous AEs
- Tardive dyskinesias (lower than other neuroleptics)
- Neuroleptic malignant syndrome
- Seizures, myocarditis
- Agranulocytosis

Weight Gain
- Problematic

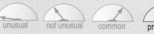
unusual　not unusual　common　problematic

Sedation
- Problematic

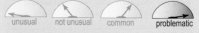
unusual　not unusual　common　problematic

What to Do About AEs
- Take at bedtime and use low dose whenever possible

- Stop drug for absolute neutrophil count below 1,000/mm^3
- Stop drug for eosinophil count over 4,000/mm^3 and do not restart until under 3,000/mm^3

Best Augmenting Agents for AEs

- Most AEs cannot be improved with an augmenting agent

DOSING AND USE

Usual Dosage Range

- Bipolar disorder/schizophrenia: 300–450 mg/day
- Psychosis in PD/DLB: 25–100 mg/day

Dosage Forms

- Tablets: 12.5 mg, 25 mg, 50 mg, 100 mg
- Oral Disintegrating Tablets: 12.5 mg, 25 mg, 50 mg, 100 mg

How to Dose

- Start at 12.5 mg twice a day for acute psychosis or mania. Increase by 25–50 mg every 1–2 days until effective dose is reached
- For psychosis with PD or DLB, consider dosing all the medication at night. Start at 6.25–12.5 mg at night. Increase by 6.25–12.5 mg every 1–2 days until symptoms improve. Most patients respond to a dose of 50 mg/day or less

 Dosing Tips

- Prescriptions are given 1 week at a time (due to risk of agranulocytosis) for 6 months, then every 2 weeks
- Disintegrating tablets may be useful in PD and DLB

Overdose

- Sedation, respiratory depression, excessive salivation, seizures, arrhythmias, and death have been reported

Long-Term Use

- Safe for long-term use with appropriate monitoring

Habit Forming

- No

How to Stop

- Taper over 1–2 weeks to avoid rebound psychosis and cholinergic rebound (diarrhea, headache)

Pharmacokinetics

- Hepatic metabolism via CYP1A2, 3A4, and 2D6. Half-life 8–12 hours, peak effect at 2.5 hours

 Drug Interactions

- Use with CNS depressants (barbiturates, opiates, general anesthetics), potentiates CNS AEs
- Caffeine may increase levels
- CYP1A2 (fluvoxamine), 3A4 (ketoconazole, fluoxetine, nefazodone, duloxetine), and 2D6 (duloxetine, paroxetine) inhibitors may increase levels
- Cigarettes and other CYP1A2 inducers (phenobarbital, carbamazepine) may lower levels
- May enhance effects of antihypertensives

 Other Warnings/ Precautions

- Use with caution in patients with enlarged prostate or glaucoma
- Possible association with cardiomyopathy

Do Not Use

- Proven hypersensitivity to drug, CNS depression, myeloproliferative disorders, or granulocytopenia

SPECIAL POPULATIONS

Renal Impairment

- No dose adjustment needed

Hepatic Impairment

- Use with caution. May need to lower dose

Cardiac Impairment

- May worsen orthostatic hypotension. Use with caution

Elderly

- Start with lower doses

Children and Adolescents
• Efficacy and safety unknown

 Pregnancy
• Category B. PD and DLB are uncommon in women of childbearing age. Use only if benefit outweighs risks

Breast Feeding
• Probably excreted in breast milk based on animal studies. Use while breast feeding is generally not recommended

THE ART OF NEUROPHARMACOLOGY

Potential Advantages
• Most effective drug for refractory psychosis associated with PD or DLB. Effective at relatively low doses, with very low risk of drug-induced parkinsonism or tardive dyskinesias. Minimal prolactin elevation

Potential Disadvantages
• Safety and need for frequent monitoring
• Sedation and weight gain

Primary Target Symptoms
• Psychosis

 Pearls
• Clozapine was formerly the first-line agent for psychosis with PD, but now often a second-line agent due to risk of agranulocytosis. Quetiapine is now the most commonly used drug. Other atypical neuroleptics may also be effective but often cause motor AEs
• Was previously believed useful in treating psychosis in patients with Alzheimer's dementia, but subsequently shown to worsen cognitive function with significant AEs
• Very effective, but dangerous, antipsychotic. Reduces suicide in schizophrenia

 Suggested Reading

Essali A, Al-Haj Haasan N, Li C, Rathbone J. Clozapine versus typical neuroleptic medication for schizophrenia. Cochrane Database Syst Rev 2009;(1):CD000059.

Lauterbach EC. The neuropsychiatry of Parkinson's disease. Minerva Med 2005; 96(3):155–73.

Lieberman JA. Maximizing clozapine therapy: managing side effects. J Clin Psychiatry 1998; 59 (Suppl 3):38–43.

Poewe W. When a Parkinson's disease patient starts to hallucinate. Pract Neurol 2008; 8(4):238–41.

Zahodne LB, Fernandez HH. Pathophysiology and treatment of psychosis in Parkinson's disease: a review. Drugs Aging 2008; 25(8):665–82.

CYCLOBENZAPRINE

THERAPEUTICS

Brands
- Flexeril, Fexmid, Amrix, Apo-Cyclobenzaprine

Generic?
Yes (except once-daily form)

Class
- Skeletal muscle relaxant, centrally acting

Commonly Prescribed for
(FDA approved in bold)
- **Muscle spasm**
- Neck pain/lower back pain
- Myofascial pain
- Fibromyalgia

How the Drug Works
- A tricyclic compound with actions similar to tricyclic antidepressants. Blocks serotonin and norepinephrine reuptake pumps and has anticholinergic effects. Acts within the CNS at the brainstem, not at the spinal cord, neuromuscular junction or skeletal muscle level. Reduces tonic somatic motor activity

How Long Until It Works
- Pain – May work within hours but maximal effect occurs in 4–14 days

If It Works
- Titrate to most effective tolerated dose

If It Doesn't Work
- Increase to highest tolerated dose. If ineffective, consider alternative medications or other modalities

Best Augmenting Combos for Partial Response or Treatment-Resistance
- Use other centrally acting muscle relaxants with caution due to potential additive CNS depressant effect
- Combine with non-pharmacologic treatments such as exercise/physical therapy, massage, heat/ice or acupuncture

Tests
- Consider checking ECG for QTc prolongation at baseline and when increasing dose

ADVERSE EFFECTS (AEs)

How Drug Causes AEs
- Anticholinergic and antihistaminic properties are causes of most common AEs

Notable AEs
- Dry mouth, dizziness, fatigue, constipation, weakness, sweating, and nausea are most common. Somnolence is more common with the intermediate-acting form

Life-Threatening or Dangerous AEs
- Orthostatic hypotension, tachycardia, QTc prolongation, and rarely death
- Increased intraocular pressure
- Paralytic ileus, hyperthermia
- Rare activation of mania or suicidal ideation
- Rare worsening of existing seizure disorders

Weight Gain
- Not unusual

Sedation
- Common

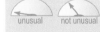

What to Do About AEs
- For somnolence or fatigue, change to once-daily formulation or decrease dose. For any serious AEs, discontinue

Best Augmenting Agents for AEs
- Most AEs cannot be improved by use of augmenting agent

DOSING AND USE

Usual Dosage Range
- 15–30 mg per day

Dosage Forms
- Tablets: 5, 7.5, 10 mg
- Extended-release capsules: 15, 30 mg

How to Dose
- Start at 5 mg 3 times a day and increase as tolerated (for best effect) to 7.5 or 10 mg

3 times day. The extended-release capsule should be taken 4–6 hours before bedtime

 Dosing Tips

- Take the largest dose in the evening to avoid somnolence with the immediate-release form. The extended-release capsule peaks at about 6–8 hours. Taking the extended-release form just before bedtime can lead to excess fatigue before awakening. Peak concentrations are greater when taking with food

Overdose

- Cardiac arrhythmias and ECG changes; death can occur. CNS depression and tachycardia are most common. Convulsions or severe hypotension are less common. Least commonly, agitation, ataxia, tremor, vomiting, or coma can occur. Patients should be hospitalized. Sodium bicarbonate can treat arrhythmias and hypotension. Treat shock with vasopressors, oxygen, or corticosteroids

Long-Term Use

- Not studied but probably safe

Habit Forming

- No

How to Stop

- Not usually tapered but may cause withdrawal similar to tricyclic antidepressants (insomnia, nausea, headache) after extended use

Pharmacokinetics

- Metabolized by CYP450 system, especially CYP3A4, 1A2 and to a lesser extent 2D6 and excreted as glucuronides via the kidney. All forms take 3–4 days to reach steady state and at usual doses exhibit linear pharmacokinetics

 Drug Interactions

- Use with anticholinergics can increase AEs (i.e., risk of ileus)
- May enhance effects of CNS depressants
- Use with MAOI, such as rasagiline or selegiline, can cause hypertensive crisis, seizures, or death

- May alter effects of antihypertensive medications, such as guanethidine (blocking effect)
- Use with tramadol may increase seizure risk

Do Not Use

- Proven hypersensitivity to drug or other tricyclic antidepressants
- Contraindicated with MAO inhibitors
- In acute recovery after myocardial infarction or uncompensated heart failure
- In conjunction with antiarrhythmics that prolong QTc interval

SPECIAL POPULATIONS

Renal Impairment

- Use with caution. May need to lower dose

Hepatic Impairment

- Increased plasma concentrations with moderate-severe liver dysfunction. Use with caution at low doses if at all

Cardiac Impairment

- Do not use in patients with recent myocardial infarction, severe heart failure, a history of QTc prolongation, or orthostatic hypotension

Elderly

- Plasma levels are higher and may be at greater risk of AEs. Use with caution, especially over age 65

 Children and Adolescents

- Not studied in children under age 15

 Pregnancy

- Category B. Use only if there is a clear need

Breast Feeding

- Unknown if excreted in breast milk. Do not use

THE ART OF NEUROPHARMACOLOGY

Potential Advantages

- Effective antispasmodic with effectiveness in acute muscle spasm and pain. Low risk of addiction/dependence compared to carisoprodol. Available as once-daily dose

Potential Disadvantages

- Sedation can be problematic, especially with immediate-acting form. Not effective for spasticity due to CNS disorders, i.e., multiple sclerosis

Primary Target Symptoms

- Muscle spasm, pain

Pearls

- Similar to tricyclic antidepressant class in structure, pharmacology and AEs. In long-standing pain disorders such as migraine, chronic neck pain, or fibromyalgia, consider using tricyclic antidepressants for long-term treatment
- Do not use for spasticity related to CNS disorders, including MS, spinal cord injury, and cerebral palsy. Baclofen or tizanidine are more effective agents for these conditions
- Usually used as a short-term adjunctive agent (2–6 weeks) for acute muscle spasm and pain. No longer-term studies have been done, but due to similarities with tricyclic antidepressants, probably safe to use for months or years

Suggested Reading

Carette S, Bell MJ, Reynolds WJ, Haraoui B, McCain GA, Bykerk VP, Edworthy SM, Baron M, Koehler BE, Fam AG, et al. Comparison of amitriptyline, cyclobenzaprine, and placebo in the treatment of fibromyalgia. A randomized, double-blind clinical trial. Arthritis Rheum 1994;37(1):32–40.

Chou R, Peterson K, Helfand M. Comparative efficacy and safety of skeletal muscle relaxants for spasticity and musculoskeletal conditions: a systematic review. J Pain Symptom Manage 2004;28(2):140–75.

See S, Ginzburg R. Choosing a skeletal muscle relaxant. Am Fam Physician 2008;78(3):365–70.

Toth PP, Urtis J. Commonly used muscle relaxant therapies for acute low back pain: a review of carisoprodol, cyclobenzaprine hydrochloride, and metaxalone. Clin Ther 2004;26(9):1355–67. Review.

CYCLOPHOSPHAMIDE

THERAPEUTICS

Brands
- Revimmune, Cytoxan, Neosar, Endoxan, Procytox

Generic?
Yes

Class
- Immunosuppressant, immunomodulator

Commonly Prescribed for
(FDA approved in bold)
- **Treatment of malignancies, including lymphomas (lymphocytic, mixed-cell type, histiocytic, Burkitt's, and Hodgkin's disease), disseminated neuroblastoma, ovarian adenocarcinoma and breast**
- Other malignancies: bronchogenic, small-cell lung, endometrial, prostate, testicular, and sarcomas
- Mycosis fungoides
- **"Minimal change" nephrotic syndrome in children**
- Myasthenia gravis (MG)
- Multiple sclerosis (MS) (relapsing remitting)
- Polymyositis and dermatomyositis
- Multifocal motor neuropathy
- Vasculitis including Wegener's granulomatosis, polyarteritis nodosa
- Rheumatoid arthritis
- Systemic lupus erythematosus
- Bone marrow transplantation

How the Drug Works
- An alkylating agent and non-specific cell-cycle inhibitor with metabolites that interfere with the growth of rapidly proliferating normal and malignant cells, most likely by cross-linking of tumor cell DNA

How Long Until It Works
- Within a week, but effect on neurological diseases may take months

If It Works
- MG: May allow improvement in symptoms or reduction in dose or discontinuation of corticosteroids or other agents
- MS: May reduce relapses and new lesions on MRI

- Other disorders: Improves symptoms (weakness, sensory changes) and clinical markers of the disease

If It Doesn't Work
- Usually used as a disease-modifying agent in refractory cases when first-line agents have failed

Best Augmenting Combos for Partial Response or Treatment-Resistance
- Often used in combination with other agents depending on the disease in question, such as corticosteroids for vasculitis or MG and plasma exchange for multifocal motor neuropathy

Tests
- Obtain complete blood counts regularly during treatment to determine WBC and platelet counts. Examine urine for red cells (hemorrhagic cystitis)

ADVERSE EFFECTS (AEs)

How Drug Causes AEs
- Immunosuppression, lymphopenia, and risk of secondary neoplasia

Notable AEs
- Nausea and vomiting, anorexia, abdominal pain, diarrhea, darkening of the skin/nails, alopecia, delay in wound healing, and lethargy. Hemorrhagic cystitis is common but preventable with the detoxifying agent mesna. May cause sterility (usually temporary) in women (amenorrhea is common) and men (decreased sperm count and increased gonadotropin levels)

Life-Threatening or Dangerous AEs
- Leukopenia occurs in all patients and is dose-related, less commonly thrombocytopenia and anemia. Recovery from leukopenia begins 7–10 days after cessation of therapy
- Severe congestive heart failure due to hemorrhagic myocarditis or myocardial necrosis

• Increases risk of new malignancy, usually several years after treatment – bladder, myeloproliferative or lymphoproliferative are most common
• Interstitial pulmonary fibrosis

Weight Gain
• Unusual

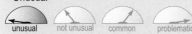

unusual   not unusual   common   problematic

Sedation
• Unusual

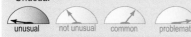

unusual   not unusual   common   problematic

What to Do About AEs
• Treat infections appropriately and reduce dose if possible

Best Augmenting Agents for AEs
• Hydration or mensa should be used to prevent hemorrhagic cystitis

DOSING AND USE

Usual Dosage Range
• Oral: 1–5 mg/kg/day adjusted based on white blood cell count
• IV: 1–3 g/m^2 not to exceed 85 mg/kg

Dosage Forms
• Tablets: 25 or 50 mg
• Injection: 75 mg mannitol/100 mg cyclophosphamide or 82 mg bicarbonate/ 100 mg cyclophosphamide in 100, 200, or 500 mg and 1 or 2 g vials

How to Dose
• Oral: Start at 2–3 mg/kg/day and adjust to maintain a white blood cell count between 2500–4000/mm^3 and lymphocyte count below 1000/mm^3. For more significant leukopenia or other AEs, patients may skip doses
• IV: Many different regimens exist. 40–50 mg/kg over 2–5 days every 3–4 weeks, 10–15 mg/kg every 7–10 days, or 3–5 mg/kg twice weekly are examples. In neurological disorders, a typical regimen is 1–3 g/m^2, given over an 8 day period on days 1, 2, 4, 6 and 8, equally divided. The 4th and 5th doses are given only if the WBC is greater than 3500/mm^3. Obtain a complete blood

count before each dose. Alternatively give a total dose of 1 g/m^2 every 4–5 weeks

 Dosing Tips
• Optimal availability with oral formulation when taken without food. With IV administration, give adequate hydration and treat nausea if necessary

Overdose
• Unknown

Long-Term Use
• Usually used on a short-term basis for refractory disorders

Habit Forming
• No

How to Stop
• No need to taper but monitor for recurrence of neurological disorder

Pharmacokinetics
• Peak action of metabolites at 2–3 h and half-life 3–12 h. Hepatic metabolism to active metabolites and renal excretion

 Drug Interactions
• Allopurinol and thiazide diuretics increase its myelosuppressive effects, potentially increasing AEs
• Phenobarbital and cloramphenicol may decrease effectiveness
• Can increase anticoagulant effect, cardiotoxicity from doxorubicin, and neuromuscular blockade of succinylcholine
• May decrease digoxin serum levels and antimicrobial effects of fluroquinolones

Do Not Use
• Known hypersensitivity to the drug or severely depressed bone marrow function

SPECIAL POPULATIONS

Renal Impairment
• No known effects

Hepatic Impairment
• No known effects

Cardiac Impairment
• Can cause cardiac toxicity, especially at high doses. Use with caution

Elderly
• No known effects. Use with caution

Children and Adolescents
• Effectiveness and safety are unknown. Rarely used due to long-term AEs

Pregnancy
• Category D. Use contraception during treatment to avoid pregnancy

Breast Feeding
• Do not breast feed while on drug

THE ART OF NEUROPHARMACOLOGY

Potential Advantages
• Useful for many refractory autoimmune neurological disorders when usual first-line disease-modifying agents fail

Potential Disadvantages
• Multiple AEs complicate use

Primary Target Symptoms
• Preventive treatment of complications from diseases, such as MG or MS

Pearls
• Appears to be effective in MG. Patients experienced increased strength and decreased prednisone doses at 12 months in 1 study. Treatment consisted of pulse doses 500 mg/m^2 monthly for 6 months
• In 1 study, a 1-time treatment with cyclophosphamide (1–12 g based on level of leukopenia over 1–2 weeks) in relapsing MS resulted in decreased relapse rates. Not a proven treatment for MS but may be considered in refractory cases
• Used in combination with corticosteroids for refractory cases of systemic or CNS vasculitis, such as polyarteritis nodosa. Treatment consists of IV cyclophosphamide until remission (usually at least 6 and up to 12 pulses) and then patients are transitioned to maintenance therapy (azothioprine or methotrexate.) Cyclophosphamide is used in most cases of systemic Wegener's granulomatosis, either orally or intravenously. Pulse doses are given every 3–4 weeks at a dose of 0.5 to 0.7 g/m^2
• In polymyositis and dermatomyositis, usually used in cases refractory to corticosteroids and azothioprine. Assess treatment success by following muscle strength and creatine kinase levels
• In multifocal motor neuropathy, intravenous cyclophosphamide is used for 6 months in cases refractory to intravenous immune globulin and often combined with plasma exchange. Follow clinical improvement and reduction of anti-GM1 antibodies

---

Suggested Reading

Gladstone DE, Brannagan TH 3rd, Schwartzman RJ, Prestrud AA, Brodsky I. High dose cyclophosphamide for severe refractory myasthenia gravis. J Neurol Neurosurg Psychiatry 2004;75(5):789–91.

Hart IK, Sathasivam S, Sharshar T. Immunosuppressive agents for myasthenia gravis. Cochrane Database Syst Rev 2007;(4): CD005224.

Hengstman GJ, van den Hoogen FH, van Engelen BG. Treatment of the inflammatory myopathies: update and practical recommendations. Expert Opin Pharmacother 2009;10(7):1183–90.

Neuhaus O, Kieseier BC, Hartung HP. Immunosuppressive agents in multiple sclerosis. Neurotherapeutics 2007;4(4):654–60.

Schwartzman RJ, Simpkins N, Alexander GM, Reichenberger E, Ward K, Lindenberg N, Topolsky D, Crilley P. High-dose cyclophosphamide in the treatment of multiple sclerosis. CNS Neurosci Ther 2009;15(2):118–27.

CYCLOSPORINE
(Ciclosporin)

THERAPEUTICS

Brands
- Gengraf, Neoral, Sandimmune, Cicloral

Generic?
Yes

Class
- Immunosuppressive agent, immunomodulator

Commonly Prescribed for
(FDA approved in bold)
- **Prophylaxis of organ rejection in patients with allogenic 1 kidney, liver, and heart transplants**
- **Rheumatoid arthritis**
- **Psoriasis**
- Myasthenia gravis (MG)
- Leukemias refractory to routine treatment
- Aplastic anemia
- Ulcerative colitis

How the Drug Works
- Specifically and reversibly inhibits T-lymphocytes, especially T-helper cells. Also inhibits lymphokine production and release, including interleukin-2

How Long Until It Works
- Most patients with MG improve 1–2 months after starting treatment, but maximum improvement takes 6 or more months

If It Works
- Decrease dose of corticosteroids. Gradually reduce to the minimum dose needed to maintain clinical improvement

If It Doesn't Work
- Consider alternative disease-modifying therapy or thymectomy

Best Augmenting Combos for Partial Response or Treatment-Resistance
- Often used with corticosteroids (prednisone), especially in the initial stages of treatment

Tests
- Obtain baseline CBC, magnesium, potassium, uric acid, lipids, blood urea nitrogen, and creatinine. Measure trough levels 1 month after starting determine dosing. Measure creatinine every 2–4 weeks for the first few months, then monthly, and then every 2–3 months when stable or when new medications are added. Measure CBC, uric acid, potassium and lipids every 2 weeks for the first 3 months, then monthly. Monitor blood pressure frequently (at least monthly)

ADVERSE EFFECTS (AEs)

How Drug Causes AEs
- Uncertain

Notable AEs
- Hypertension, hirsutism, cramps, diarrhea, infection, hypomagnesemia
- Tremor, convulsions, paresthesias

Life-Threatening or Dangerous AEs
- Renal failure. Elevations of BUN and creatinine are common and are dose-related. Nephrotoxicity occurs in over 20% of patients
- Thrombocytopenia and microangiopathic hemolytic anemia
- Hyperkalemia
- Hepatotoxicity, usually in 1st month of therapy

Weight Gain
- Unusual

Sedation
- Not unusual

What to Do About AEs
- Renal function generally improves with dose reductions. Creatinine should be below 150% of baseline. Reduce dose by 25–50% for laboratory abnormalities

Best Augmenting Agents for AEs
- Most cannot be improved

DOSING AND USE

Usual Dosage Range
- MG – 200–600 mg/day in 2 divided doses

Dosage Forms
- Capsules: 25 mg, 100 mg
- Oral Solution: 100 mg/mL
- Injection: 50 mg/mL

How to Dose
- Start at dose of 4–6 mg/kg per day in 2 doses per day about 12 hours apart
- Adjust dose for a trough level of 75–150 ng/mL every month

 Dosing Tips
- Take at about the same times daily, with or without food

Overdose
- There is minimal experience with overdose. Forced emesis is of value up to 2 hours after ingestion

Long-Term Use
- Safe for long-term use

Habit Forming
- No

How to Stop
- Taper slowly, as MG symptoms may worsen

Pharmacokinetics
- Incompletely absorbed from GI tract. Most drug is metabolized in the liver by the CYP-450 3A4 enzyme. Peak effect is 3.5 hours for Sandimmune formulation and 1.5–2 hours for Neoral and Gengraf. Half-life is 19 hours for Sandimmune and 8.4 hours for Neoral and Gengraf

 Drug Interactions
- Concomitant NSAID use can worsen hypertension and renal disease
- Avoid medications, such as orlistat, that decrease absorption
- CYP3A4 inhibitors reduce metabolism and can increase levels and toxicity. Drugs that increase levels include verapamil, diltiazem, ketoconazole, fluconazole, azithromycin, erythromycin, allopurinol, oral contraceptives, colchicine, and amiodarone
- Corticosteroids, fluroquinolones (ciprofloxacin), metoclopramide, and bromocriptine, beta-blockers can also increase levels
- HIV protease inhibitors likely also increase levels
- SSRIs that are CYP3A4 inhibitors, such as fluvoxamine or fluoxetine, may increase levels and toxicity
- CYP3A4 inducers, such as phenytoin, phenobarbital, carbamazepine, rifampin, and St. John's wort, may decrease levels
- Use with potassium-sparing drugs, including ACE inhibitors and angiotensin II receptor antagonists, can cause hyperkalemia
- May cause myopathy or rhabdomyolysis with HMG-CoA reductase inhibitors
- Decreases concentrations of methotrexate and sirolimus
- Grapefruit juice can increase concentrations and should be avoided

 Other Warnings/ Precautions
- Patients with malabsorption may have difficulty reaching therapeutic levels
- Vaccines may be less effective and patients should be given live vaccines due to risks of illness

Do Not Use
- Hypersensitivity to drug or components, uncontrolled hypertension, new-onset renal failure or malignancy

SPECIAL POPULATIONS

Renal Impairment
- Renal function commonly worsens on drug. Monitor function closely

Hepatic Impairment
- Liver transplant patients are more likely to develop encephalopathy. Use with caution

Cardiac Impairment
- May cause new-onset or worsen existing hypertension

Elderly

• More prone to development of systolic hypertension and renal failure. Use with caution

Children and Adolescents

• Poorly studied but no unusual AEs have been observed in children as young as 6 months

Pregnancy

• Category C. Embryotoxic and fetotoxic in animals. Complications such as prematurity, low birth weight, preeclampsia or eclampsia and fetal losses, are common in the pregnancies of women on cyclosporine. Do not use for treatment of MG during pregnancy

Breast Feeding

• Excreted in breast milk. Discontinue the drug or bottle feed

---

THE ART OF NEUROPHARMACOLOGY

Potential Advantages

• Fairly effective disease-modifying agent in MG

Potential Disadvantages

• Multiple AEs and need for frequent monitoring by physicians familiar with immunosuppressive therapy

Primary Target Symptoms

• To improve weakness, visual problems, respiratory symptoms associated with MG

Pearls

• In small clinical trials, improved strength and lowered antireceptor antibody titers, allowing lowering of corticosteroid doses in MG
• Prevents opening of mitochondrial permeability pore, which inhibits the release of cytochrome c, a stimulator of apoptosis. This may be protective and could prevent complications of head injury and neurodegenerative diseases
• Intrathecal cyclosporine is under investigation for the treatment of amyotrophic lateral sclerosis

---

Suggested Reading

Appel SH, Stewart SS, Appel V, Harati Y, Mietlowski W, Weiss W, Belendiuk GW. A double-blind study of the effectiveness of cyclosporine in amyotrophic lateral sclerosis. Arch Neurol 1988;45(4):381–6.

Ciafaloni E, Nikhar NK, Massey JM, Sanders DB. Retrospective analysis of the use of cyclosporine in myasthenia gravis. Neurology 2000; 55(3):448–50.

Hart IK, Sathasivam S, Sharshar T. Immunosuppressive agents for myasthenia gravis. Cochrane Database Syst Rev 2007;(4): CD005224.

Hatton J, Rosbolt B, Empey P, Kryscio R, Young B. Dosing and safety of cyclosporine in patients with severe brain injury. J Neurosurg 2008; 109(4):699–707.

Lavrnic D, Vujic A, Rakocevic-Stojanovic V, Stevic Z, Basta I, Pavlovic S, Trikic R, Apostolski S. Cyclosporine in the treatment of myasthenia gravis. Acta Neurol Scand 2005; 111(4):247–52.

THERAPEUTICS

Brands
• Periactin, Cypromar, Periavit, Pyrohep

Generic?
Yes

Class
• Antihistamine

Commonly Prescribed for
(FDA approved in bold)
• **Hypersensitivity reactions**
• Migraine prophylaxis (children and adults)
• Tension-type headache prophylaxis
• Nightmares/post-traumatic stress disorder

How the Drug Works
• Antihistamine and anticholinergic activity. 5-HT2$_{A/C}$ receptor antagonist and perhaps a calcium-channel blocker. The relative importance of each action in headache prophylaxis is unclear. Prevention of cortical spreading depression may be the mechanism of action for all migraine preventive drugs

How Long Until It Works
• Migraines may decrease in as little as 2 weeks, but can take up to 2 months to see full effect

If It Works
• Migraine – goal is a 50% or greater decrease in migraine frequency or severity. Consider tapering or stopping if headaches remit for more than 6 months or if considering pregnancy

If It Doesn't Work
• Increase to highest tolerated dose
• Migraine: address other issues, such as medication-overuse, other coexisting medical disorders, such as anxiety, and consider changing to another agent or adding a second agent

Best Augmenting Combos for Partial Response or Treatment-Resistance
Migraine: For some patients with migraine, low-dose polytherapy with 2 or more drugs may be better tolerated and more effective than high-dose monotherapy. May use in combination with AEDs, antidepressants, natural products, and non-medication treatments, such as biofeedback, to improve headache control

Tests
• Monitor weight during treatment

ADVERSE EFFECTS (AEs)

How Drug Causes AEs
• Most are related to antihistamine and anticholinergic activity

Notable AEs
• Sedation, dizziness, dry mouth, postural hypotension, photosensitivity, and weight gain

Life-Threatening on Dangerous AEs
• Bradycardia, ECG changes, including QTc prolongation
• Hypersensitivity reactions

Weight Gain
• Problematic

Sedation
• Common

What to Do About AEs
• Lower dose or switch to another agent. For serious AEs, do not use

Best Augmenting Agents for AEs
• No treatment for most AEs other than lowering dose or stopping drug

DOSING AND USE

Usual Dosage Range
• 8–32 mg/day

Dosage Forms
• Tablets: 4 mg
• Syrup: 2 mg/5mL

How to Dose
- Migraine/tension-type headache: Initial dose is usually 2 mg at night. Increase by 2 mg every 3–7 days in 3 divided doses until beneficial or AEs develop

Dosing Tips
- Take the largest dose at night to minimize drowsiness

Overdose
- CNS depression is most common, but hypotension, cardiac collapse or ECG changes, and respiratory depression may occur. Anticholinergic effects include fixed pupils, flushing, and hyperthermia Convulsions indicate poor prognosis. Protect against aspiration, correct electrolyte disturbances and acidosis, and give activated charcoal with a cathartic. Give diazepam for convulsions and consider physostigmine for central anticholinergic effects

Long-Term Use
- Safe for long-term use

Habit Forming
- No

How to Stop
- No need to taper, but migraine often returns after stopping

Pharmacokinetics
- Peak levels at 1–2 hours, duration 4–6 hours. Hepatic metabolism with renal excretion of metabolites and some unchanged drug

Drug Interactions
- MAO inhibitors, ketoconazole, and erythromycin may increase plasma levels and toxicity
- Cyproheptadine may lower effectiveness of SSRIs due to serotonin antagonism
- May diminish expected pituitary adrenal response to metyrapone
- Excess sedation with other CNS depressants (alcohol, barbiturates) can occur

Other Warnings/ Precautions
- Avoid in patients with respiratory disease such as sleep apnea or chronic obstructive pulmonary disease

Do Not Use
- Hypersensitivity to drug, angle-closure glaucoma, bladder neck obstruction, patients using MAO inhibitors, symptomatic prostatic hypertrophy

SPECIAL POPULATIONS

Renal Impairment
- No known effects

Hepatic Impairment
- May reduce metabolism. Titrate more slowly

Cardiac Impairment
- Rarely causes arrhythmias and ECG changes. Use with caution

Elderly
- More likely to experience AEs, especially anticholinergic. Avoid using for headache prophylaxis

Children and Adolescents
- Drug is used most often for pediatric headache disorders, but may decrease alertness or produce paradoxical excitation

Pregnancy
- Category B. Use only if potential benefit outweighs risk to the fetus

Breast Feeding
- Unknown if excreted in breast milk. Patient should not breast feed while on drug

THE ART OF NEUROPHARMACOLOGY

Potential Advantages
- Commonly used pediatric migraine preventive, especially for younger children

Potential Disadvantages
- No large studies that demonstrate effectiveness and many AEs that limit use

Primary Target Symptoms
- Headache frequency and severity

 Pearls
- In 1 study, superior to placebo but inferior to methysergide

- Antiserotonin effects are most likely responsible for effectiveness, but can cause depression despite previously successful treatment when used with SSRIs
- Antagonism of 5-HT2$_A$ receptors suggests usefulness in the treatment of serotonin syndrome and monoamine oxidase inhibitor toxicity

 Suggested Reading

Graudins A, Stearman A, Chan B. Treatment of the serotonin syndrome with cyproheptadine. J Emerg Med 1998; 16(4):615–9.

Lewis DW, Yonker M, Winner P, Sowell M. The treatment of pediatric migraine. Pediatr Ann 2005;34(6):448–60.

Meythaler JM, Roper JF, Brunner RC. Cyproheptadine for intrathecal baclofen withdrawal. Arch Phys Med Rehabil 2003;84(5):638–42.

Peroutka SJ, Allen GS. The calcium antagonist properties of cyproheptadine: implications for antimigraine action. Neurology 1984; 34(3):304–9.

DANTROLENE

THERAPEUTICS

Brands
- Dantrium, Dantamacrin, Dantrolen

Generic?
Yes

Class
- Neuromuscular drug; skeletal muscle relaxant, direct acting

Commonly Prescribed for
(FDA approved in bold)
- **Chronic spasticity**
- **Malignant hyperthermia (MT)**
- Exercise-induced muscle pain
- Heat stroke
- Neuroleptic malignant syndrome

How the Drug Works
- Dantrolene produces relaxation by interfering with the release of calcium from the sarcoplasmic reticulum, weakening muscle contraction, and reversing the hypermetabolic process of MT

How Long Until It Works
- Pain – hours-days

If It Works
- Discontinue use once MT symptoms remit. For chronic spasticity, continue to use with standard precautions

If It Doesn't Work
- For spasticity, increase to highest tolerated dose. If ineffective, stop after 45 days and consider alternative treatments. In MT cases, stop all anesthetics

Best Augmenting Combos for Partial Response or Treatment-Resistance
- For focal spasticity, i.e., post-stroke spasticity, botulinum toxin is often more effective and is better tolerated
- Use other centrally acting muscle relaxants with caution due to potential synergistic CNS depressant effect
- 100% oxygen, cold gastric lavage, cooling blankets, and cold intravenous fluids may be useful in MT

Tests
- Obtain baseline liver function studies then do periodically

ADVERSE EFFECTS (AEs)

How Drug Causes AEs
- Some are related to CNS depression, others hepatic disease

Notable AEs
- Fatigue, diarrhea, drowsiness, weakness, rash, labile blood pressure, confusion/depression, abdominal cramps, crystalluria, chills, and fever. Thrombophlebitis

Life-Threatening or Dangerous AEs
- Hepatotoxicity is not rare even after only short-term use, especially in patients that are females, over 35, taking multiple medications or taking dose greater than 800 mg
- Less common: heart failure, pulmonary edema and hematologic abnormalities have been reported

Weight Gain
- Unusual

Sedation
- Problematic

What to Do About AEs
- If symptoms of hepatotoxicity develop (clinically or based on elevated hepatic enzymes), discontinue drug. For sedation, lower the dose and titrate more slowly. Do not let patient drive or perform hazardous tasks

Best Augmenting Agents for AEs
- Most AEs cannot be improved by an augmenting agent

DOSING AND USE

Usual Dosage Range
Spasticity: 75–300 mg/day in divided doses
MT: 1–10 mg/kg per day

Dosage Forms
• Capsules: 25, 50 and 100 mg
• Infusion: 20 mg/vial (with 3 g mannitol)

How to Dose
• Oral: Start at 25 mg daily. Increase dose every 7 days and change to 3 times daily, dosing as follows: 25 mg, 50 mg and 100 mg. Wait at least 7 days between dose increases to assess response. If increasing a dose does not produce added benefit, then decrease to the previous lower dose. For MT, give 4–8 mg/kg in 3–4 divided doses for 1–2 days before surgery. If needed following a crisis, give for 1–3 days to prevent recurrence
• Injection: Preoperatively give 2.5 mg/kg about 1 ¼ hours before anticipated anesthesia. For recognized MT, give minimum of 1 mg/kg (usually 2) as an intravenous bolus until symptoms improve or a maximum of 10 mg/kg

Overdose
• Weakness, lethargy, coma, vomiting, diarrhea

Long-Term Use
• Safety with long-term use not established

Habit Forming
• No

How to Stop
• No need to taper

Pharmacokinetics
• Hepatic metabolism. Half-life of 8–9 hours on average, with peak levels at 4–5 hours
• Some drug is protein bound. Excreted in feces and urine as active drug and metabolites

 Drug Interactions
• Use with other CNS depressants can worsen sedation
• Hepatotoxicity more common in women on oral estrogens
• Use with verapamil can cause hyperkalemia or myocardia depression

• Use with vecuronium may potentiate neuromuscular block
• Warfarin and clofibrate lower plasma protein binding of drug
• May affect concentrations of CYP450 3A4 medications

 Other Warnings/ Precautions
• At high doses carcinogenic in animals, although not proven in humans
• Patients who rely on spasticity to sustain upright posture and balance in walking should not use

Do Not Use
• Hypersensitivity to the drug or active hepatic disease

SPECIAL POPULATIONS

Renal Impairment
• No known effects

Hepatic Impairment
• Do not use

Cardiac Impairment
• May worsen existing heart failure, change blood pressure, or produce tachycardia. Use with caution

Elderly
• Very susceptible to AEs, including hepatotoxicity. Titrate carefully and use with extreme caution

 Children and Adolescents
• Children over age 5 may use, but potential for carcinogenesis with long-term use. Titrate as follows: 0.5 mg/kg once daily for 7 days, then 0.5 mg/kg 3 times daily for 1 day, then 1 mg/kg 3 times daily for 1 day, then 2 mg/kg 3 times daily

 Pregnancy
• Category C. Use only if benefits of medication outweigh risks

Breast Feeding
• Do not use

THE ART OF NEUROPHARMACOLOGY

Potential Advantages
- Most effective medication in the treatment of MT

Potential Disadvantages
- Multiple serious AEs, including hepatic toxicity and sedation, along with lack of long-term data make it a second-line agent for the treatment of chronic spasticity

Primary Target Symptoms
- Spasticity, pain, fever

Pearls
- The introduction of dantrolene reduced mortality of MT from about 70% to 10%
- Drug works best for MT if given early in the setting of illness
- The dose and usage of dantrolene for treatment of neuroleptic malignant syndrome (1 mg/kg, up to 10 mg/kg) is similar to that of acute MT, but is of unproven effectiveness

Suggested Reading

Dressler D, Benecke R. Diagnosis and management of acute movement disorders. J Neurol 2005;252(11):1299–306.

Saulino M, Jacobs BW. The pharmacological management of spasticity. J Neurosci Nurs 2006;38(6):456–9.

Velamoor VR, Swamy GN, Parmar RS, Williamson P, Caroff SN. Management of suspected neuroleptic malignant syndrome. Can J Psychiatry 1995;40(9): 545–50.

Verrotti A, Greco R, Spalice A, Chiarelli F, Iannetti P. Pharmacotherapy of spasticity in children with cerebral palsy. Pediatr Neurol 2006;34(1):1–6.

3,4-DIAMINOPYRIDINE

THERAPEUTICS

Brands
• Amifampridine

Generic?
Yes

Class
• Cholinergic agonist, potassium channel blocker, neuromuscular drug

Commonly Prescribed for
(FDA approved in bold)
• Lambert-Eaton myasthenic syndrome (LEMS)
• Congenital myasthenia gravis (CMG)
• Multiple sclerosis (MS)

 How the Drug Works
• Potassium channel blocker. Reduces flow of potassium across nerve terminal membranes and increases calcium influx with prolongation of action potential. This promotes presynaptic release of acetylcholine and may improve weakness and autonomic dysfunction

How Long Until It Works
• About 20 minutes, but maximum effect might take a few days

If It Works
• Continue to use to reduce symptoms of LEMS or CMG at lowest required dose. In LEMS, disease-modifying treatments, such as plasma exchange, intravenous immune globulin, corticosteroids, or immunosuppressives, are useful
• Identifying malignancy such as small-cell lung cancer is essential

If It Doesn't Work
• LEMS – Treat with immunologic therapy. Removal of neoplasm may improve symptoms
• CMG – Establish the type. Presynaptic forms may respond to 3, 4 diaminopyridine. Acetylcholinesterase inhibitors may improve or worsen symptoms, depending on the disorder

 Best Augmenting Combos for Partial Response or Treatment-Resistance
• May be combined with pyridostigmine, which increases the available amount of acetylcholine for receptor binding and may allow reduction of dose

Tests
• Obtain baseline CBC, electrolytes, glucose, BUN, creatinine, liver function tests. Repeat monthly for 3 months, then every 6 months while on treatment

ADVERSE EFFECTS (AEs)

How Drug Causes AEs
• Some AEs are related to acetylcholine release, others are unknown

Notable AEs
• Paresthesias, perioral numbness, insomnia, abdominal pain

 Life-Threatening or Dangerous AEs
• Seizures, delirium – most common at doses of 100 mg or greater

Weight Gain
• Unusual

unusual   not unusual   common   problematic

Sedation
• Unusual

unusual   not unusual   common   problematic

What to Do About AEs
• Lower dose, supplement with pyridostigmine in LEMS. For first seizure, lower dose or discontinue and evaluate for metastatic brain tumor. For recurrent seizure, discontinue

Best Augmenting Agents for AEs
• Cannot be improved with augmenting agents

DOSING AND USE

Usual Dosage Range
- 15–80 g/day

Dosage Forms
- Tablets: 5 mg

How to Dose
- Start at 10 mg PO 3–4 times daily or as tolerated. Increase every 1–2 weeks by 5 mg until maximum benefit, up to 80 mg/day. For suboptimal benefit in LEMS, add pyridostigmine

 ### Dosing Tips
- Dose requirements may change over time. Periodically attempt to lower dose

Overdose
- Seizures and encephalopathy have been reported

Long-Term Use
- Requires frequent monitoring for hematologic or renal complications

Habit Forming
- No

How to Stop
- No need to taper, but LEMS symptoms may worsen

Pharmacokinetics
- Bioavailability 30%

 ### Drug Interactions
- No significant drug interactions due to lack of metabolism
- Do not combine with acetylcholinesterase inhibitors other than pyridostigmine

Do Not Use
- Hypersensitivity to drug

SPECIAL POPULATIONS

Renal Impairment
- No known effects

Hepatic Impairment
- No known effects

Cardiac Impairment
- No known effects

Elderly
- Unknown

 ### Children and Adolescents
- Unknown

 ### Pregnancy
- Unknown. Use only if benefits of medication outweigh risks

Breast Feeding
- Unknown if excreted in breast milk. Do not use

THE ART OF NEUROPHARMACOLOGY

Potential Advantages
- Fewer AEs than other symptomatic agents for LEMS

Potential Disadvantages
- Does not alter disease outcome in LEMS. Limited availability

Primary Target Symptoms
- Weakness associated with LEMS, CMG, or MG

 ### Pearls
- Unlike MG, LEMS is a presynaptic disorder of neuromuscular transmission. LEMS is an autoimmune disease with antibodies directed against the voltage-gated calcium channels. LEMS is usually associated with small-cell lung cancer
- Not approved in the US but available on a compassionate-use basis
- Effective in the majority of LEMS patients, with or without malignancy
- In studies improved both strength and resting compound muscle amplitude

- Pyridostigmine or other acetylcholinesterase inhibitors alone are usually not effective in LEMS
- CMG is a group of disorders that are genetic – immunotherapy is not effective, so symptomatic treatment is the rule. Ptosis or ophthalmoplegia are common and age of presentation is variable. Some variants may respond to acetylcholinesterase inhibitors
- In small clinical trials, appears effective for improving motor symptoms and fatigue in MS. Experimental studies suggest enhancement of excitatory synaptic transmission
- Compared to 4-aminopyridine, more effective with fewer AEs due to lack of CNS penetration in LEMS, but 4-aminopyridine may be superior for treating MS symptoms
- May be beneficial in the treatment of downbeat nystagmus

 Suggested Reading

Bever CT Jr, Anderson PA, Leslie J, Panitch HS, Dhib-Jalbut S, Khan OA, Milo R, Hebel JR, Conway KL, Katz E, Johnson KP. Treatment with oral 3,4 diaminopyridine improves leg strength in multiple sclerosis patients: results of a randomized, double-blind, placebo-controlled, crossover trial. Neurology 1996;47(6):1457–62.

Engel AG. The therapy of congenital myasthenic syndromes. Neurotherapeutics 2007; 4(2):252–7.

Maddison P, Newsom-Davis J. Treatment for Lambert-Eaton myasthenic syndrome. Cochrane Database Syst Rev 2005;(2):CD003279.

Oh SJ, Claussen GG, Hatanaka Y, Morgan MB. 3,4-Diaminopyridine is more effective than placebo in a randomized, double-blind, crossover drug study in LEMS. Muscle Nerve 2009; 40(5):795–800.

Polman CH, Bertelsmann FW, de Waal R, van Diemen HA, Uitdehaag BM, van Loenen AC, Koetsier JC. 4-Aminopyridine is superior to 3,4-diaminopyridine in the treatment of patients with multiple sclerosis. Arch Neurol 1994; 51(11):1136–9.

Rucker JC. Current treatment of nystagmus. Curr Treat Options Neurol 2005;7(1):69–77.

DIAZEPAM

THERAPEUTICS

Brands
• Valium, Diastat, Dialar, Diazemuls, Rimapam, Stesolid, Tensium, Valclair, Alupram, Solis, Atensine, Evacalm

Generic?
Yes

Class
• Benzodiazepine, antiepileptic drug (AED)

Commonly Prescribed for
(FDA approved in bold)
• **Seizure disorders. Adjunctively and to control bouts of increased seizure activity**
• **Anxiety disorders**
• **Acute alcohol withdrawal**
• **Muscle relaxant**
• **Preoperative medication**
• Status epilepticus
• Tetanus
• Insomnia
• Agitation
• Stiff person syndrome
• Spasticity due to upper motor neuron disorders
• Irritable bowel syndrome
• Panic attacks
• Nausea and vomiting (from chemotherapy)
• Emergency treatment of preeclampsia
• Dystonia
• Vertigo
• Opioid or other drug withdrawal
• Acute mania in bipolar disorder

How the Drug Works
• Benzodiazepines bind to and potentiate the effect of GABA-A receptors, boosting chloride conductance through GABA-regulated channels, and other inhibitory neurotransmitters. There are at least 2 benzodiazepine receptors, 1 of which is associated with sleep mechanisms, the other with memory, sensory and cognitive functions. They act at spinal cord, brainstem, cerebellum, and limbic and cortical areas

How Long Until It Works
• Works quickly (minutes-hours depending on formulation) in the treatment of seizures, acute anxiety, drug withdrawal, and muscle relaxation. In patients with chronic disorders such as spasticity, dystonia or generalized anxiety it may take weeks to determine optimal dose for maximal therapeutic benefit

If It Works
• Seizures – rectal diazepam is used intermittently as an adjunctive for patients with known epilepsy with increased seizure frequency. Intravenous diazepam is used for status epilepticus in conjunction with intravenous maintenance anticonvulsants. In patients with epilepsy who benefit from oral diazepam as an adjunctive medication, consider tapering the medication after 2 years without seizures, depending on the type of epilepsy
• Spasticity – used as an adjunct medication. The cause of spasticity usually determines the duration of use. For acute muscle spasm, change to as needed use 1–3 weeks after onset
• Anxiety – generally used on a short-term basis. Consider adding an SSRI or SNRI for long-term treatment

If It Doesn't Work
• Epilepsy: For acute use only. Status epilepticus is a medical emergency requiring immediate medical attention. After using diazepam, start maintenance AEDs such as phenytoin and evaluate for cause of worsening seizures
• Spasticity: If not effective change to another agent
• Anxiety: Consider a secondary cause, mania or substance abuse. Change to another agent or add an augmenting agent

Best Augmenting Combos for Partial Response or Treatment-Resistance
• Epilepsy: often used in combination with other AEDs for optimal control but sedation can increase
• Spasticity: tizanidine, baclofen, and other CNS depressants may be used
• Anxiety: SSRI, SNRIs or tricyclic antidepressants are helpful for chronic anxiety. In most cases it is best to avoid combining with other benzodiazepines
• Insomnia: may be combined with low-dose tricyclic antidepressants (amitriptyline), or tetracyclics (trazodone, mirtazapine)

Tests
• None required

How Drug Causes AEs
• Actions on benzodiazepine receptors including augmentation of inhibitory neurotransmitter effects

Notable AEs
• Most common: sedation, fatigue, depression, weakness, ataxia, nystagmus, confusion, and psychomotor retardation
• Less common: bradycardia, anorexia, hypotonia, and anterograde amnesia

 Life-Threatening or Dangerous AEs

• CNS depression and decreased respiratory drive, especially in combination with opiates, barbiturates, or alcohol
• Rare blood dyscrasias or liver function abnormalities
• With injection there is a 1.7% risk of serious AEs, such as hypotension, respiratory and cardiac arrest

Weight Gain
• Unusual

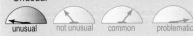

Sedation
• Common

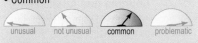

What to Do About AEs
• May decrease or remit in time as tolerance develops
• Lower the total dose and take more at bedtime
• For severe, life-threatening AEs administer flumazenil to reverse effects

Best Augmenting Agents for AEs
• Most AEs cannot be improved by adding an augmenting agent

Usual Dosage Range
• Epilepsy: 2–10 mg 2–4 times daily
• Muscle spasm: 2–10 mg 3–4 times daily
• Panic/anxiety disorders: 2–10 mg 2–4 times daily

Dosage Forms
• Tablets: 2, 5, and 10 mg
• Oral Solution: 5 mg per mL
• Rectal Gel: 2, 5 and 10 mg
• Injection: 5 mg/mL

How to Dose
• Epilepsy: Used as adjunct in chronic epilepsy. Start at 2 mg 2–3 times daily and increase as tolerated to effective dose over days to weeks to maximum 10 mg 3–4 times daily
• Bouts of increased seizures in patients with epilepsy: Dose based on age and weight. In patients 12 or older, give rectal diazepam 5 mg if 14–27 kg, 10 mg if 28–50 kg, 15 mg 51–75 mg and 20 mg to patients 76 kg or more
• Status Epilepticus: 0.15–0.25 mg/kg in adults. Usually given 2–5 mg/min. IV or IM injection if no IV access available. After initial 5 or 10 mg, repeat every 10–15 minutes up to maximum of 30 mg in adults if seizures do not remit
• Spasticity: Start at 2 mg at bedtime. Increase by 2–5 mg every few days as tolerated to most effective/best tolerated dose
• Panic disorder: Start at 2 mg 2–3 times daily. Increase over 1–2 weeks as tolerated to most effective dose. Maximum 10 mg 4 times a day

 Dosing Tips
• Children usually require higher doses per body weight for acute seizure control
• Rectal administration or injections are useful for acute seizures including exacerbations in patients with chronic epilepsy
• Assess need to continue treatment in all disorders

Overdose
• Confusion, drowsiness, decreased reflexes, incoordination, and lethargy are common. Ataxia, hypotension, coma, and death are rare. Coma and respiratory or circulatory

depression are rare when used alone. Use with other CNS depressants (such as alcohol, opioids or barbiturates) place patients at greater risk for severe AEs. Induce vomiting and use supportive measures along with gastric lavage or ipecac and in severe cases forced diuresis

- Flumazenil, an antagonist, reverses effect of diazepam
- Physostigmine can reverse some AEs but either can provoke seizures in patients with epilepsy

Long-Term Use

- Safe for long-term use with appropriate monitoring

Habit Forming

- Schedule IV drug with risk of tolerance and dependence. Dependence is common after 6 weeks or more of use. Patients with a history of drug or alcohol abuse have an increased risk of dependency

How to Stop

- Taper slowly. Abrupt withdrawal can cause seizures, even in patients without epilepsy. Seizures can occur over a week after stopping drug
- Taper 1–2 mg/day every 3 days to reduce risk of withdrawal. Once at a lower dose, decrease speed of taper to as little as 1–2 mg/week or less. Slow tapers are especially recommended for patient on diazepam for many months or years
- Monitor for re-emergence of disease symptoms (seizures, muscle spasm, or anxiety)

Pharmacokinetics

- Peak plasma level at 0.5–2 hours and elimination half-life 20–80 hours. 98% protein bound. Mostly metabolized by CYP3A4 isoenzyme. Highly lipid soluble with good CNS penetration

 Drug Interactions

- Alcohol and other CNS depressants (barbiturates, opioids) increase CNS AEs
- Ranitidine may reduce GI absorption
- Inhibitors of hepatic metabolism (i.e., oral contraceptives, fluoxetine, isoniazid, ketoconazole, propranolol, valproic acid, metoprolol) can increase diazepam levels

- Antacids may alter the rate of absorption
- May increase serum concentrations of digoxin and phenytoin, leading to toxicity

 Other Warnings/ Precautions

- May cause drowsiness and impair ability to drive or perform tasks that require alertness
- Rare reports of death in patients with severe pulmonary impairment

Do Not Use

- Patients with a proven allergy to diazepam or any benzodiazepine. Significant liver disease or narrow angle-closure glaucoma

SPECIAL POPULATIONS

Renal Impairment

- Metabolites are renally excreted. Use with caution

Hepatic Impairment

- Do not use in patients with significant liver dysfunction

Cardiac Impairment

- No known effects

Elderly

- May clear drug more slowly and have lower dose requirement. Use lower doses than in younger adults

 Children and Adolescents

- For bouts of increased seizures in epilepsy, dose by age and weight Age 2–5: 5 mg 6–11 kg, 10 mg 12–22 kg, 15 mg 23–33 kg and 20 mg 34–44 kg. Age 6–11: 5 mg 10–18 kg, 10 mg 19–37 kg, 15 mg 38–55 kg and 20 mg 56 kg and up
- Status epilepticus: 0.1–1.0 mg/kg total dose at 2–5 mg/min
- Used in children as young as 6 months (oral) and neonates under 30 days of age (injection)
- Paradoxical excitement and rage may occur in psychiatric patients and hyperactive children

Pregnancy

- Risk category D. Drug crosses placenta, and drug and its metabolites may accumulate. May increase risk of fetal malformations and infants can experience withdrawal. Use during labor can cause "floppy infant" syndrome with hypotonia, lethargy, and sucking difficulties
- Consider changing to another AED in patients that use as a daily preventative, but can be used for status epilepticus
- Do not use for treatment of anxiety

Breast Feeding

- Drug is found in mother's breast milk and may cause accumulation of drug and metabolites. Infants may become lethargic and lose weight. Do not breast feed on drug

THE ART OF NEUROPHARMACOLOGY

Potential Advantages

- Rapid onset of action in epilepsy, spasticity, and anxiety disorders. Useful in the emergency treatment of seizures and as an adjunctive medication in spasticity disorders

Potential Disadvantages

- Not a first-line maintenance agent in most patients with epilepsy. Development of tolerance and CNS depression often problematic. Significant potential for abuse due to quick onset of action compared to clonazepam

Primary Target Symptoms

- Seizure frequency and severity
- Pain in spasticity disorders or dystonia
- Reduction in anxiety

Pearls

- Useful for treatment of acute seizures including status epilepticus, but patients typically require loading of a longer-lasting AED such as phenytoin
- A first-line agent for symptoms in stiff person syndrome, but not curative
- In cases of acute vertigo, works to suppress vestibular function and improve symptoms. Treat every 4–6 hours with 5–10 mg

---

Suggested Reading

Abbruzzese G. The medical management of spasticity. Eur J Neurol 2002;9 (Suppl 1):30–4; discussion 53–61.

Cesarani A, Alpini D, Monti B, Raponi G. The treatment of acute vertigo. Neurol Sci 2004;25 (Suppl 1):S26–30.

Okoromah CN, Lesi FE. Diazepam for treating tetanus. Cochrane Database Syst Rev 2004;(1): CD003954.

Rey E, Tréluyer JM, Pons G. Pharmacokinetic optimization of benzodiazepine therapy for acute seizures. Focus on delivery routes. Clin Pharmacokinet 1999; 36(6):409–24.

Treiman DM. The role of benzodiazepines in the management of status epilepticus. Neurology 1990;40 (5 Suppl 2):32–42.

DIHYDROERGOTAMINE (DHE)

THERAPEUTICS

Brands
• Migranal, DHE-45, Dihydergot

Generic?
Yes

 Class
• Ergot

Commonly Prescribed for
(FDA approved in bold)
• **Acute migraine treatment**
• **Acute cluster headache treatment**
• Status migrainosus

 How the Drug Works
• Agonism of 5-HT1$_B$ and $_D$ receptors similar to triptans, but with additional actions at 5-HT1$_F$ 5-HT1$_A$ and 5-HT2$_A$ receptors. Also acts at norepinephrine (inhibits reuptake) and dopamine (including D2 and D3) receptors
• Effectiveness and vasoconstrictive effects are likely related to agonism of 5-HT1$_B$ and $_D$ receptors. Blocking the transmission of pain signals from the trigeminal nerve to the trigeminal nucleus caudalis and preventing release of inflammatory neuropeptides is more likely the reason for effectiveness rather than vasoconstriction. Unlike triptans, can reverse central sensitization

How Long Until It Works
• Migraine/cluster- within 1–2 hours

If It Works
• Continue to take as needed. Patients taking acute treatment more than 2 days/week are at risk for medication-overuse headache, especially if they have migraine

If It Doesn't Work
• Treat early in the attack (before severe pain)
• Change to another agent

 Best Augmenting Combos for Partial Response or Treatment-Resistance
• Migraine: Non-steroidal anti-inflammatory drugs (NSAIDs) or antiemetics are often used to augment response

• Cluster: Oxygen (high-flow)
• Status migrainosus: Combine with neuroleptics, ketorolac, diphenhydramine, intravenous valproate, intravenous magnesium, hydrate and start preventive treatment

Tests
• Monitor blood pressure – especially after intravenous administration

ADVERSE EFFECTS (AEs)

How Drug Causes AEs
• Actions on serotonin receptors cause vasoconstriction, nausea

Notable AEs
• Nausea, dizziness, paresthesias, chest or throat tightness
• Muscle pains, coldness, pallor, and cyanosis of digits
• Hypertension
• Altered taste, rhinitis (nasal spray), injection site reaction (IM)

 Life-Threatening or Dangerous AEs
• Ergotism, cardiac (acute myocardial infarction, arrhythmia) or cerebrovascular events (hemorrhagic or ischemic stroke) are all rare

Weight Gain
• Unusual

unusual not unusual common problematic

Sedation
• Unusual

unusual not unusual common problematic

What to Do About AEs
• Lower dose for nausea, stop for serious AEs

Best Augmenting Agents for AEs
• Pretreat before using (especially intravenously) with antiemetics

DOSING AND USE

Usual Dosage Range
- IV/IM up to 3 mg/day
- Nasal spray – up to 2 kits (4 mg each)/day

Dosage Forms
- Nasal spray: 4 mg/mL
- Injection: 1 mg/mL

How to Dose
- IV: Give 0.1–1 mg 3–4 times daily as needed, usually for status migrainosus. Start with a test dose of 0.5 mg in adults. Reduce dose for significant nausea (more than 10 minutes) after dose. If tolerated and pain not relieved, increase to 1 mg dose. Give a maximum 3 mg/day. Give up to 21 mg for status migrainosus over 7 days
- IM: Give 0.5–1 mg as needed, up to 3 mg/day
- Nasal spray: Give 1 spray (0.5 mg) in each nostril, repeat in 10–15 minutes up to twice a day

 Dosing Tips
- Push IV form slowly over 3 or more minutes to avoid nausea
- Pretreatment with antiemetics is recommended for IV administration, but may not be necessary with IM or nasal spray. Pretreat with antiemetics (metoclopramide, droperidol, prochlorperazine) 30 minutes before DHE
- In patients with risk factors for coronary artery disease, give the first dose in a medical setting

Overdose
- Ergotamine poisoning may cause abdominal pain, nausea, vomiting, paresthesias, edema, muscle pain, cold hands and feet, and hypertension or hypotension. Confusion, depression, convulsions and gangrene may occur. Unclear if DHE poses similar risks

Long-Term Use
- Appears safe, but monitor blood pressure and vascular risk factors with extended use

Habit Forming
- No

How to Stop
- No need to taper

Pharmacokinetics
- Very low oral bioavailability (about 1%). Nasal spray has 40% bioavailability. Peak plasma level 30 minutes after IM injection, 45 minutes after SC injection, and less than 1 hour after intranasal use. Hepatic metabolism, mostly excreted in bile

 Drug Interactions
- Use with caution with other vasoconstrictive agents, such as other ergot alkaloids or triptans
- Do not administer with potent CYP3A4 inhibitors, including macrolide antibiotics (erythromycin, clarithromycin), HIV protease or reverse transcriptase inhibitors (delaviridine, ritonavir, nelfinavir, indinavir) or azole antifungals (ketoconazole, itraconazole, voriconazole). Less potent inhibitors 3A4 inhibitors include saquinavir, nefazodone, fluconazole, fluoxetine, fluvoxamine, grapefruit juice and clotrimazole
- Nicotine may predispose to vasoconstriction
- May decrease effectiveness of nitrates

Do Not Use
- Uncontrolled hypertension, coronary artery vasospasm (Prinzmetal angina), pregnancy, breast feeding, coronary arterial disease, or hypersensitivity to ergots

SPECIAL POPULATIONS

Renal Impairment
- Risks unknown. May be prone to hypertension and cardiac AEs

Hepatic Impairment
- Safety and effect of significant disease on drug metabolism unknown. Avoid in patients with severe disease

Cardiac Impairment
- Do not use in patients with uncontrolled hypertension or coronary artery disease

Elderly

- No known effects, but ensure safety before use (normal blood pressure, no coronary artery disease)

 ## Children and Adolescents

- Not studied in children but likely safe

 ## Pregnancy

- Category X. Associated with developmental toxicity and has oxytocic properties

Breast Feeding

- Likely excreted in breast milk. Do not breast feed after using

---

THE ART OF NEUROPHARMACOLOGY

Potential Advantages

- Effective in status migrainosus, with low risk for medication overuse and fewer AEs than ergotamine. Effective in preventing migraine recurrence

Potential Disadvantages

- Compared to triptans: not available as oral form, as effective in episodic migraine and acute cluster compared with sumatriptan injection but more AEs

Primary Target Symptoms

- Headache pain, nausea, photo- and phonophobia

 ## Pearls

- An ergotamine derivative with better safety profile than other ergots: less arterial constriction, less nausea and emesis, less oxytocic, and less likely to produce ergotism and gangrene
- Safety with other potentially vasoconstrictive drugs (i.e., triptans) is unknown. In general do not use within 24 hours of triptans
- Compared with sumatriptan injection, less effective for cluster headache and less rapid onset of action, but with lower rates of headache recurrence
- May be useful in the setting of acute medication overuse. Medication overuse from opioids, barbiturates, or triptans can lead to treatment refractoriness
- An orally inhaled DHE (Levadex) will soon be available for acute migraine with efficacy comparable to IV treatment

---

 ## Suggested Reading

Pringsheim T, Howse D. In-patient treatment of chronic daily headache using dihydroergotamine: a long-term follow-up study. Can J Neurol Sci 1998;25(2):146–50.

Raskin NH. Repetitive intravenous dihydroergotamine as therapy for intractable migraine. Neurology 1986;36(7):995–7.

Saper JR, Silberstein SD. Pharmacology of dihydroergotamine and evidence for efficacy and safety in migraine. Headache 2006;46 (Suppl 4): S171–81.

Winner P, Ricalde O, Le Force B, Saper J, Margul B. A double-blind study of subcutaneous dihydroergotamine vs subcutaneous sumatriptan in the treatment of acute migraine. Arch Neurol 1996; 53(2):180–4.

DIPYRIDAMOLE AND ASPIRIN

Brands
• Aggrenox

Generic?
Yes

Class
• Antiplatelet agent

Commonly Prescribed for
(FDA approved in bold)
• **To reduce risk of recurrent transient ischemic attack (TIA) or ischemic stroke (IS) due to thrombosis**
• Adjunctive prophylaxis of thromboembolism after cardiac valve replacement (adjunctive with warfarin: use dipyridamole only)

 ## How the Drug Works
• Aspirin: By acetylating cyclo-oxygenase-1 and 2 (cox-1), aspirin inhibits thromboxane synthetase, reducing synthesis of thromboxane A2, a prostaglandin derivative that is a potent vasoconstrictor and inducer of platelet aggregation
• Dipyridamole: Inhibits (1) thromboxane synthetase, (2) the cellular reuptake of adenosine into platelets, endothelial cells, and erythrocytes and adenosine deaminase, which both increase extracellular adenosine levels leading to stimulation of platelet adenylate cyclase and inhibition of platelet aggregation, and (3) phosphodiesterase, augmenting the effect of endothelium-derived relaxing factor (nitric oxide)

How Long Until It Works
• 1–2 hours. Inhibits platelet aggregation for the life of the platelet (7–10 days)

If It Works
• Continue to use

If It Doesn't Work
• Only reduces risk of MI or IS. Warfarin is superior for cardiogenic stroke. Control all IS risk factors such as smoking, hyperlipidemia, and hypertension. For acute events, admit patients for treatment and diagnostic testing

 ## Best Augmenting Combos for Partial Response or Treatment-Resistance
• Combinations with other antiplatelet agents are not recommended

Tests
• None required

How Drug Causes AEs
• Antiplatelet effects increase bleeding risk. Effects on nitric oxide may produce headache

Notable AEs
• Headache, abdominal pain, dyspepsia, nausea/vomiting, diarrhea, arthralgias, hypotension, epistaxis

 ## Life-Threatening or Dangerous AEs
• GI, intracranial, or intraocular bleeding. Rare hepatic failure

Weight Gain
• Unusual

unusual   not unusual   common   problematic

Sedation
• Unusual

unusual   not unusual   common   problematic

What to Do About AEs
• For significant GI or intracranial bleeding, stop drug. For intolerable headaches, switch to 1 capsule at bedtime and low-dose aspirin in the morning for 1 week (headaches usually resolve in 1 week or less)

Best Augmenting Agents for AEs
• Proton pump inhibitors reduce risk of GI bleeding

DOSING AND USE

Usual Dosage Range
- 200 mg extended-release dipyridamole/ 25 mg aspirin twice daily

Dosage Forms
- Capsules: 200 mg extended-release dipyridamole/25 mg aspirin

How to Dose
- 1 capsule twice daily

 ### Dosing Tips
- Taking with food decreases absorption and reduces GI AEs

Overdose
- Aspirin: Respiratory alkalosis resulting in tachypnea, nausea, hypokalemia, tinnitus, thrombocytopenia, and easy bruising early. Can lead to pulmonary edema, respiratory failure, renal failure, and coma
- Dipyridamole: Flushing, sweating, restlessness, dizziness and a feeling of weakness can occur. Less commonly tachycardia and hypotension

Long-Term Use
- Safe for long-term use

Habit Forming
- No

How to Stop
- No need to taper

Pharmacokinetics
- Aspirin: Half-life is about 20 minutes. > 99% protein binding. Hepatic metabolism and renal excretion
- Dipyridamole: Peak levels at 2 hours. Hepatic metabolism into a glucuronide metabolite that is mostly excreted via bile into feces. Plasma half-life 13.6 hours

 ### Drug Interactions
Aspirin:
- Alcohol increases risk of GI ulceration and may prolong bleeding time
- Urinary acidifiers (ascorbic acid, methionine) decrease secretion and increase drug effect
- Antacids and urinary alkalinizers may decrease drug effect
- Carbonic anhydrase inhibitors may increase risk of salicylate intoxication, and aspirin may displace acetazolamide from protein binding sites leading to toxicity
- Activated charcoal decreases aspirin absorption and effect
- Corticosteroids may increase clearance and decrease serum levels
- Use with heparin or oral anticoagulants has an additive effect and can increase bleeding risks
- Aspirin may cause unexpected hypotension after treatment with nitroglycerin
- Use with NSAIDs may decrease NSAID serum levels and increases risk of GI AEs
- May displace valproic acid from binding sites and increase pharmacologic effects
- May blunt effectiveness of beta-blockers and angiotensin-converting enzyme inhibitors
- May decrease effect of loop diuretics and spironolactone
- Increases drug levels of methotrexate
- Reduces the uricosuric effects of probenecid and sulfinpyrazone
Dipyridamole:
- Increases plasma levels and cardiac effects of adenosine
- May decrease effect of cholinesterase inhibitors, such as pyridostigmine, which may worsen symptoms of myasthenia gravis

 ### Other Warnings/ Precautions
- The use of aspirin or other salicylates in children or teens with influenza or chicken pox may be associated with Reye's syndrome. Symptoms include vomiting and lethargy that may progress to delirium or coma
- Aspirin intolerance is not rare, especially in asthmatics. Symptoms include bronchospasm, angioedema, severe rhinitis or shock

Do Not Use
- Known hypersensitivity to salicyclates, NSAIDs or dipyridamole, acute asthma or hay fever, severe anemia or blood coagulation defects, children or teenagers with chicken pox or flu symptoms

Renal Impairment
• Use with caution with significant disease. May temporarily worsen renal function

Hepatic Impairment
• Use with caution in patients with significant disease, including those with hypoprothrombinemia or vitamin K deficiency. Hepatotoxicity may occur

Cardiac Impairment
• Use with caution in patients with severe coronary artery disease, including recent myocardial infarction or angina. The vasodilatory effect of dipyridamole can aggravate chest pain. May exacerbate hypotension if present. The low dose of aspirin in the combination product may not provide adequate treatment for cardiac indications

Elderly
• No known effects

 Children and Adolescents
• Not studied in children younger than age 12. Do not use in setting of chicken pox or flu symptoms

 Pregnancy
• Category B (dipyridamole) /D (aspirin). Crosses the placenta and is associated with anemia, ante- or post-partum hemorrhage, prolonged gestation and labor, and constriction of ductus arteriosus. Do not use, especially in 3rd trimester

Breast Feeding
• Both products excreted in breast milk in low concentrations. Risk to infants is unknown

Potential Advantages
• Highly effective medication for IS prevention

Potential Disadvantages
• Low aspirin doses may not provide adequate prophylaxis against cardiac disease. Cost

Primary Target Symptoms
• Prevention of the neurological complications that result from ischemic stroke

 Pearls
• First-line drug for secondary prevention of IS along with clopidogrel and aspirin
• Compared to clopidogrel, may be less effective in patients with peripheral vascular disease
• Stop 1 week before any surgical procedure, given its effect on platelet function
• Headache is a common AE that may raise concerns in the setting of recent IS. When starting drug, inform patients that headache is common in the first week of treatment
• This dipyridamole and aspirin combination is more effective than 25 mg aspirin twice daily, but it is unclear if it is more effective than higher aspirin doses

DIPYRIDAMOLE AND ASPIRIN (continued)

 Suggested Reading

Diener HC, Sacco RL, Yusuf S, Cotton D, Ounpuu S, Lawton WA, Palesch Y, Martin RH, Albers GW, Bath P, Bornstein N, Chan BP, Chen ST, Cunha L, Dahlöf B, De Keyser J, Donnan GA, Estol C, Gorelick P, Gu V, Hermansson K, Hilbrich L, Kaste M, Lu C, Machnig T, Pais P, Roberts R, Skvortsova V, Teal P, Toni D, VanderMaelen C, Voigt T, Weber M, Yoon BW; Prevention Regimen for Effectively Avoiding Second Strokes (PRoFESS) study group. Effects of aspirin plus extended-release dipyridamole versus clopidogrel and telmisartan on disability and cognitive function after recurrent stroke in patients with ischaemic stroke in the Prevention Regimen for Effectively Avoiding Second Strokes (PRoFESS) trial: a double-blind, active and placebo-controlled study. Lancet Neurol 2008;7(10):875–84.

Lenz T, Wilson A. Clinical pharmacokinetics of antiplatelet agents used in the secondary prevention of stroke. Clin Pharmacokinet 2003;42(10):909–20.

Redman AR, Ryan GJ. Aggrenox((R)) versus other pharmacotherapy in preventing recurrent stroke. Expert Opin Pharmacother 2004;5(1):117–23.

Serebruany VL, Malinin AI, Sane DC, Jilma B, Takserman A, Atar D, Hennekens CH. Magnitude and time course of platelet inhibition with Aggrenox and Aspirin in patients after ischemic stroke: the AGgrenox versus Aspirin Therapy Evaluation (AGATE) trial. Eur J Pharmacol 2004;499(3):315–24.

Usman MH, Notaro LA, Nagarakanti R, Brahin E, Dessain S, Gracely E, Ezekowitz MD. Combination antiplatelet therapy for secondary stroke prevention: enhanced efficacy or double trouble? Am J Cardiol 2009;103(8):1107–12.

DONEPEZIL

THERAPEUTICS

Brands
• Aricept, Aricept Evess, Memorit

Generic?
No

Class
• Cholinesterase inhibitor

Commonly Prescribed for
(FDA approved in bold)
• **Alzheimer dementia (AD) (mild, moderate or severe)**
• Vascular dementia
• Mild cognitive impairment
• Dementia with Lewy bodies (DLB)
• HIV dementia
• Autism
• Attention deficit hyperactivity disorder (ADHD)

How the Drug Works
• Increases the concentration of acetylcholine through reversible, non-competitive inhibition of acetylcholinesterase, which increases availability of acetylcholine. A deficiency of cholinergic function is felt to be important in producing the signs and symptoms of AD. May interfere with amyloid deposition
• Although symptoms of AD can improve, donepezil does not prevent disease progression

How Long Until It Works
• Typically 2–6 weeks at a given dose, but effect is best observed over a period of months

If It Works
• Continue to use but symptoms of dementia usually continue to worsen

If It Doesn't Work
• Non-pharmacologic measures are the basis of dementia treatment. Maintain regular schedules and routines. Avoid prolonged travel, unnecessary medical procedures or emergency room visits, crowds, and large social gatherings
• Limit drugs with sedative properties such as opioids, hypnotics, Antiepileptic drugs and tricyclic antidepressants
• Consider adjusting dose

• Treat other disorders which can worsen symptoms such as hyperglycemia or urinary difficulties

Best Augmenting Combos for Partial Response or Treatment-Resistance
• Addition of the NMDA receptor antagonist memantine may be beneficial. In 1 study donepezil plus memantine reduced the rate of progression compared to those taking donepezil alone
• Treat depression or apathy, if present, with SSRIs. Avoid tricyclic antidepressants in demented patients due to risk of confusion
• For significant confusion and agitation avoid neuroleptics (especially in Lewy Body dementia) to avoid the risk of neuroleptic malignant syndrome. Atypical antipsychotics (risperidone, quetiapine, olanzapine, clozapine) can be used instead

Tests
• None required

ADVERSE EFFECTS (AEs)

How Drug Causes AEs
• Acetylcholinesterase inhibition in the CNS and PNS

Notable AEs
• GI AEs (nausea, diarrhea, anorexia and weight loss) are most common
• Fatigue, depression, dizziness, muscle cramps and sleep disturbances

Life-Threatening or Dangerous AEs
• Rarely bradycardia or heart block causing syncope. Generalized convulsions. Increases gastric acid secretions which can predispose to GI bleeding

Weight Gain
• Unusual

unusual   not unusual   common   problematic

• Weight loss is more common

Sedation
• Unusual

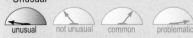

unusual   not unusual   common   problematic

What to Do About AEs
• In patients with dementia, determining if AEs are related to medication or another medical condition can be difficult. For CNS side effects, discontinuation of non-essential centrally acting medications may help. If a bothersome AE is clearly drug-related then lower the dose (especially for GI AEs) or discontinue donepezil

Best Augmenting Agents for AEs
• Most AEs do not respond to adding other medications

DOSING AND USE

Usual Dosage Range
• 5–10 mg at night

Dosage Forms
• Tablets, regular or orally disintegrating: 5, 10 mg
• Oral Solution: 1 mg/mL

How to Dose
• Start at 5 mg in the evening. Increase to 10 mg in 4–6 weeks if needed. If AEs occur, titrate more slowly

 Dosing Tips
• Slow titration can reduce AEs. Food does not affect absorption

Overdose
• Symptoms of cholinergic crisis can occur: nausea/vomiting, hypotension, diaphoresis, convulsions, bradycardia/collapse. May cause muscle weakness and respiratory failure. Atropine with an initial dose of 1–2 mg IV is a potential antidote

Long-Term Use
• Safe for long-term use. Effectiveness may decrease over time as the dementing illness progresses

Habit Forming
• No

How to Stop
• Abrupt discontinuation can produce rapid worsening of dementia symptoms, memory and behavioral disturbances. Taper slowly

Pharmacokinetics
• Metabolized by CYP-450 isoenzymes 2D6 and 3A4. Elimination half-life is 70 hours but peak effect at 3–4 hours. About 17% of drug is excreted unchanged in urine. Linear pharmacokinetics. Protein binding 96%

 Drug Interactions
• Increases the effect of anesthetics. Stop donepezil before surgery
• Anticholinergics interfere with effect of drug
• Other cholinesterase inhibitors, cholinergic agonists (bethanechol) and neuromuscular blockers (such as succinylcholine) may cause a synergistic effect
• CYP-450 3A4 and 2D6 inhibitors (ketoconazole, quinidine) increase donepezil concentrations and inducers (carbamazepine, phenobarbital, phenytoin, rifampin, dexamethasone) reduce concentrations
• Bradycardia may occur when used with beta-blockers

Do Not Use
• Hypersensitivity to the drug or piperidine derivatives (including meperidine and fentanyl)

SPECIAL POPULATIONS

Renal Impairment
• No known effects

Hepatic Impairment
• Patients with severe disease have 20% reduced clearance. This may not be clinically significant

Cardiac Impairment
• Significant heart block, bradycardia and syncope are rare but have been reported

Elderly
- No known effects

Children and Adolescents
- Not studied. AD does not occur in children. May be useful for ADHD as adjunctive treatment

Pregnancy
- Category C. Use only if benefits of medication outweigh risks

Breast Feeding
- Unknown if excreted in breast milk. Do not use

THE ART OF NEUROPHARMACOLOGY

Potential Advantages
- Proven effectiveness for AD, even with severe dementia. Low risk of the hepatotoxicity seen with other acetylcholinesterases (tacrine), and lower GI AEs (nausea, anorexia) than rivastigmine. Once-daily dosing

Potential Disadvantages
- Cost and minimal effectiveness. Sleep disturbances such as insomnia are more common than with other AD treatments. Does not prevent progression of AD or other dementia

Primary Target Symptoms
- Confusion, agitation, memory, performing activities of daily living

Pearls
- May be used in combination with memantine with good effect, but combining with other cholinesterase inhibitors is not recommended
- In most clinical trials, medication treatments for AD patients had a similar rate of benefit
- May be useful for both behavioral problems in AD (delusion, anxiety and apathy for example) as well as memory disturbance
- May delay the need for nursing home placement
- Shown to be effective for the cognitive and behavioral symptoms (agitation, apathy, hallucinations) of DLB
- When changing from 1 cholinesterase inhibitor to another, avoid a washout period which could precipitate clinical deterioration
- May help treat dementia in Down's syndrome, which has similar pathology as AD
- Most open-label studies of donepezil for ADHD did not demonstrate benefit, and AEs were common. For treatment of Tourette's in children with coexisting ADHD, donepezil appears to reduce tics, but AEs are problematic

Suggested Reading

Bentué-Ferrer D, Tribut O, Polard E, Allain H. Clinically significant drug interactions with cholinesterase inhibitors: a guide for neurologists. CNS Drugs 2003;17(13):947–63.

Birks J, Harvey RJ. Donepezil for dementia due to Alzheimer's disease. Cochrane Database Syst Rev 2006;(1):CD001190.

Downey D. Pharmacologic management of Alzheimer disease. J Neurosci Nurs 2008; 40(1):55–9.

Porsteinsson AP, Grossberg GT, Mintzer J, Olin JT; Memantine MEM-MD-12 Study Group. Memantine treatment in patients with mild to moderate Alzheimer's disease already receiving a cholinesterase inhibitor: a randomized, double-blind, placebo-controlled trial. Curr Alzheimer Res 2008;5(1):83–9.

Schmitt FA, van Dyck CH, Wichems CH, Olin JT; for the Memantine MEM-MD-02 Study Group. Cognitive response to memantine in moderate to severe Alzheimer disease patients already receiving donepezil: an exploratory reanalysis. Alzheimer Dis Assoc Disord 2006;20(4):255–62.

Stahl SM. The new cholinesterase inhibitors for Alzheimer's disease, Part 1: their similarities are different. J Clin Psychiatry 2000;61(10):710–11.

DROPERIDOL

THERAPEUTICS

Brands
• Inapsine

Generic?
Yes

 Class
• Antiemetic, antipsychotic

Commonly Prescribed for
(FDA approved in bold)
• **Antiemetic**
• Migraine (acute)
• Chemotherapy-induced nausea and vomiting

 How the Drug Works
• Antidopaminergic, with mild alpha-1 adrenergic blockade and sedative effects

How Long Until It Works
• Migraine, nausea in less than 10 minutes

If It Works
• Use at lowest required dose
• Monitor QT corrected (QTc) interval

If It Doesn't Work
• Change to another agent

 Best Augmenting Combos for Partial Response or Treatment-Resistance
• For migraine, can be used with dihydroergotamine or NSAIDs

Tests
• Obtain ECG to monitor QTc

ADVERSE EFFECTS (AEs)

How Drug Causes AEs
• Hypotension and dizziness are related to alpha-blockade, and abnormal movement AEs are related to dopamine blocking effects

Notable AEs
• Drowsiness, hypotension, tachycardia, chills

• Dystonia, akathisia, restlessness, anxiety
• Less common: elevated blood pressure, apnea, muscular rigidity

 Life-Threatening or Dangerous AEs
• QTc prolongation and torsade de pointes have been reported, especially with higher doses

Weight Gain
• Unusual

Sedation
• Common

What to Do About AEs
• Lowering dose or changing to another antiemetic improves most AEs
• Use with caution in patients if QTc is above 450 (females) or 440 (males). Lower dose or change to another agent. Do not administer droperidol with QTc greater than 500
• For patients on daily intravenous therapy, continue to monitor with daily ECG, especially as dose increases

Best Augmenting Agents for AEs
• Give fluids to avoid hypotension and dizziness
• Give anticholinergics (diphenhydramine or benztropine) for extrapyramidal reactions

DOSING AND USE

Usual Dosage Range
• 0.625–2.5 mg every 6–8 hours

Dosage Forms
• Injection: 2.5 mg/mL

How to Dose
• After ensuring no QTc prolongation, give 0.625–2.5 mg as a single dose every 6–8 hours intravenously or as intramuscular injection

Dosing Tips

- In hospitalized patients, start with lower dose to ensure no QTc prolongation occurs and drug well-tolerated and increase as needed to effective dose
- Check ECG daily while receiving treatment

Overdose

- Sedation, hypotension, extrapyramidal reactions, and arrhythmias, including QTc prolongation

Long-Term Use

- Safe for long-term use with appropriate monitoring

Habit Forming

- No

How to Stop

- No need to taper

Pharmacokinetics

- Onset of action in 3–10 minutes and peak levels at 30 minutes. Half-life 2.2 hours. Hepatic metabolism and excreted mostly as metabolites in urine and feces

 Drug Interactions

- Use with CNS depressants (barbiturates, opiates, general anesthetics) potentiates CNS AEs
- Epinephrine may worsen hypotension due to alpha-1 adrenergic blockade by droperidol
- Use with some forms of conduction anesthesia (spinal anesthesia, peridural anesthetics) can cause hypotension or peripheral vasodilation due to sympathetic blockade
- Fentanyl and droperidol may induce hypertension due to alterations in sympathetic pathway

⚠ Other Warnings/ Precautions

Risk factors for QTc prolongation include:
- Significant bradycardia (less than 50 bpm)
- Cardiac disease
- Treatment with class I and III antiarrhythmics
- Treatment with monoamine oxidase (MAO) inhibitors

- Treatment with medications known to prolong QTc intervals
- Electrolyte imbalance (hypokalemia, hypomagnesemia), as seen with some diuretics

Do Not Use

- Hypersensitivity to drug, QTc prolongation, including long QT syndrome

Renal Impairment

- Unknown effects. Use with caution

Hepatic Impairment

- Use with caution. May need to lower dose

Cardiac Impairment

- May worsen orthostatic hypotension. Avoid using in patients with arrhythmia

Elderly

- May be more sensitive to CNS AEs

 Children and Adolescents

- Appears safe in children over age 2. Reduce dose to 1 or 1.5 mg in young children

 Pregnancy

- Category C. Use only if benefit outweighs risks

Breast Feeding

- Unknown if found in breast milk. Use while breast feeding is generally not recommended

Potential Advantages

- Highly effective drug in the treatment of refractory migraine

Potential Disadvantages

- Need to monitor QTc interval. Extrapyramidal reactions

Primary Target Symptoms
• Headache, nausea

Pearls
• Effective in refractory migraine and status migrainosus. Often combined with dihydroergotamine, given about 30 minutes after droperidol

• Combine with diphenhydramine, 25–50 mg, to reduce rate of akathisia and dystonic reactions
• Black-box warning due to risk of QTc prolongation and death, but with appropriate ECG monitoring and doses under 10 mg/day, this is extremely rare. Patients with QTc above 500 are at greatest risk

Suggested Reading

Evans RW, Young WB. Droperidol and other neuroleptics/antiemetics for the management of migraine. Headache 2003;43(7):811–3.

Nuttall GA, Eckerman KM, Jacob KA, Pawlaski EM, Wigersma SK, Marienau ME, Oliver WC, Narr BJ, Ackerman MJ. Does low-dose droperidol administration increase the risk of drug-induced QT prolongation and torsade de pointes in the general surgical population? Anesthesiology 2007;107(4):531–6.

Silberstein SD, Young WB, Mendizabal JE, Rothrock JF, Alam AS. Acute migraine treatment with droperidol: A randomized, double-blind, placebo-controlled trial. Neurology 2003;60(2): 315–21.

Wang SJ, Silberstein SD, Young WB. Droperidol treatment of status migrainosus and refractory migraine. Headache 1997; 37(6):377–82.

Brands

• Cymbalta, Xeristar, Yentreve, Ariclaim

Generic?

No

Class

• Serotonin and norepinephrine reuptake inhibitor (SNRI), antidepressant

Commonly Prescribed for

(FDA approved in bold)

• **Major depressive disorder**
• **Generalized anxiety disorder**
• **Fibromyalgia**
• **Diabetic peripheral neuropathic pain (PDN)**
• Migraine prophylaxis
• Tension-type headache prophylaxis
• Other painful peripheral neuropathies
• Cancer pain (neuropathic)
• Stress urinary incontinence

How the Drug Works

• Blocks serotonin and noradrenergic reuptake pumps, increasing their levels within hours, but antidepressant effects take weeks. Effect is more likely related to adaptive changes in serotonin and norepinephrine receptors systems
• Weakly blocks dopamine reuptake pump (dopamine transporter)

How Long Until It Works

• Fibromyalgia – as little as 2 weeks, but may take up to 3 months
• Migraine – effective in as little as 2 weeks, but can take up to 10 weeks on a stable dose to see full effect
• Tension-type headache prophylaxis – effective in 4–8 weeks
• Neuropathic pain – usually some effect within 4 weeks
• Diabetic neuropathy – may have significant improvement with high doses within 6 weeks
• Depression – 2 weeks but up to 2 months for full effect

If It Works

• Fibromyalgia- the goal is to reduce pain intensity and symptoms, reduce

use of analgesics and improve quality of life
• Migraine – goal is a 50% or greater reduction in migraine frequency or severity. Consider tapering or stopping if headaches remit for more than 6 months or if considering pregnancy
• Tension-type headache – goal is 50% or greater reduction of days with headache, duration or intensity. Consider tapering or stopping if headaches remit for more than 6 months or if considering pregnancy
• Diabetic neuropathy – the goal is to reduce pain intensity and reduce use of analgesics, but usually does not produce remission. Continue to monitor for AEs and maintain strict glycemic control
• Depression – continue to use and monitor for AE. May continue for 1 yr following first depression episode or indefinite if >1 episode of depression

If It Doesn't Work

• Increase to highest tolerated dose
• Fibromyalgia, migraine and tension-type headache: address other issues, such as medication-overuse, other coexisting medical disorders, such as anxiety, and consider changing to another agent or adding a second agent
• Neuropathic pain: either change to another agent or add a second agent

Best Augmenting Combos for Partial Response or Treatment-Resistance

• Fibromyalgia: SNRIs such as milnacipran and/or AEDs, such as gabapentin, pregabalin, are agents that may be useful in managing fibromyalgia. May also use in combination with natural products and non-medication treatments, such as biofeedback or physical therapy, to improve pain control
• Migraine: For some patients, low-dose polytherapy with 2 or more drugs may be better tolerated and more effective than high-dose monotherapy. May use in combination with AEDs, antihypertensives, natural products, and non-medication treatments, such as biofeedback, to improve headache control

• Neuropathic pain: AEDs, such as gabapentin, pregabalin, carbamazepine, and capsaicin, mexiletine are agents used for neuropathic pain. Opioids are appropriate for long-term use in some cases but require careful monitoring

Tests

• Check blood pressure at baseline and when increasing dose

ADVERSE EFFECTS (AEs)

How Drug Causes AEs

• By increasing serotonin and norepinephrine on non-therapeutic responsive receptors throughout the body. Most AEs are dose-dependent and time-dependent

Notable AEs

• Orthostatic hypotension and syncope usually within the first week of use, constipation, dry mouth, sweating, diarrhea, fatigue, loss of appetite, nausea, weight loss, hypertension, headache, asthenia, dizziness, insomnia, somnolence

Life-Threatening or Dangerous AEs

• Serotonin syndrome
• Hepatotoxicity
• Rare activation of mania, depression, or suicidal ideation
• Rare worsening of coexisting seizure disorders

Weight Gain

• Not unusual

unusual   not unusual   common   problematic

Sedation

• Not unusual

unusual   not unusual   common   problematic

What to Do About AEs

• For minor AEs, lower dose, titrate slower, or switch to another agent. For serious AEs, lower dose and consider stopping, taper to avoid withdrawal

Best Augmenting Agents for AEs

• Try magnesium for constipation

DOSING AND USE

Usual Dosage Range

• 20–120 mg/ day once daily

Dosage Forms

• Oral capsule, delayed release: 20 mg, 30 mg, 60 mg

How to Dose

• Initial dose 20–30 mg taken daily. Effective range from 20–120 mg/day, but doses over 60 mg may not provide additional benefit except in headache prevention

Dosing Tips

• Start at a low dose, usually 20 mg or 30 mg, and titrate up every few days as tolerated. Low doses may be effective for pain but higher doses are often superior. Dividing doses as 2 times daily dosing may be recommended in initiating therapy for depression (i.e., 20 mg BID)

Overdose

• Serotonin syndrome, somnolence, seizures, vomiting, death can occur. No specific antidote

Long-Term Use

• Safe for long-term use with monitoring of blood pressure

Habit Forming

• No

How to Stop

• Taper slowly (e.g., 50% reduction every 3–4 days until discontinuation, slower if withdrawal symptoms emerge during taper or for patients with well-controlled pain disorders) to avoid withdrawal symptoms or pain disorder relapse

Pharmacokinetics

• Metabolized via oxidation by CYP2D6 and CYP1A2. Duloxetine is a secondary amine and a weak inhibitor of these isoenzymes. Half-life 12 hr

Drug Interactions

• CYP2D6 inhibitors (duloxetine, paroxetine, fluoxetine, bupropion) cimetidine, and

valproic acid can increase drug concentration
- Concomitant use of potent CYP1A2 inhibitors (fluvoxamine, cimetidine, quinolone antimicrobials [eg, ciprofloxacin, enoxacin]) should be avoided
- Serotonin release by platelets is important for maintaining hemostasis. Combined use of SSRIs or SNRIs (such as duloxetine) and NSAIDs, and/or drugs that affect anticoagulation has been associated with an increased risk of bleeding
- CYP2D6 and 1A2 enzyme inducers, such as rifamycin, nicotine, phenobarbital, can lower levels
- May cause serotonin syndrome when used within 14 days of MAO inhibitors
- May increase risk of cardiotoxicity and arrhythmia when used with tricyclic antidepressants

 Other Warnings/ Precautions
- May increase risk of seizure
- Patients should be observed closely for clinical worsening, suicidality, and unusual changes in behavior in known or unknown bipolar disorder

Do Not Use
- Proven hypersensitivity to drug
- Concurrently with MAOI; allow at least 14 days between discontinuation of an MAOI and initiation of duloxetine hydrochloride or at least 5 days between discontinuation of duloxetine hydrochloride and initiation of an MAOI
- In patient with uncontrolled narrow angle-closure glaucoma
- In patients taking thioridazine
- In patients overusing alcohol (increases risk of liver failure)

SPECIAL POPULATIONS

Renal Impairment
- Not recommended for patients with severe renal function impairment (creatinine clearance less than 30mL/min) or end-stage renal disease

Hepatic Impairment
- Not recommended for patients with hepatic function impairment

Elderly
- No adjustments necessary based on age

 Children and Adolescents
- Although duloxetine is often used off-label for children, safety and efficacy not established. Use with caution. Patient should be observed closely for clinical worsening, suicidality, and unusual changes in behavior, in known or unknown bipolar disorder. Parents should be informed and advised of the risks

 Pregnancy
- Category C. Generally not recommended for the treatment of headache or neuropathic pain during pregnancy. Neonates exposed to duloxetine or other SNRIs or SSRIs late in the third trimester have developed complications necessitating extended hospitalizations, respiratory support, and tube feeding. Respiratory distress, cyanosis, apnea, seizures, temperature instability, feeding difficulty, vomiting, hypoglycemia, hypotonia, hyperreflexia, tremor, jitteriness, irritability, and constant crying consistent with a toxic effect of the drug or drug discontinuation syndrome have been reported

Breast Feeding
- Duloxetine is found in breast milk and use while breast feeding is not recommended

THE ART OF NEUROPHARMACOLOGY

Potential Advantages
- Effective in the treatment of multiple pain disorders and for comorbid depression, anxiety. Less sedation than tertiary amine TCAs (i.e., amitriptyline). Less hypertension than other SNRIs (venlafaxine)

Potential Disadvantages
- Patients with decreased liver function or elevated transaminases

Primary Target Symptoms

- Neuropathic pain
- Pain caused by fibromyalgia
- Headache frequency, duration, and intensity

Pearls

- Number needed to treat is 6 for 50% pain relief in fibromylagia and PDN
- Higher potency at both serotonin and norepinephrine reuptake sites than milnacipran or venlafaxine
- The presence of anxiety may be a positive predictor in treatment with duloxetine as a headache prophylaxis

- May provide benefits in chronic pain similar to TCA without the antihistamine, and strong anticholinergic AEs (e.g., sedation, orthostatic hypotension, etc.)
- AEs are usually dose-dependent
- Dosages higher than 60 mg may provide additional therapeutic responses in the management of PDN or fibromyalgia, but may result in increased AEs
- Duloxetine can often precipitate mania in patients with bipolar disorder. Use with caution

Suggested Reading

Choy EH, Mease PJ, Kajdasz DK, Wohlreich MM, Crits-Christoph P, Walker DJ, Chappell AS. Safety and tolerability of duloxetine in the treatment of patients with fibromyalgia: pooled analysis of data from five clinical trials. Clin Rheumatol 2009;28(9):1035–44.

Karpa KD, Cavanaugh JE, Lakoski JM. Duloxetine pharmacology: profile of a dual monoamine modulator. CNS Drug Rev 2002;8(4):361–76.

Quilici S, Chancellor J, Löthgren M, Simon D, Said G, Le TK, Garcia-Cebrian A, Monz B. Meta-analysis of duloxetine vs. pregabalin and gabapentin in the treatment of diabetic peripheral neuropathic pain. BMC Neurol 2009;9:6.

Taylor AP, Adelman JU, Freeman MC. Efficacy of duloxetine as a migraine preventive medication: possible predictors of response in a retrospective chart review. Headache 2007;47(8):1200–3.

EDROPHONIUM

THERAPEUTICS

Brands
• Enlon, Reversol, Tensilon, Enlon-Plus

Generic?
Yes

Class
• Cholinesterase inhibitor, peripheral

Commonly Prescribed for
(FDA approved in bold)
• **Myasthenia gravis (MG) – diagnostic test**
• Curare antagonist (to reverse respiratory depression)

How the Drug Works
• Improves symptoms of MG by preventing the metabolism of acetylcholine by cholinesterase. This improves neuromuscular transmission in MG

How Long Until It Works
• Less than 1 minute

If It Works
• Usually assists with the differential diagnosis of MG. Pyridostigmine is used for long-term treatment

If It Doesn't Work
• If no effect with the 10 mg dose, question the diagnosis of MG

Tests
• None

ADVERSE EFFECTS (AEs)

How Drug Causes AEs
• Pro-cholinergic properties of the drug

Notable AEs
• Diarrhea, abdominal cramps, nausea, increased salivation, miosis, increased bronchial secretions, worsening of bronchial asthma, fasciculations, muscle weakness, and diaphoresis

Life-Threatening or Dangerous AEs
• Bradycardia – possibly leading to hypotension – is most common

Weight Gain
• Unusual

unusual not unusual common problematic

Sedation
• Unusual

unusual not unusual common problematic

What to Do About AEs
• Give atropine to treat airway obstruction from bronchial secretions

Best Augmenting Agents for AEs
• Not applicable

DOSING AND USE

Usual Dosage Range
• MG – 10 mg in adults

Dosage Forms
• Injection: 10 mg/mL

How to Dose
• In adults, give 0.2 mL (2 mg) within 15–30 seconds. If no reaction occurs after 45 seconds, give the remaining 8 mg. Discontinue the test if any cholinergic reactions and monitor for any clinical changes
• Alternatively give 10 mg intramuscularly. In patients with hypersensitivity (cholinergic reaction), wait 30 minutes and give a lower dose (2 mg) to rule out a false-negative reaction

Dosing Tips
• Not applicable

Overdose
• Not applicable

Long-Term Use
• Not applicable

Habit Forming
• Not applicable

How to Stop
• Not applicable

Pharmacokinetics
• Onset of action <1 min IV and 2–10 min IM. Peak plasma levels <7 min IV and 5–20 min IM. Eliminated through the kidneys and excreted in urine

Drug Interactions
• Do not combine with other cholinesterase inhibitors
• May increase neuromuscular blocking effects of succinylcholine

Do Not Use
• Known hypersensitivity to the cholinesterase inhibitors. Mechanical intestinal or urinary obstruction

SPECIAL POPULATIONS

Renal Impairment
• Markedly increases half-life and plasma clearance

Hepatic Impairment
• No known effects

Cardiac Impairment
• Use with caution in patients with arrhythmias, hypotension, or bradycardia

Elderly
• May be more prone to cardiac events, such as bradycardia

Children and Adolescents
• Safe for use. For children 34 kg or less, give 1 mg and if no response in 45 seconds give another 4 mg. For children over 34 kg give the adult dose (up to 10 mg)

Pregnancy
• Category C. Use only if benefits of medication outweigh risks

Breast Feeding
• Unknown if excreted in breast milk. Do not use

THE ART OF NEUROPHARMACOLOGY

Potential Advantages
• Helpful in the diagnosis of MG. Rapid onset of action

Potential Disadvantages
• Not a long-term treatment. Need to give in a monitored setting due to risk of AEs

Primary Target Symptoms
• To improve weakness, visual problems, respiratory symptoms associated with MG

Pearls
• When using to diagnose MG, pick a specific testable symptom to measure before administration, such as muscle strength or extraocular eye movements
• Can differentiate between myasthenic and cholinergic crisis in established MG. Give 1–2 mg 1 hour after last dose of the agent used to treat MG (usually pyridostigmine). If muscle strength (ptosis, diplopia, dysphagia, respiration, limb strength) improves, then myasthenic crisis is confirmed. Decreased muscle strength, fasciculations, and severe pro-cholinergic AEs (lacrimation, diaphoresis, salivation, nausea) confirm cholinergic crisis. Cholinergic crisis is rare in patients with MG taking typically prescribed doses of cholinesterase-inhibitor medication

Suggested Reading

Aquilonius SM, Hartvig P. Clinical pharmacokinetics of cholinesterase inhibitors. Clin Pharmacokinet 1986;11(3):236–49.

Ing EB, Ing SY, Ing T, Ramocki JA. The complication rate of edrophonium testing for suspected myasthenia gravis. Can J Ophthalmol 2000;35(3):141–4; discussion 145.

Scherer K, Bedlack RS, Simel DL. Does this patient have myasthenia gravis? JAMA 2005; 293(15):1906–14.

THERAPEUTICS

Brands
• Relpax, Relert

Generic?
No

 Class
• Triptan

Commonly Prescribed for
(FDA approved in bold)
• Migraine

 How the Drug Works
• Selective 5-HT1 receptor agonist, working predominantly at the B, D and F receptor subtypes. Effectiveness may be due to blocking the transmission of pain signals from the trigeminal nerve to the trigeminal nucleus caudalis and preventing release of inflammatory neuropeptides rather than just causing vasoconstriction

How Long Until It Works
• 1 hour or less

If It Works
• Continue to take as needed. Patients taking acute treatment more than 2 days/week are at risk for medication-overuse headache, especially if they have migraine

If It Doesn't Work
• Treat early in the attack – triptans are less likely to work after the development of cutaneous allodynia, a marker of central sensitization
• For patients with partial response or reoccurrence, add an NSAID
• Change to another agent

 Best Augmenting Combos for Partial Response or Treatment-Resistance
• NSAIDs or neuroleptics are often used to augment response

Tests
• None required

ADVERSE EFFECTS (AEs)

How Drug Causes AEs
• Direct effect on serotonin receptors

Notable AEs
• Tingling, flushing, sensation of burning, vertigo, sensation of pressure, palpitations, heaviness, nausea

 Life-Threatening or Dangerous AEs
• Rare cardiac events including acute MI, cardiac arrhythmias, and coronary artery vasospasm have been reported with eletriptan

Weight Gain
• Unusual

Sedation
• Unusual

What to Do About AEs
• In most cases, only reassurance is needed. Lower dose, change to another triptan or use an alternative headache treatment

Best Augmenting Agents for AEs
• Treatment of nausea with antiemetics is acceptable. Other AEs improve with time

DOSING AND USE

Dosage Forms
• Tablets: 20 and 40 mg

How to Dose
• Tablets: Most patients respond best at 40 mg oral dose. Give 1 pill at the onset of an attack and repeat in 2 hours for a partial response or if headache returns. 80 mg is also effective but associated with more AEs. Maximum 80 mg/day. Limit 10 days per month

Dosing Tips
• Treat early in attack

Overdose
• May cause hypertension, cardiovascular symptoms. Other possible symptoms include seizure, tremor, extremity erythema, cyanosis or ataxia. For patients with angina, perform ECG and monitor for ischemia for at least 20 hours

Long-Term Use
• Monitor for cardiac risk factors with continued use

Habit Forming
• No

How to Stop
• No need to taper. Patients who overuse triptans often experience withdrawal headaches lasting up to several days

Pharmacokinetics
• Half-life about 4 hours. Tmax 2 hours. Bioavailability is 50%. Metabolized by CYP3A4 enzyme. 85% protein binding

 Drug Interactions
• Theoretical interactions with SSRI/SNRI. It is unclear that triptans pose any risk for the development of serotonin syndrome in clinical practice
• Concurrent propranolol use slightly increases peak concentrations

Do Not Use
• Within 24 hours of ergot-containing medications such as dihydroergotamine
• Patients with proven hypersensitivity to eletriptan, known cardiovascular disease, uncontrolled hypertension, or Prinzmetal's angina
• Eletriptan was not studied in patients with hemiplegic and basilar migraine
• May worsen symptoms in ischemic bowel disease
• Do not use within 72 hours of CYP3A4 inhibitors: ketoconazole, erythromycin, fluconazole, and verapamil

Renal Impairment
• Concentration increases in those with severe renal impairment (creatinine clearance less than 2 mL/min). May be at increased cardiovascular risk

Hepatic Impairment
• Drug metabolism decreased with hepatic disease. Do not use with severe hepatic impairment

Cardiac Impairment
• Do not use in patients with known cardiovascular or peripheral vascular disease

Elderly
• May be at increased cardiovascular risk

 Children and Adolescents
• Safety and efficacy have not been established
• Triptan trials in children were negative, due to higher placebo response

 Pregnancy
• Category C. Use only if potential benefit outweighs risk to the fetus. Migraine often improves in pregnancy, and other acute agents (opioids, neuroleptics, prednisone) have more proven safety

Breast Feeding
• Eletriptan is found in breast milk. Use with caution

THE ART OF NEUROPHARMACOLOGY

Potential Advantages
• Effective and long-lasting, even compared to other oral triptans. May be drug of choice for patients with severe, long-lasting migraines. Less risk of abuse than opioids or barbiturate-containing treatments

Potential Disadvantages
• Cost, potential for medication-overuse headache. More AEs at 80 mg dose than other triptans

Primary Target Symptoms

- Headache pain, nausea, photo- and phonophobia

Pearls

- Early treatment of migraine is most effective
- Very effective, even compared to other triptans. Best sustained pain-free response among the triptans
- May not be effective when taking during aura, before headache begins
- In patients with "status migrainosus" (migraine lasting more than 72 hours) neuroleptics and DHE are more effective

- Triptans were not originally studied for use in the treatment of basilar or hemiplegic migraine
- Patients taking triptans more than 10 days/month are at increased risk of medication-overuse headache which is less responsive to treatment
- May have more AEs than other triptans
- Chest and throat tightness are usually benign and may be related to esophageal spasm rather than cardiac ischemia. These symptoms occur more commonly in patients without cardiac risk factors

Suggested Reading

Dodick D, Lipton RB, Martin V, Papademetriou V, Rosamond W, MaassenVanDenBrink A, Loutfi H, Welch KM, Goadsby PJ, Hahn S, Hutchinson S, Matchar D, Silberstein S, Smith TR, Purdy RA, Saiers J; Triptan Cardiovascular Safety Expert Panel. Consensus statement: cardiovascular safety profile of triptans (5-HT agonists) in the acute treatment of migraine. Headache. 2004;44(5):414–25.

Ferrari MD, Roon KI, Lipton RB, Goadsby PJ. Oral triptans (serotonin 5-HT(1B/1D) agonists) in acute migraine treatment: a meta-analysis of 53 trials. Lancet. 2001;358(9294):1668–75.

Gladstone JP, Gawel M. Newer formulations of the triptans: advances in migraine management. Drugs. 2003;63(21):2285–305.

Goadsby PJ, Zanchin G, Geraud G, de Klippel N, Diaz-Insa S, Gobel H, Cunha L, Ivanoff N, Falques M, Fortea J. Early vs. non-early intervention in acute migraine-'Act when Mild (AwM)'. A double-blind, placebo-controlled trial of almotriptan. Cephalalgia. 2008;28(4):383–91.

Goldstein JA, Massey KD, Kirby S, Gibson M, Hettiarachchi J, Rankin AJ, Jackson NC. Effect of high-dose intravenous eletriptan on coronary artery diameter. Cephalalgia. 2004;24(7):515–21.

ENTACAPONE

THERAPEUTICS

Brands
• Comptan, Stalevo

Generic?
No

 Class
• Antiparkinson agent

Commonly Prescribed for
(FDA approved in bold)
• **Parkinsonism, including Parkinson's disease (PD)**

 How the Drug Works
• Highly selective peripherally acting inhibitor of catechol-O-methyltransferase (COMT), an important enzyme in dopamine metabolism. Use with levodopa/carbidopa enables more levodopa to enter the brain and prevents the end-of-dose wearing-off seen in PD. Entacapone has less activity on COMT in the brain, meaning the drug is not considered centrally active

How Long Until It Works
• PD – hours-weeks

If It Works
• PD – a majority (58%) of patients taking 800 mg or more per day of levodopa will lower levodopa dose, on average by 25% of the total after starting entacapone

If It Doesn't Work
• If end-of-dose wearing-off does not improve with entacapone and levodopa, decrease the dosing interval, add a dopamine agonist, monoamine oxidase B (MAO-B) inhibitor or consider neurosurgical options. For sudden, unpredictable wearing–off, consider apomorphine

 Best Augmenting Combos for Partial Response or Treatment-Resistance
• Entacapone is used only as an adjunctive medication in PD with levodopa
• For dyskinesias, lower dose of levodopa or add a dopamine agonist

• Younger patients with bothersome tremor: anticholinergics may help
• For severe motor fluctuations and/or dyskinesias with good "on" time, functional neurosurgery is an option
• Amantadine may help suppress dyskinesias, although benefit is often short-lived
• Depression is common in PD and may respond to low dose SSRIs
• Cognitive impairment/dementia is common in mid-late stage PD and may improve with acetylcholinesterase inhibitors

Tests
• None required

ADVERSE EFFECTS (AEs)

How Drug Causes AEs
• COMT inhibition increases the level and duration of action of levodopa

Notable AEs
• (Entacapone alone) Diarrhea (usually mild-moderate), dyspnea, weakness. May increase levodopa-related AEs such as dyskinesias, nausea, orthostatic hypotension, and hallucinations

 Life-Threatening or Dangerous AEs
• Rare cases of rhabdomyolysis, unclear if related to entacapone. It is unclear if non-ergot medications such as entacapone that increase dopaminergic activity predispose to the fibrotic complications (i.e., pleural thickening, retroperitoneal fibrosis) seen with ergot agonists

Weight Gain
• Unusual

 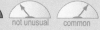
unusual · not unusual · common · problematic

Sedation
• Unusual

unusual · not unusual · common · problematic

What to Do About AEs
• Many AEs are related to increase in levodopa effect. Reduce levodopa dose. Take after meals to reduce nausea. This may reduce the

peak dose and AEs, but delays effect and reduces effectiveness

Best Augmenting Agents for AEs

- For nausea, increase dose of carbidopa relative to levodopa
- Lower levodopa dose and use amantadine or a dopamine agonist to reduce dyskinesias
- Orthostatic hypotension: adjust dose or stop antihypertensives, add dietary salt, and consider fludrocortisone or midodrine
- Urinary incontinence: reducing PM fluids, voiding schedules, oxybutynin, desmopressin nasal spray, hyoscyamine sulfate, urological evaluation

DOSING AND USE

Usual Dosage Range

- 600–1600 mg/day

Dosage Forms

- Entacapone tablets: 200 mg
- As carbidopa/levodopa/entacapone tablets (Stalevo): 12.5/50/200, 25/100/200 and 37.5/150/200

How to Dose

- Add 200 mg to each dose of levodopa or change to combination carbidopa/levodopa/entacapone to maximum of 1600 mg (8 doses) per day

 Dosing Tips

- Food does not affect the absorption of entacapone, but since it is dosed with levodopa, take before meals for best effect. Distributing protein throughout the day may help avoid fluctuations in PD. Low protein meals may reduce "wearing-off."

Overdose

- Little clinical experience, but theoretically can produce inability to metabolize endogenous and exogenous catecholamines. Immediate gastric drug lavage and activated charcoal is recommended. Hemodialysis is unlikely to remove due to protein binding

Long-Term Use

- Safe for long-term use. Effectiveness may decrease over time

Habit Forming

- No

How to Stop

- Stopping abruptly may worsen symptoms of PD, especially if levodopa is also discontinued. This may cause confusion, rigidity, and hyperpyrexia, as seen in neuroleptic malignant syndrome

Pharmacokinetics

- Rapidly absorbed, with maximum effect in 1 hour and lasts about 8 hours. Hepatic metabolism and glucuronidation. Highly protein bound. Excreted through bile

 Drug Interactions

- Monoamine oxidase (MAO) inhibitors are also important in the metabolism of catecholamines. Do not use with non-selective MAO inhibitors, but can use with the MAO-B selective inhibitors used in PD (rasagiline, selegiline)
- Drugs that interfere with biliary excretion or glucuronidation (probenecid, cholestyramine, erythromycin, rifampin, ampicillin, chloramphenicol) will increase the effect of entacapone
- Entacapone can increase the effect of all drugs metabolized by COMT, such as epinephrine, norepinephrine, dopamine, dobutamine, methyldopa, apomorphine, isoproterenol, isoetherine, bitolterol. This can lead to increased heart rates, arrhythmia and increases in blood pressure

 Other Warnings/ Precautions

- Nephrotoxic and associated with renal tubular adenomas at high doses in mice, unknown if this occurs in humans

Do Not Use

- Patients with known hypersensitivity to the drug, non-selective MAO inhibitors, patients with significant biliary disorders

SPECIAL POPULATIONS

Renal Impairment
- No known effects

Hepatic Impairment
- Effect of drug is approximately double in patients with alcoholism or hepatic impairment. Use with caution

Cardiac Impairment
- Use with caution in patients with known arrhythmias

Elderly
- Safe for use

Children and Adolescents
- Not studied in children (PD is rare)

Pregnancy
- Category C. Use only if benefit of medication may outweigh risks

Breast Feeding
- Concentration in breast milk unknown. Breast feeding is not recommended

THE ART OF NEUROPHARMACOLOGY

Potential Advantages
- Allows patients to lower dose or lengthen dosing intervals of levodopa. Fairly well tolerated. Unlike tolcapone, is not centrally acting and no risk of fulminant hepatic failure

Potential Disadvantages
- Not useful as monotherapy for PD. May increase levodopa AEs. Cost

Primary Target Symptoms
- PD – end-of-dose wearing-off

 Pearls
- Has effectively replaced tolcapone as the COMT inhibitor of choice for the treatment of PD
- Extends clinical effect of levodopa by 30–45 minutes and improves motor scores by about 16%
- A useful alternative to dopamine agonists for patients experiencing AEs, such as sudden-onset sleep or impulse control disorders. Less likely to cause hallucinations

---

Suggested Reading

Hauser RA, Zesiewicz TA. Advances in the pharmacologic management of early Parkinson disease. Neurologist 2007;13 (3):126–32.

Leegwater-Kim J, Waters C. Role of tolcapone in the treatment of Parkinson's disease. Expert Rev Neurother 2007;7(12):1649–57.

Linazasoro G, Kulisevsky J, Hernández B; Spanish Stalevo Study Group. Should levodopa dose be reduced when switched to Stalevo? Eur J Neurol 2008; 15(3):257–61.

Müller T, Kolf K, Ander L, Woitalla D, Muhlack S. Catechol-O-methyltransferase inhibition improves levodopa-associated strength increase in patients with Parkinson disease. Clin Neuropharmacol 2008;31(3):134–40.

Olanow CW, Stern MB, Sethi K. The scientific and clinical basis for the treatment of Parkinson disease. Neurology 2009;72 (21 Suppl 4): S1–136.

Seeberger LC, Hauser RA. Levodopa/ carbidopa/entacapone in Parkinson's disease. Expert Rev Neurother 2009;9(7):929–40.

ETHOSUXIMIDE

THERAPEUTICS

Brands
• Zarontin, Emeside

Generic?
Yes

 Class
• Antiepileptic drug (AED)

Commonly Prescribed for
(FDA approved in bold)
• **Absence (petit mal) epilepsy**

 How the Drug Works
• There are multiple proposed mechanisms of action, and it is uncertain which of these give the drug its effectiveness
• Blocks or modulates T-type calcium channels
• Modulates sodium channel function
• May alter glutamate or GABA levels
• Proven to suppress paroxysmal 3-hertz spike and slow wave discharges on EEG

How Long Until It Works
• Seizures – should decrease by 2 weeks

If It Works
• Seizures – goal is the remission of seizures. Continue as long as effective and well-tolerated. Consider tapering and slowly stopping after 2 years without seizures, depending on the type of epilepsy

If It Doesn't Work
• Increase to highest tolerated dose
• Epilepsy: consider changing to another agent or adding a second agent

 Best Augmenting Combos for Partial Response or Treatment-Resistance
• Epilepsy: Often used in combination when more than 1 type of epilepsy exists. Effective in combination with valproate for absence seizures but this can cause interactions and change levels of drug. Lamotrigine is another option

Tests
• Blood counts, urinalysis, and liver function tests at baseline and on a periodic basis

ADVERSE EFFECTS (AEs)

How Drug Causes AEs
• CNS AEs are probably caused by effects on calcium or sodium channels

Notable AEs
• Sedation, ataxia, dizziness, headache, blurred vision, insomnia
• Nausea, vomiting, cramps, anorexia, abdominal pain, constipation
• Increased urinary frequency, muscle weakness, periorbital edema, pruritus

 Life-Threatening or Dangerous AEs
• Rare blood dyscrasias including leuckopenia, eosinophilia, pancytopenia
• Rare cases of systemic lupus erythematosus
• Severe dermatologic manifestations including Stevens-Johnson syndrome, erythema multiforme

Weight Gain
• Unusual

unusual · not unusual · common · problematic

Sedation
• Common

unusual · not unusual · common · problematic

What to Do About AEs
• Check blood counts for any signs of systemic infection
• Lower dose or change to another agent

Best Augmenting Agents for AEs
• Most AEs cannot be improved with the use of an augmenting agent

DOSING AND USE

Usual Dosage Range
• 250–1500 mg/day

Dosage Forms
- 250 mg tablets or syrup 250 mg/5 mL

How to Dose
- Start at 250 mg/day once daily or in 2 divided doses. Increase by 250 mg every 4–7 days to goal dose

 Dosing Tips
- If GI upset occurs take with food or milk
- Very young children (age 3 or less) are more likely to require twice-daily dosing

Overdose
- Acute: CNS depression with coma and respiratory depression. Confusion, hypotension, flaccid muscles, absent reflexes
- Chronic: Skin rash, hematuria, confusion, ataxia, depression, dizziness

Long-Term Use
- Safe for long-term use

Habit Forming
- No

How to Stop
- Taper slowly
- Abrupt withdrawal can lead to seizures
- Patients with childhood absence epilepsy (onset before age 12) have a high rate of remission and little risk of grand mal seizures. Patients with juvenile absence (onset age 12 or later) have a higher risk of relapse with drug withdrawal

Pharmacokinetics
- Hepatic metabolism mostly by P450 system. Renal excretion
- Half-life is 30 hours in children, 40–60 in adults
- Bioavailability is 95–100%

 Drug Interactions
- Increases levels of phenytoin
- Decreases levels of primidone and phenobarbital
- Valproate can either increase or decrease ethosuximide levels

- Enzyme-inducing drugs including phenytoin, carbamazepine, phenobarbital, and rifampin lower ethosuximide levels

 Other Warnings/ Precautions
- CNS AEs increase when used with other CNS depressants
- Systemic symptoms such as fever, flu-like symptoms, swelling of eyelids along with any dermatologic changes require immediate evaluation
- Rare reports of psychiatric abnormalities including auditory hallucinations, depression, suicidal behavior, and psychosis

Do Not Use
- Patients with a proven allergy to succinimides

SPECIAL POPULATIONS

Renal Impairment
- Use with extreme caution

Hepatic Impairment
- Use with extreme caution

Cardiac Impairment
- No known effects

 Children and Adolescents
- Approved for use in children 3 and older
- Ages 3–6: 250 mg/day
- Ages 6 and up: 500 mg/day
- Increase dose by 250 mg every 4–7 days until seizures are well controlled or side effects occur. Usual maximum dose 1500 mg/day

 Pregnancy
- Risk category C. Risks of stopping medication must outweigh risk to fetus for patients with epilepsy
- Supplementation with 0.4 mg of folic acid before and during pregnancy is recommended

Breast Feeding
- Generally recommendations are to discontinue drug or bottle feed
- Monitor infant for sedation, poor feeding, or irritability

THE ART OF NEUROPHARMACOLOGY
Potential Advantages
- Effective for absence seizures
- Avoids risk of hepatotoxicity

Potential Disadvantages
- Not effective for most types of epilepsy
- Valproate is more likely to be effective in atypical absence epilepsy

Primary Target Symptoms
- Seizure frequency and severity

 Pearls
- Effective in the treatment of absence seizures (equivalent to valproate)
- One of 3 succinimides used in epilepsy. The others are phensuximide and methsuximide
- May increase risk of generalized tonic-clonic seizures in some individuals with absence seizures
- Useful in animal models for treating neuropathic pain and hyperalgesia

 Suggested Reading

Flatters SJ, Bennett GJ. Ethosuximide reverses paclitaxel- and vincristine-induced painful peripheral neuropathy. Pain 2004;109 (1–2):150–61.

Gomora JC, Daud AN, Weiergraber M, Perez-Reyes E. Block of cloned human T-type calcium channels by succinimide antiepileptic drugs. Mol Pharmacol 2001;60(5):1121–32.

Posner EB, Mohamed K, Marson AG. Ethosuximide, sodium valproate or lamotrigine for absence seizures in children and adolescents.

Cochrane Database Syst Rev 2005;(4): CD003032.

Sayer RJ, Brown AM, Schwindt PC, Crill WE. Calcium currents in acutely isolated human neocortical neurons. J Neurophysiol 1993;69 (5):1596–606.

Schmitt B, Kovacevic-Preradovic T, Critelli H, Molinari L. Is ethosuximide a risk factor for generalized tonic-clonic seizures in absence epilepsy? Neuropediatrics 2007;38(2):83–7.

THERAPEUTICS

Brands
• Felbatol, Taloxa

Generic?
Yes

Class
• Antiepileptic drug (AED)

Commonly Prescribed for
(FDA approved in bold)
• **Complex partial seizures (adjunctive)**
• **Partial and generalized seizures associated with Lennox-Gastaut syndrome (children)**
• Infantile spasms (West syndrome)

How the Drug Works
• The exact mechanism of action in epilepsy is unknown, but putative mechanisms include changes in binding at GABA and benzodiazepine receptors and blockade of NMDA-activated glutamate receptors

How Long Until It Works
• Seizures – 2 weeks

If It Works
• Seizures – goal is the decrease or remission of seizures. Continue as long as effective and well-tolerated

If It Doesn't Work
• Increase to highest tolerated dose. If not effective discontinue

Best Augmenting Combos for Partial Response or Treatment-Resistance
• Epilepsy: generally used in combination with other agents for severe epilepsy

Tests
• Obtain liver function testing and CBC before starting, and monitor frequently – especially in the first months after initiating treatment
• Repeat liver function testing whenever new medications are added

ADVERSE EFFECTS (AEs)

How Drug Causes AEs
• CNS AEs may be caused by binding changes at GABA, benzodiazepine or NMDA receptors
• Aplastic anemia may be related to a reactive metabolite, 2-phenylpropenal

Notable AEs
• Most common: Anorexia, vomiting, insomnia, headache, dizziness, somnolence
• Less common: Rash, acne, edema, rhinitis, otitis media, diplopia, abnormal taste or vision

Life-Threatening or Dangerous AEs
• Liver failure, often with rapid onset (2–4 weeks)
• Aplastic anemia, often fatal and usually beginning 5–30 weeks after starting treatment

Weight Gain
• Unusual

unusual   not unusual   common   problematic

Sedation
• Common

unusual   not unusual   common   problematic
• Usually dose related

What to Do About AEs
• Most AEs resolve with reduction in dose
• For serious AEs discontinue drug

Best Augmenting Agents for AEs
• Most do not respond to an augmenting agent

DOSING AND USE

Usual Dosage Range
• 2400–3600 mg/day

Dosage Forms
• Tablets: 400 mg, 600 mg
• Suspension: 600 mg/5 mL

How to Dose
• Start at 400 mg 3 times daily. Increase dose every 2 weeks by 600 mg/day until taking

2400 mg/day 3–4 times daily and up to 3600 mg/day if tolerated and needed based on clinical response. Reduce dose of concomitant AEDs by 20–30% in the first week, then by one-third at 2 weeks

 Dosing Tips
- Most AEs associated with felbamate resolve with lowering doses of concomitant AEDs
- Food does not affect absorption

Overdose
- GI distress and tachycardia have been reported with high doses

Long-Term Use
- Routine CBC and liver function testing are mandatory

Habit Forming
- No

How to Stop
- Taper slowly, as abrupt withdrawal can lead to seizures in patients with epilepsy

Pharmacokinetics
- Peak plasma levels at 1–4 hours with plasma half-life of 20–23 hours. About 50% of drug is metabolized, the remainder is excreted unchanged in urine. Bioavailability is 90%

 Drug Interactions
- CYP2C19 inhibitor which may increase levels of many common medications (propranolol, warfarin, indomethacin, proton pump inhibitors)
- Phenytoin, phenobarbital, and carbamazepine increase clearance and lower levels
- Increases valproate and phenytoin levels and lowers carbamazepine levels
- May decrease effectiveness of oral contraceptives, but usually not to a relevant degree

⚠ **Other Warnings/ Precautions**
- Contains small amount of animal carcinogens

Do Not Use
- Hypersensitivity to drug, any active liver disease or blood dyscrasias

Renal Impairment
- Clearance is reduced and half-life prolonged. Lower dose and use with caution

Hepatic Impairment
- Do not use

Cardiac Impairment
- No known effects

Elderly
- No known effects

 Children and Adolescents
- Approved for use in children with Lennox-Gastaut ages 2–14
- Start at 15 mg/kg/day in 3–4 divided doses daily and reduce dose of present AEDs by 20%. Increase by 15 mg/kg/day weekly until clinical effect or at 45 mg/kg/day

 Pregnancy
- Risk category C
- Supplementation with 0.4 mg of folic acid before and during pregnancy is recommended

Breast Feeding
- Drug is present in breast milk. Breast feeding is not recommended

THE ART OF NEUROPHARMACOLOGY

Potential Advantages
- Broad-spectrum and effective AED. Useful in refractory epilepsy

Potential Disadvantages
- Risk of aplastic anemia and liver failure

Primary Target Symptoms
- Seizure frequency and severity

Pearls

- Relatively well-tolerated, broad-spectrum and effective AED, but idiosyncratic AE of liver failure and aplastic anemia have made it a drug only for refractory patients. The rate of aplastic anemia is about 100–250 times the risk for the disorder in the general population

- Flurofelbamate is a drug in development that may have similar efficacy, when compared to felbamate, with a lower risk of serious AEs
- The patient or guardian must read and sign an informed consent before felbamate can be prescribed

Suggested Reading

Hancock EC, Cross HH. Treatment of Lennox-Gastaut syndrome. Cochrane Database Syst Rev 2009; (3):CD003277.

Harden CL. Therapeutic safety monitoring: what to look for and when to look for it. Epilepsia 2000;41 (Suppl 8):S37–44.

Pellock JM. Felbamate. Epilepsia 1999;40 (Suppl 5):S57–62.

Rogawski MA. Diverse mechanisms of antiepileptic drugs in the development pipeline. Epilepsy Res 2006;69(3):273–94.

Tsao CY. Current trends in the treatment of infantile spasms. Neuropsychiatr Dis Treat 2009;5:289–99.

FLUNARIZINE

Brands
- Sibelium

Generic?
Yes

Class
- Antihypertensive, calcium channel blocker, antihistamine

Commonly Prescribed for
(FDA approved in bold)
- Migraine prophylaxis
- Vasospasm in subarachnoid hemorrhage
- Adjunctive drug for epilepsy
- Vertigo
- Alternating hemiplegia of childhood
- Tourette's syndrome
- Tinnitus

How the Drug Works
- Migraine/cluster: Proposed prior mechanisms included inhibition of smooth muscle contraction preventing arterial spasm and hypoxia, prevention of vasoconstriction or platelet aggregation, and alterations of serotonin release and uptake
- Prevention of cortical spreading depression may be the mechanism of action for all migraine preventives
- May also interact with other neurotransmitters, and may inhibit the synthesis and release of nitric oxide
- The drug also appears to act by blocking dopamine D2 receptors in a manner similar to antipsychotics

How Long Until It Works
- Migraines may decrease in as little as 2 weeks, but can take up to 2 months to see full effect

If It Works
- Migraine – goal is a 50% or greater decrease in migraine frequency or severity. Consider tapering or stopping if headaches remit for more than 6 months or if patient considering pregnancy

If It Doesn't Work
- Increase to highest tolerated dose

- Migraine: address other issues, such as medication-overuse, other coexisting medical disorders, such as anxiety, and consider changing to another agent or adding a second agent

 Best Augmenting Combos for Partial Response or Treatment-Resistance
- Migraine: For some patients with migraine, low-dose polytherapy with 2 or more drugs may be better tolerated and more effective than high-dose monotherapy. May use in combination with AEDs, antidepressants, natural products, and non-medication treatments, such as biofeedback, to improve headache control

Tests
- Monitor ECG for PR interval

How Drug Causes AEs
- Direct effects of calcium receptor antagonism and other CNS receptors
- Antihistaminic properties likely cause weight gain and sedation. D2 blockade can cause movement disorders

Notable AEs
- Sedation, depression, weight gain are most problematic
- Nausea, dry mouth, gingival hyperplasia, weakness, muscle aches, and abdominal pain can occur

 Life-Threatening or Dangerous AEs
- Severe depression in a minority
- Extrapyramidal side effects and parkinsonism

Weight Gain
- Problematic

unusual — not unusual — common — problematic

Sedation
- Common

unusual — not unusual — common — problematic

What to Do About AEs
- Lower dose or switch to another agent. For serious AEs, do not use

Best Augmenting Agents for AEs
- Lower dose to 5 mg

DOSING AND USE

Usual Dosage Range
- 5–10 mg/day

Dosage Forms
- Tablets: 5 mg, 10 mg

How to Dose
- Migraine: Initial dose is usually 10 mg at night. Start at 5 mg in sensitive patients. The dose is generally not increased for migraine prophylaxis

 Dosing Tips
- Take at night to minimize drowsiness

Overdose
- Sedation, weakness, confusion, or agitation may occur. Cardiac AEs, such as bradycardia or tachycardia, have been reported

Long-Term Use
- Safe for long-term use

Habit Forming
- No

How to Stop
- No need to taper, but migraine often returns after stopping

Pharmacokinetics
- Peak levels at 2–4 hours and more than 90% protein bound. More metabolites are excreted in bile and elimination half-life is about 18 days

 Drug Interactions
- Enzyme inducers such as phenytoin, rifampin may increase clearance and lower levels
- Use with beta-blockers can be synergistic and bradycardia, AV conduction disturbance may occur

- May increase risk of GI bleeding with NSAIDs
- May increase levels of carbamazepine
- Excess sedation with other CNS depressants (alcohol, barbiturates) can occur

 Other Warnings/ Precautions
- Similar to antipsychotics (D2 receptor blockers) may increase prolactin levels

Do Not Use
- Sick sinus syndrome, greater than first-degree heart block
- Severe CHF, cardiogenic shock, severe left ventricular dysfunction, hypotension
- History of depression, parkinsonism, or porphyria

SPECIAL POPULATIONS

Renal Impairment
- No known effects

Hepatic Impairment
- Flunarizine is highly metabolized by the liver. Start with lower dose and use with caution

Cardiac Impairment
- Do not use in acute shock, severe CHF, hypotension, and greater than first-degree heart block

Elderly
- May be more likely to experience AEs (sedation)

 Children and Adolescents
- Appears to be effective in pediatric migraine at a dose of 5 mg daily

 Pregnancy
- Category C (all calcium channel blockers). Use only if potential benefit outweighs risk to the fetus

Breast Feeding
- Drug is found in breast milk at high concentrations. Do not breast feed on drug

THE ART OF NEUROPHARMACOLOGY

Potential Advantages

- Effective in both pediatric and adult migraine prophylaxis and possibly effective in epilepsy and schizophrenia

Potential Disadvantages

- Sedation and weight gain can limit use. Not available in the US

Primary Target Symptoms

- Headache frequency and severity
- Seizure frequency and severity
- Hemiplegic attacks

 Pearls

- Effective in reducing migraine frequency at rates comparable to other agents (propranolol, pizotifen)
- There have been investigations of using flunarizine for epilepsy, but the effect was weak and AEs were significant
- Unlike many calcium-channel blockers, it does not alter heart rate and is a poor antihypertensive
- Generally more effective than other calcium-channel blockers for migraine prophylaxis, but not available in many countries, including the US

 Suggested Reading

Ciancarelli I, Tozzi-Ciancarelli MG, Di Massimo C, Marini C, Carolei A. Flunarizine effects on oxidative stress in migraine patients. Cephalalgia 2004;24 (7):528–32.

Hoppu K, Nergårdh AR, Eriksson AS, Beck O, Forssblad E, Boréus LO. Flunarizine of limited value in children with intractable epilepsy. Pediatr Neurol 1995;13(2):143–7.

Lewis DW, Yonker M, Winner P, Sowell M. The treatment of pediatric migraine. Pediatr Ann 2005;34(6):448–60.

Neville BG, Ninan M. The treatment and management of alternating hemiplegia of childhood. Dev Med Child Neurol 2007;49 (10):777–80.

Silberstein SD. Preventive migraine treatment. Neurol Clin 2009;27(2):429–43.

FLUOXETINE

Brands
• Prozac, Sarafem, Fluox, Symbyax

Generic?
Yes

Class
• Selective serotonin reuptake inhibitor (SSRI), antidepressant

Commonly Prescribed for
(FDA approved in bold)
• **Major depressive disorder (MDD)**
• **Generalized anxiety disorder (GAD)**
• **Obsessive-compulsive disorder**
• **Premenstrual dysphoric disorder**
• **Bulimia nervosa**
• **Panic disorder**
• **Bipolar depression [in combination with olanzapine (Symbyax)]**
• Migraine prophylaxis
• Chronic daily headache (CDH)
• Hot flashes
• Pain in peripheral neuropathies
• Post-traumatic stress disorder
• Raynaud phenomenon

How the Drug Works
• Blocks serotonin reuptake pumps, increasing their levels within hours, but antidepressant effects take weeks. Effect is likely related to adaptive changes in serotonin receptor systems and desensitization of serotonin 1A receptors
• Weakly blocks dopamine and norepinephrine reuptake pumps, and has antagonist properties at serotonin 2C receptors which may increase norepinephrine and dopamine neurotransmission

How Long Until It Works
• Migraine/CDH, neuropathic pain – effective in as little as 2 weeks, but can take up to 10 weeks on a stable dose to see full effect

If It Works
• Migraine/CDH – goal is a 50% or greater reduction in migraine frequency or severity. Consider tapering or stopping if headaches remit for more than 6 months or if considering pregnancy

• Neuropathic pain – the goal is to reduce pain intensity and reduce use of analgesics, but usually does not produce remission

If It Doesn't Work
• Increase to highest tolerated dose
• Headache: address other issues, such as medication-overuse, other coexisting medical disorders, such as anxiety, and consider changing to another agent or adding a second agent
• Neuropathic pain: either change to another agent or add a second agent

Best Augmenting Combos for Partial Response or Treatment-Resistance
• Migraine/CDH: For some patients, low-dose polytherapy with 2 or more drugs may be better tolerated and more effective than high-dose monotherapy. May use in combination with AEDs, antihypertensives, natural products, and non-medication treatments, such as biofeedback, to improve headache control
• Neuropathic pain: AEDs, such as gabapentin, pregabalin, carbamazepine, and capsaicin, mexiletine are agents used for neuropathic pain. Opioids are appropriate for long-term use in some cases but require careful monitoring

Tests
• Not required

How Drug Causes AEs
• By increasing serotonin on non-therapeutic responsive receptors throughout the body. Most AEs are dose-dependent and time-dependent. Serotonin may decrease dopamine release, leading to emotional flattening and apathy. Increased serotonin levels may affect platelet function, increasing bleeding risks

Notable AEs
• Sexual dysfunction (erectile dysfunction, anorgasmia), sweating, insomnia or sedation, dizziness, dry mouth
• Nausea, diarrhea (usually improve with time)

Life-Threatening or Dangerous AEs

- Rare activation of mania, depression, or suicidal ideation
- Rare worsening of coexisting seizure disorders

Weight Gain

- Not unusual

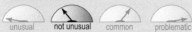

Sedation

- Unusual

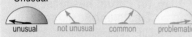

What to Do About AEs

- For minor AEs, lower dose or switch to another agent. Many AEs improve with time. For serious AEs, lower dose and consider stopping

Best Augmenting Agents for AEs

- Sexual dysfunction: bupropion, sildenafil, vardenafil, tadalafil
- Insomnia: low-dose tricyclic antidepressant, mirtazapine, trazodone, or sleep aid

DOSING AND USE

Usual Dosage Range

- 20–80 mg/ day

Dosage Forms

- Capsule: 10 mg, 20 mg, 40 mg
- Tablet: 10 mg, 15 mg, 20 mg
- Oral Solution: 20 mg/5 mL
- Delayed-release capsules: 90 mg

How to Dose

- Start at 10 or 20 mg in the morning. Increase dose by 10–20 mg every 2 weeks to goal dose based on clinical effects

 Dosing Tips

- Start at a low dose to reduce AEs and dose either once daily or with divided doses. Dosing during evenings is also well-tolerated and should be considered if it improves compliance

Overdose

- Seizures, vertigo, tremor, hypertension, tachycardia, movement disorders, and death have been reported. Most deaths occur in combination with other agents. ECG changes, including QTc prolongation, can occur

Long-Term Use

- Safe for long-term use

Habit Forming

- No

How to Stop

- May taper rapidly due to long half-life. Depression or pain may worsen

Pharmacokinetics

- Hepatic metabolism mostly via CYP450 2D6 and 3A4 to metabolites, some of them active. Half-life 2 weeks and takes 28 days to reach steady state. Peak levels at 6–8 hours. Inhibits 2D6 and 3A4

 Drug Interactions

- Tramadol increases seizure risk when used with SSRIs
- Strong CYP2D6 inhibitor. May increase levels of many drugs, including TCAs, antipsychotics, beta-blockers (metoprolol or propranolol), and codeine
- Weak-moderate CYP3A4 inhibitor. May increase levels of cyclosporine, TCAs, protease inhibitors, calcium channel blockers, benzodiazepines, some anticholesterol agents (simvastatin, atorvastatin, fluvastatin), and buspirone
- May increase risk of bleeding when used with anticoagulant or antiplatelet drugs
- May increase adverse GI effects of NSAIDs
- Lithium levels may increase or decrease
- Use with pimozide or thioridazine may cause QTc prolongation

 Other Warnings/ Precautions

- May increase risk of seizure
- Do not use in bipolar disorder unless patients are on mood-stabilizing agents

Do Not Use
- Hypersensitivity to drug
- Concurrently with monoamine oxidase (MAO) inhibitor; allow at least 2 weeks between discontinuation of an MAO inhibitor and starting fluoxetine, or at least 5 weeks between discontinuation of fluoxetine and starting MAO inhibitors
- If patient taking thioridazine or pimozide

SPECIAL POPULATIONS

Renal Impairment
- No known effects

Hepatic Impairment
- Slower elimination and clearance. Use lower doses

Elderly
- No known effects

 Children and Adolescents
- Use with caution and observe for clinical worsening, suicidality, and unusual changes in behavior. May activate known or unknown bipolar disorder
- SSRIs appear to be effective in children 8 and older but have not been studied in pediatric headache
- May decrease growth

 Pregnancy
- Category C. Generally not recommended for the treatment of headache during pregnancy. No major adverse outcomes based on pregnancy registries

Breast Feeding
- Some drug is found in breast milk but few adverse events in infants appear related

THE ART OF NEUROPHARMACOLOGY

Potential Advantages
- Well-tolerated antidepressant with long half-life. Useful in the treatment of chronic daily headache. Generic is less expensive

Potential Disadvantages
- Relatively ineffective in most pain disorders

Primary Target Symptoms
- Headache frequency, duration, and intensity
- Depression, anxiety
- Neuropathic pain

 Pearls
- For patients with significant depression or anxiety, SSRI are generally better tolerated than tricyclic antidepressants (TCAs). Attempting to use high doses of TCAs to treat both conditions may lead to AEs. Consider using an SSRI, such as fluoxetine, to treat depression and another agent to treat headache
- At doses of 20 mg twice daily, appears effective for the treatment of chronic daily headache
- In general, SSRIs have little efficacy for migraine prophylaxis but should be considered for patients with coexisting affective disorders
- Compared with other SSRIs, has a lower rate of serotonin withdrawal syndrome due to long half-life
- Serotonin syndrome is most common when combining multiple SSRIs and TCAs, MAO inhibitors or rarely dopamine agonists, amphetamines, lithium, buspirone or other psychostimulants. Triptans, which are relatively selective for 1B and 1D receptors, are unlikely to increase risk
- Studies for neuropathic treatment at doses of 20–40 mg/day have been largely negative

Suggested Reading

Mathew NT. The prophylactic treatment of chronic daily headache. Headache 2006;46(10):1552–64.

Silberstein SD. Preventive migraine treatment. Neurol Clin 2009;27(2):429–43.

Singh VP, Jain NK, Kulkarni SK. On the antinociceptive effect of fluoxetine, a selective serotonin reuptake inhibitor. Brain Res 2001;915(2):218–26.

FROVATRIPTAN

THERAPEUTICS

Brands
• Frova, Migard

Generic?
No

Class
• Triptan

Commonly Prescribed for
(FDA approved in bold)
• **Migraine**
• Menstrual migraine

How the Drug Works
• Selective 5-HT1 receptor agonist, working predominantly at the B and D receptor subtypes. Effectiveness may be due to blocking the transmission of pain signals from the trigeminal nerve to the trigeminal nucleus caudalis and preventing release of inflammatory neuropeptides rather than just causing vasoconstriction

How Long Until It Works
• 2 hours or less

If It Works
• Continue to take as needed. Patients taking acute treatment more than 2 days/week are at risk for medication-overuse headache, especially if they have migraine

If It Doesn't Work
• Treat early in the attack – triptans are less likely to work after the development of cutaneous allodynia, a marker of central sensitization
• For patients with partial response or reoccurrence, add an NSAID
• Change to another agent

Best Augmenting Combos for Partial Response or Treatment-Resistance
• NSAIDs or neuroleptics are often used to augment response

Tests
• None required

ADVERSE EFFECTS (AEs)

How Drug Causes AEs
• Direct effect on serotonin receptors

Notable AEs
• Tingling, flushing, dizziness, palpitations, muscle pain, sensation of burning, vertigo, sensation of pressure, nausea

Life-Threatening or Dangerous AEs
• Rare cardiac events including acute MI, cardiac arrhythmias, and coronary artery vasospasm have been reported with frovatriptan

Weight Gain
• Unusual

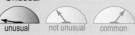

unusual   not unusual   common   problematic

Sedation
• Unusual

unusual   not unusual   common   problematic

What to Do About AEs
• In most cases, only reassurance is needed. Lower dose, change to another triptan or use an alternative headache treatment

Best Augmenting Agents for AEs
• Treatment of nausea with antiemetics is acceptable. Other AEs improve with time

DOSING AND USE

Usual Dosage Range
• 2.5 mg

Dosage Forms
• Tablets: 2.5 mg

How to Dose
• Tablets: Give 1 pill at the onset of an attack and repeat in 2 hours for a partial response or if headache returns. Maximum 7.5 mg/day. Limit 10 days per month

Dosing Tips
- Treat early in attack

Overdose
- May cause hypertension, cardiovascular symptoms. Other possible symptoms include seizure, tremor, extremity erythema, cyanosis or ataxia. For patients with angina, perform ECG and monitor for ischemia for at least 48 hours

Long-Term Use
- Monitor for cardiac risk factors with continued use

Habit Forming
- No

How to Stop
- No need to taper. Patients who overuse triptans often experience withdrawal headaches lasting up to several days

Pharmacokinetics
- Half-life about 25 hours. Tmax 3 hours. Bioavailability is 30%. Metabolized by CYP1A2 isoenzymes. 15% protein binding

Drug Interactions
- Theoretical interactions with SSRI/SNRI. It is unclear that triptans pose any risk for the development of serotonin syndrome in clinical practice
- Concurrent propranolol or fluvoxamine use increases concentrations

Do Not Use
- Within 24 hours of ergot-containing medications such as dihydroergotamine
- Patients with proven hypersensitivity to naratriptan, known cardiovascular disease, uncontrolled hypertension, or Prinzmetal's angina
- Frovatriptan was not studied in patients with hemiplegic and basilar migraine
- May worsen symptoms in ischemic bowel disease

Renal Impairment
- Concentration minimally increases with moderate-severe renal impairment – less than other triptans. Use with caution. May be at increased cardiovascular risk

Hepatic Impairment
- Do not use with severe hepatic impairment

Cardiac Impairment
- Do not use in patients with known cardiovascular or peripheral vascular disease

Elderly
- May be at increased cardiovascular risk

Children and Adolescents
- Safety and efficacy have not been established
- Triptan trials in children were negative, due to higher placebo response

Pregnancy
- Category C. Use only if potential benefit outweighs risk to the fetus. Migraine often improves in pregnancy, and other acute agents (opioids, neuroleptics, prednisone) have more proven safety

Breast Feeding
- Frovatriptan is found in breast milk. Use with caution

Potential Advantages
- Excellent tolerability and low rate of recurrence, even compared to other oral triptans. Less risk of abuse than opioids or barbiturate-containing treatments

Potential Disadvantages
- Cost, potential for medication-overuse headache. Less effective than other triptans

Primary Target Symptoms
- Headache pain, nausea, photo- and phonophobia

Pearls

- Early treatment of migraine is most effective
- Longer half-life than any other triptan but less effective
- May not be effective when taken during aura, before headache begins
- In patients with "status migrainosus" (migraine lasting more than 72 hours) neuroleptics and DHE are more effective
- Triptans were not originally studied for use in the treatment of basilar or hemiplegic migraine

- Patients taking triptans more than 10 days/month are at increased risk of medication-overuse headache which is less responsive to treatment
- Chest and throat tightness are usually benign and may be related to esophageal spasm rather than cardiac ischemia. These symptoms occur more commonly in patients without cardiac risk factors
- Useful for short-term prophylaxis of menstrual migraine at dose of 2.5 mg twice daily for up to 6 days

Suggested Reading

Ferrari MD, Roon KI, Lipton RB, Goadsby PJ. Oral triptans (serotonin 5-HT(1B/1D) agonists) in acute migraine treatment: a meta-analysis of 53 trials. Lancet 2001;358(9294):1668–75.

Gladstone JP, Gawel M. Newer formulations of the triptans: advances in migraine management. Drugs 2003;63(21):2285–305.

Silberstein SD, Berner T, Tobin J, Xiang Q, Campbell JC. Scheduled short-term prevention with frovatriptan for migraine occurring exclusively in association with menstruation. Headache 2009;49(9):1283–97.

Wenzel RG, Tepper S, Korab WE, Freitag F. Serotonin syndrome risks when combining SSRI/SNRI drugs and triptans: is the FDA's alert warranted? Ann Pharmacother 2008; 42(11):1692–6.

GABAPENTIN

Brands
- Neurontin, Gabarone, Neupentin, Neurostil

Generic?
Yes

Class
- Antiepileptic drug (AED)

Commonly Prescribed for
(FDA approved in bold)
- **Partial-onset seizures with and without secondary generalization (adjunctive for adults and children 12 and older)**
- **Partial-onset seizures in children 3 and older**
- **Pain associated with post-herpetic neuralgia**
- Neuropathic pain
- Migraine prophylaxis
- Facial pain
- Allodynia and hyperalgesia
- Fibromyalgia
- Bipolar disorder
- Generalized anxiety disorder
- Alcohol and drug withdrawal
- Insomnia

How the Drug Works
- Structural analog of gamma-aminobutyric acid (GABA) which binds at the alpha-2-delta subunit of voltage-sensitive calcium channels and reduces calcium influx. Changes calcium channel function but not as a blocker
- Reduces release of excitatory neurotransmitters, and decreases brain glutamate and glutamine levels
- Increases plasma serotonin levels
- Inactive at GABA receptors and does not affect GABA uptake or degradation

How Long Until It Works
- Seizures – 2 weeks
- Pain/Anxiety – days-weeks

If It Works
- Seizures – goal is the remission of seizures. Continue as long as effective and well-tolerated. Consider tapering and slowly stopping after 2 years without seizures, depending on the type of epilepsy
- Pain – goal is reduction of pain. Usually reduces but does not cure pain and there is recurrence off the medication. Consider tapering for conditions that may improve over time, i.e., post-herpetic neuralgia or migraine

If It Doesn't Work
- Increase to highest tolerated dose
- Epilepsy: Consider changing to another agent, adding a second agent or referral for epilepsy surgery evaluation
- Pain: If not effective in 2 months, consider stopping or using another agent

Best Augmenting Combos for Partial Response or Treatment-Resistance
- Epilepsy: No major drug interactions with other AEDs. Using in combination may worsen CNS side effects
- Neuropathic pain: Can use with tricyclic antidepressants, SNRIs, other AEDs or opiates to augment treatment response. Gabapentin usually decreases opiate use
- Anxiety: Usually used as an adjunctive agent with SSRIs, SNRIs, monoamine oxidase (MAO) inhibitors or benzodiazepines

Tests
- No regular blood tests are recommended

How Drug Causes AEs
- CNS AEs are probably caused by interaction with calcium channel function

Notable AEs
- Sedation, dizziness, fatigue, ataxia
- Weight gain, nausea, constipation, dry mouth
- Blurred vision, peripheral edema

Life-Threatening or Dangerous AEs
- None

Weight Gain
• Not unusual

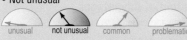

Sedation
• Common

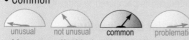

• May wear off with time but can limit titration

What to Do About AEs
• Decrease dose or take a higher dose at night to avoid sedation
• Switch to another agent

Best Augmenting Agents for AEs
• Adding a second agent unlikely to decrease AEs

DOSING AND USE

Usual Dosage Range
• Epilepsy: 900–1800 mg/day, but can use as much as 3600 mg/day
• Neuropathic pain: 300–1800 mg/day, but can use as much as 3600 mg/day

Dosage Forms
• Tablets: 100 mg, 300 mg, 400 mg, 600 mg, 800 mg
• Capsules: 100 mg, 300 mg, 400 mg
• Liquid: Oral solution 250 mg/5 mL

How to Dose
• Epilepsy (ages 12 and older): 900 mg in 3 divided doses, then increase by 300 mg every few days until at goal dose. Maximum time between doses should not exceed 12 hours
• Neuropathic pain: Start at 300 mg day 1 and increase by 300 mg every 1–3 days as tolerated to goal dose

 Dosing Tips
• Bioavailability decreases as dose increases, from 60% at 900 mg dose to 27% at 3600 mg dose
• Slow increase will improve tolerability. Increase evening dose first

• Use a slower titration for patients on other medications that can increase CNS side effects
• Twice-daily dosing may improve compliance and can be adequate for treatment of pain or anxiety. The need for 3 times a day dosing increases with higher daily doses
• Avoid taking until 2 hours after antacid administration

Overdose
• No reported deaths. Sedation, blurred vision, ataxia, slurred speech, diarrhea

Long-Term Use
• Safe for long-term use

Habit Forming
• No

How to Stop
• Taper slowly
• Abrupt withdrawal can lead to seizures in patients with epilepsy

Pharmacokinetics
• Renal excretion without being metabolized. Non-linear kinetics. Half-life 5–7 hours. Less than 3% is bound to plasma proteins

 Drug Interactions
• May increase CNS side effects of other medications
• Antacids decrease the bioavailability of gabapentin
• Cimetidine, naproxen, hydrocodone, and morphine increase the absorption of gabapentin and plasma levels

 Other Warnings/ Precautions
• Adenocarcinomas found in male rats
• Emotional liability, hostility, and thought disorder in children ages 3–12

Do Not Use
• Patients with a proven allergy to pregabalin or gabapentin

Renal Impairment

- Renal excretion means that lower dose is needed and that hemodialysis will remove
- Adjust dose based on creatinine clearance: 15 mL/min or less – 100–300 mg/day once daily, >15–29 mL/min 200–700 mg/day once daily, 30–59 mL/min 400–1400 mg/day in 2 divided doses. Patients receiving hemodialysis may require supplemental doses

Hepatic Impairment

- No known effects

Cardiac Impairment

- No known effects

Elderly

- May tolerate lower doses better. More likely to experience AEs

Children and Adolescents

- Start at 10–15 mg/kg/day in 3 divided doses. Increase every 3 days to effective dose. In children aged 3–4 usually 40 mg/kg/day and age 5 and up 25 mg/kg/day
- May be effective for benign rolandic epilepsy but not absence or generalized tonic-clonic seizures

Pregnancy

- Risk category C. Some teratogenicity in animal studies. Patients taking for pain or anxiety should generally stop before considering pregnancy
- Supplementation with 0.4 mg of folic acid before and during pregnancy is recommended

Breast Feeding

- Some drug is found in mother's breast milk
- Generally recommendations are to discontinue drug or bottle feed
- Monitor infant for sedation, poor feeding, or irritability

Potential Advantages

- Safe and wide therapeutic index
- Proven efficacy for multiple types of pain as well as epilepsy
- Relatively low side effects and drug interactions compared to older AEDs

Potential Disadvantages

- Dosing 3 times a day. Sedation. Difficult titration to therapeutic dose
- Non-linear kinetics mean bioavailability decreases with dose; higher doses may be well tolerated but may not improve efficacy
- Not effective for primary generalized seizures

Primary Target Symptoms

- Seizure frequency and severity
- Pain
- Anxiety

 Pearls

- Gabapentin is effective for migraine prevention, but only at higher doses (1800 to 3600 mg). Low doses are not proven effective
- May be effective in the treatment of allodynia (pain in response to a normally non-painful stimulus) and hyperalgesia (exaggerated response to painful stimuli)
- Multiple potential uses for pain relief, such as pain after burn injury, post-operative pain, reducing opioid requirements in cancer, pain and spasticity in multiple sclerosis, and most forms of neuropathic pain
- 300 mg of gabapentin is about the same as 50 mg of pregabalin, but at higher doses this ratio often does not apply
- Appears to enhance slow-wave delta sleep – adding to effect in pain disorders
- The majority of gabapentin use is for off-label conditions
- Can treat fibromyalgia at doses of 1200 mg to 2400 mg/day
- Used off-label for bipolar disorder, but found ineffective in recent trials

Suggested Reading

Backonja M, Glanzman RL. Gabapentin dosing for neuropathic pain: evidence from randomized, placebo-controlled clinical trials. Clin Ther 2003;25(1):81–104.

Bazil CW, Battista J, Basner RC. Gabapentin improves sleep in the presence of alcohol. J Clin Sleep Med 2005;1(3):284–7.

Berry JD, Petersen KL. A single dose of gabapentin reduces acute pain and allodynia in patients with herpes zoster. Neurology 2005; 65(3):444–7.

Gilron I, Bailey JM, Tu D, Holden RR, Jackson AC, Houlden RL. Nortriptyline and gabapentin, alone and in combination for neuropathic pain: a double-blind, randomised controlled crossover trial. Lancet 2009;374(9697):1252–61.

Häuser W, Bernardy K, Uçeyler N, Sommer C. Treatment of fibromyalgia syndrome with gabapentin and pregabalin – a meta-analysis of randomized controlled trials. Pain 2009; 145(1–2):69–81.

Silberstein SD. Preventive migraine treatment. Neurol Clin 2009;27(2):429–43.

GALANTAMINE

THERAPEUTICS

Brands
• Razadyne, Reminyl

Generic?
No

Class
• Cholinesterase inhibitor

Commonly Prescribed for
(FDA approved in bold)
• **Alzheimer dementia (AD) (mild or moderate)**
• Dementia with Lewy Bodies (DLB)
• Vascular dementia

How the Drug Works
• Increases the concentration of acetylcholine through reversible inhibition of metabolism by acetylcholinesterase enzyme, which increases availability of acetylcholine. A deficiency of cholinergic function is felt to be important in producing the signs and symptoms of AD
• May also modulate nicotine receptors, increasing acetylcholine release
• May interfere with amyloid deposition
• Although symptoms of AD can improve, galantamine does not prevent disease progression

How Long Until It Works
• Typically 2–6 weeks at a given dose, but effect is best observed over a period of months

If It Works
• Continue to use but symptoms of dementia usually worsen over time

If It Doesn't Work
• Change to another cholinesterase inhibitor or NMDA-antagonist (memantine)
• Non-pharmacologic measures are the basis of dementia treatment. Maintain regular schedules and routines. Avoid prolonged travel, unnecessary medical procedures or emergency room visits, crowds, and large social gatherings
• Limit drugs with sedative properties such as opioids, hypnotics, antiepileptic drugs and tricyclic antidepressants

• Treat other disorders which can worsen symptoms such as hyperglycemia or urinary difficulties

Best Augmenting Combos for Partial Response or Treatment-Resistance
• Addition of the NMDA receptor antagonist memantine may be useful
• Treat depression or apathy, if present, with SSRIs. Avoid tricyclic antidepressants in demented patients due to risk of confusion
• For significant confusion and agitation avoid neuroleptics (especially in Lewy Body dementia) because of the risk of neuroleptic malignant syndrome. Atypical antipsychotics (risperidone, quetiapine, olanzapine, clozapine) can be used instead

Tests
• None required

ADVERSE EFFECTS (AEs)

How Drug Causes AEs
• Acetylcholinesterase inhibition in the CNS and PNS

Notable AEs
• GI AEs (nausea/vomiting, diarrhea, anorexia and weight loss) are most common. Fatigue, headache, and dizziness

Life-Threatening or Dangerous AEs
• Rarely bradycardia or heart block, causing syncope

Weight Gain
• Unusual

unusual   not unusual   common   problematic
• Weight loss is more common

Sedation
• Unusual

unusual   not unusual   common   problematic

What to Do About AEs
• In patients with dementia, determining if AEs are related to medication or another medical condition can be difficult. For CNS side

effects, discontinuation of non-essential centrally acting medications may help. If a bothersome AE is clearly drug-related then lower the dose (especially for GI AEs), titrate more slowly or discontinue

Best Augmenting Agents for AEs
• Most AEs do not respond to adding other medications

DOSING AND USE

Usual Dosage Range
• 16–24 mg/day in 2 divided doses for immediate-release formulations or once daily for ER capsules

Dosage Forms
• Tablets: 4, 8, 12 mg
• Oral Solution: 4 mg/mL in a 100 mL pipette
• Capsules (extended-release): 8, 16 and 24 mg

How to Dose
• (Immediate release): Start at 4 mg twice a day. Increase to 8 mg twice daily after a minimum of 4 weeks. After another 4 weeks can attempt to increase to 12 mg twice daily
• (Extended release): Start at 8 mg daily. Increase to 16 mg after a minimum of 4 weeks. After another 4 weeks can attempt to increase to 24 mg daily based on assessment of tolerability and clinical benefit

Dosing Tips
• Slow titration can reduce AEs. Food delays time to peak effect

Overdose
• Symptoms of cholinergic crisis can occur: nausea/vomiting, salivation, hypotension, diaphoresis, convulsions, bradycardia/collapse. May cause muscle weakness and respiratory failure. Atropine with an initial dose of 1–2 mg IV is an antidote

Long-Term Use
• Safe for long-term use. Effectiveness may decrease over time as the dementing illness progresses

Habit Forming
• No

How to Stop
• Abrupt discontinuation can produce worsening of dementia symptoms, memory and behavioral disturbances. Taper slowly

Pharmacokinetics
• Mainly hepatic metabolism via CYP2D6 and 3A4 isoenzymes. Maximum effect at 1 hour. About 7% of the population are 2D6 poor metabolizers. These patients excrete a larger percentage unchanged in urine and may need a lower dose. Bioavailability is 90% and plasma protein binding 18%

Drug Interactions
• Increases the effect of anesthetics such as succinylcholine. Stop before surgery
• Anticholinergics interfere with effect of drug
• Cimetidine may increase bioavailability
• Other cholinesterase inhibitors and cholinergic agonists (bethanechol) may cause a synergistic effect
• CYP2D6 and 3A4 inhibitors, including ketoconazole, cimetidine, paroxetine and erythromycin, may increase the concentration and effect of galantamine
• Bradycardia may occur when used with beta-blockers

Do Not Use
• Hypersensitivity to the drug

SPECIAL POPULATIONS

Renal Impairment
• For patient with moderate impairment use 16 mg/day. If severe impairment do not use

Hepatic Impairment
• For moderate impairment use 16 mg/day. If severe impairment (Child-Pugh score 10–15), do not use

Cardiac Impairment
• Syncope has been reported. Use with caution in patients with bradyarrhythmias

Elderly
• Slightly higher concentrations than in younger subjects

Children and Adolescents
• Not studied. AD does not occur in children

Pregnancy
• Category B. Use only if benefits of medication outweigh risks

Breast Feeding
• Unknown if excreted in breast milk. Do not use

THE ART OF NEUROPHARMACOLOGY

Potential Advantages
• Proven effectiveness for AD. Low risk of hepatotoxicity compared to other acetylcholinesterases (tacrine). Relatively low non-GI AEs, even compared to other AD medications. Available as once daily in ER form

Potential Disadvantages
• Cost and minimal effectiveness. Does not prevent progression of AD or other dementia

Primary Target Symptoms
• Confusion, agitation, memory, performing activities of daily living

 Pearls
• May be used in combination with memantine with good effect, but combining with other cholinesterase inhibitors is not recommended
• In most clinical trials, all approved medications for AD had a similar rate of benefit
• May be useful for both behavioral problems in AD (delusion, anxiety and apathy) as well as memory disturbance
• PD patients may benefit from lower doses than in AD (less than 6 mg/day)
• Actions at nicotinic receptors may enhance release of acetylcholine and other neurotransmitters, improving attention and behaviors
• The effect of galantamine is not dramatic, but patients with DLB might show more benefit
• May be useful for cognitive decline in Down's syndrome

 Suggested Reading

Ballard CG, Chalmers KA, Todd C, McKeith IG, O'Brien JT, Wilcock G, Love S, Perry EK. Cholinesterase inhibitors reduce cortical Abeta in dementia with Lewy bodies. Neurology 2007; 68(20):1726–9.

Bentué-Ferrer D, Tribut O, Polard E, Allain H. Clinically significant drug interactions with cholinesterase inhibitors: a guide for neurologists. CNS Drugs 2003;17(13):947–63.

Bhasin M, Rowan E, Edwards K, McKeith I. Cholinesterase inhibitors in dementia with Lewy bodies: a comparative analysis. Int J Geriatr Psychiatry 2007;22(9):890–5.

Downey D. Pharmacologic management of Alzheimer disease. J Neurosci Nurs 2008; 40(1):55–9.

Edwards K, Royall D, Hershey L, Lichter D, Hake A, Farlow M, Pasquier F, Johnson S. Efficacy and safety of galantamine in patients with dementia with Lewy bodies: a 24-week open-label study. Dement Geriatr Cogn Disord 2007;23(6):401–5.

Olin J, Schneider L. Galantamine for Alzheimer's disease. Cochrane Database Syst Rev 2002;(3): CD001747.

Stahl SM. The new cholinesterase inhibitors for Alzheimer's disease, Part 1: their similarities are different. J Clin Psychiatry 2000;61(10):710–11.

GLATIRAMER ACETATE

THERAPEUTICS

Brands
• Copaxone, Copolymer 1

Generic?
No

Class
• Immunosuppressive agent, immunomodulator

Commonly Prescribed for
(FDA approved in bold)
• **For reduction of relapses in patients with relapsing-remitting multiple sclerosis. (RRMS)**
• Clinically isolated syndromes (CIS)

How the Drug Works
• By modifying the immune processes responsible in part for the development of MS. Glatiramer is a mixture of 4 amino acids thought to approximate the antigenic structure of myelin basic protein (MBP). Experimentally competes with CNS MBP for presentation to T cells
• Inducer of specific T 2 helper-type cells that express anti-inflammatory cytokines

How Long Until It Works
• At least 6 months

If It Works
• Continue to use until RRMS becomes progressive

If It Doesn't Work
• Change to an interferon, reconsider the diagnosis of RRMS, and consider using natalizumab or mitoxantrone, especially for secondary progressive MS

Best Augmenting Combos for Partial Response or Treatment-Resistance
• Acute attacks are often treated with glucocorticoids, especially if there is functional impairment due to vision loss, weakness, or cerebellar symptoms
• Treat common clinical symptoms with appropriate medication for spasticity (baclofen, tizanidine), neuropathic pain, and fatigue (modafinil)

• For patients with RRMS refractory to glatiramer, (measured by clinical relapses and MRI accumulation of lesions) consider changing to interferon-beta, natalizumab, or mitoxantrone. Other options, which are experimental, include monthly methylprednisolone, pulse cyclophosphamide, and other immunosuppressants
• Combination therapy may have a role, but has not been proven more effective than monotherapy. There is an ongoing clinical trial looking at combination treatment with avonex and copaxone

Tests
• None required

ADVERSE EFFECTS (AEs)

How Drug Causes AEs
• Except for injection site reactions, the cause of AEs (i.e., chest pain) seen with glatiramer use are unclear

Notable AEs
• Chest pain, usually immediately post-injection, is common and typically lasts less than a minute, with no associated ECG changes or adverse consequences. This usually starts about 1 month after initiation of treatment
• About 10% of patients experience immediate post-injection reactions, including anxiety, flushing, dyspnea, throat constriction, and urticaria
• Injection site reactions including erythema, induration, pain, pruritus, welts, inflammation, or hemorrhage
• Fever, neck pain, migraine, agitation, anxiety, sweating, and weight gain are slightly more common in treated patients

Life-Threatening or Dangerous AEs
• None

Weight Gain
• Not unusual

unusual   not unusual   common   problematic

Sedation
• Unusual

unusual   not unusual   common   problematic

What to Do About AEs
• The chest pain and post-injection reactions do not require any specific treatment and are self-limiting but may cause distress for the patient. If AEs are bothersome enough, consider changing to another disease-modifying agent

Best Augmenting Agents for AEs
• Most AEs cannot be improved with an augmenting agent

Drug Interactions
• In general, do not combine with other immunosuppressant medications

Other Warnings/ Precautions
• In theory, can interfere with normal immune function. No evidence of this to date

Do Not Use
• Known hypersensitivity to the drug or to mannitol

DOSING AND USE

Usual Dosage Range
• 20 mg daily

Dosage Forms
• Injection: 20 mg/mL (premixed injection)

How to Dose
• Self inject at a site in the arms, abdomen, hips or thighs
• Also available as an autoinjector

 Dosing Tips
• Remove from refrigerator for 20 minutes to allow solution to warm to room temperature before injecting

Overdose
• No information available

Long-Term Use
• Safe for long-term use

Habit Forming
• No

How to Stop
• No need to taper

Pharmacokinetics
• Some drug metabolized locally and some enters the lymphatic circulation and regional lymph nodes. It is unclear how much drug reaches the systemic circulation

SPECIAL POPULATIONS

Renal Impairment
• No known effects

Hepatic Impairment
• No known effects

Cardiac Impairment
• No known effects

Elderly
• No known effects

 Children and Adolescents
• Not studied in initial trials, but has been used since with AEs similar to those of adults. Disease-modifying therapy appears to have benefit in reducing long-term cognitive and physical disability from RRMS; it is reasonable to offer treatment early in the disease course

 Pregnancy
• Category B. Use in pregnancy only if clearly needed. In most cases, it is discontinued and steroids are used for acute relapses during pregnancy

Breast Feeding
• Unknown if excreted in breast milk. Use with caution

THE ART OF NEUROPHARMACOLOGY

Potential Advantages

- Excellent treatment option for RRMS. Lower incidence of AEs compared to interferons (including flu-like symptoms, depression, fever, myalgias, and liver function abnormalities). Neutralizing antibodies do not occur

Potential Disadvantages

- Probably not effective for most progressive forms of MS and not always effective in RRMS. Cost. Injection site reactions. Most number of injections per year

Primary Target Symptoms

- Decrease in relapse rates, delay/prevention of disability, and slower accumulation of lesions on MRI imaging

Pearls

- MRI studies and clinical experience demonstrate that RRMS usually changes over time into secondary progressive MS, which has a more degenerative than inflammatory course. There is no evidence for using glatiramer in any progressive form of MS, but could be useful for some patients who have an inflammatory component and acute relapses
- One large study suggested that glatiramer was ineffective for primary progressive MS
- Early treatment of RRMS with disease-modifying therapies is superior to placebo. Given that early intervention leads to better outcome in RRMS, consider using glatiramer for patients with clearly defined, clinically isolated syndromes, especially if there is MRI evidence of progression

Suggested Reading

Patten SB, Williams JV, Metz LM. Anti-depressant use in association with interferon and glatiramer acetate treatment in multiple sclerosis. Mult Scler 2008;14(3):406–11.

Perumal J, Filippi M, Ford C, Johnson K, Lisak R, Metz L, Tselis A, Tullman M, Khan O. Glatiramer acetate therapy for multiple sclerosis: a review. Expert Opin Drug Metab Toxicol 2006; 2(6):1019–29.

Stuart WH. Combination therapy for the treatment of multiple sclerosis: challenges and opportunities. Curr Med Res Opin 2007; 23(6):1199–208.

Wingerchuk DM. Current evidence and therapeutic strategies for multiple sclerosis. Semin Neurol 2008;28(1):56–68.

Ytterberg C, Johansson S, Andersson M, Olsson D, Link H, Holmqvist LW, von Koch L. Combination therapy with interferon-beta and glatiramer acetate in multiple sclerosis. Acta Neurol Scand 2007;116(2):96–9.

GUANFACINE

THERAPEUTICS

Brands
- Tenex, Intuniv

Generic?
Yes (except extended release)

Class
- Antiadrenergic, alpha-2 agonist

Commonly Prescribed for
(FDA approved in bold)
- **Hypertension**
- Gilles de la Tourette syndrome (GTS)
- Tics
- Attention deficit hyperactivity disorder (ADHD)
- Neuropathic pain
- Opioid detoxification
- Alcohol withdrawal
- Hypertensive "urgency"
- Post-traumatic stress disorder

How the Drug Works
- Alpha-2 adrenergic agonist. Reduces sympathetic output from CNS, which decreases cardiac output, peripheral vascular resistance, and blood pressure
- Specifically targets alpha-2 receptors in the brainstem vasomotor center, decreasing presynaptic calcium levels and the release of norepinephrine
- Its effect in GTS and ADHD may be due to actions at the level of the prefrontal cortex

How Long Until It Works
- Hypertension, withdrawal – less than 2 hours
- GTS – weeks to months

If It Works
- In neurologic disorders, such as tics, continue to assess effect of the medication to see if it is still needed

If It Doesn't Work
- GTS/tics – Neuroleptics are often effective, but their use should be reserved for patients with significant social isolation or embarrassment

Best Augmenting Combos for Partial Response or Treatment-Resistance
- In hypertension, combine with treatments less likely to cause orthostasis

(angiotensin-converting enzyme inhibitors, diuretics)
- Tics and GTS symptoms may change over time. Many patients improve with age. Behavioral and psychological therapy are useful, and education and reassurance are all that is needed in mild cases
- Identify and treat comorbid conditions such as ADHD or obsessive-compulsive disorder

Tests
- Monitor blood pressure and pulse

ADVERSE EFFECTS (AEs)

How Drug Causes AEs
- Related to alpha-2 adrenergic agonist effect – hypotension and sedation

Notable AEs
- Dry mouth, drowsiness, dizziness, constipation, weakness, headache, depression, paresthesia, dermatitis, impotence, and syncope

Life-Threatening or Dangerous AEs
- Bradycardia and syncope. Rapid withdrawal can cause rebound hypertension with increased catecholamine levels

Weight Gain
- Unusual

unusual · not unusual · common · problematic

Sedation
- Not unusual

unusual · not unusual · common · problematic

What to Do About AEs
- Lower the dose and take the highest dose in the evening. Many AEs (especially sedation) improve with time

Best Augmenting Agents for AEs
- Most AEs cannot be improved by an augmenting agent

DOSING AND USE

Usual Dosage Range
- 0.5–2 mg/day at night or in 2 divided doses
- Extended release: up to 4 mg at night

Dosage Forms
- Tablets: 1 mg, 2 mg
- Extended release: 1 mg, 2 mg, 3 mg, 4 mg

How to Dose
- Hypertension: start with 1 mg at night. If effect less than desired, increase to 1 mg twice daily or 2 mg at night
- GTS/tics, ADHD: Start at 0.5 mg per day. Increase by 0.5 mg every 3–4 days as needed and tolerated. Average dose is 1.5 mg/day. Most patients take the entire dose at night

Dosing Tips
- Start at bedtime only, and if well tolerated (little sedation) can divide doses
- Rebound hypertension usually occurs 2–4 days after discontinuation

Overdose
- Hypotension, bradycardia, drowsiness, and lethargy have been reported. Consider gastric lavage for large quantities

Long-Term Use
- Safe, but tolerance to antihypertensive effects is common

Habit Forming
- No

How to Stop
- Taper slowly to avoid rebound tachycardia and hypertension. Other withdrawal symptoms may include nervousness and anxiety

Pharmacokinetics
- Half-life is 17 hours, but shorter in younger patients. The peak effect is at 1–4 hours Bioavailability is 80%, with about half of the drug metabolized into inactive metabolites and the other excreted unchanged in urine

Drug Interactions
- Use with other CNS depressants increases sedation

- CYP-450 enzyme inducers (phenytoin, phenobarbital) lower elimination half-life and plasma levels. Increase daily dose and dose more frequently

Other Warnings/ Precautions
- Do not discontinue perioperatively and monitor blood pressure closely
- Skin rash (exfoliative) has been reported

Do Not Use
- Known hypersensitivity

SPECIAL POPULATIONS

Renal Impairment
- Clearance is reduced but has little clinical effect. Consider using a lower dose

Hepatic Impairment
- No known effects

Cardiac Impairment
- Avoid using in patients with known coronary artery disease, conduction disturbances, recent myocardial infarction, or cerebrovascular events

Elderly
- No known effects

Children and Adolescents
- Children may be more sensitive to CNS AEs than adults. Doses for GTS and tics are similar to adults, but titrate more slowly. Consider giving the entire oral dose at night

Pregnancy
- Category B. Use only if there is a clear need

Breast Feeding
- Likely excreted in breast milk. Do not use

THE ART OF NEUROPHARMACOLOGY

Potential Advantages
- Fewer AEs than neuroleptics in the treatment of GTS and tic disorders. Less somnolence than clonidine

Potential Disadvantages

- Less effective than neuroleptics for GTS or tics. Hypotension and rebound hypertension may limit use

Primary Target Symptoms

- Tics, attention-deficit, and hyperactivity

 Pearls

- The first decision in the treatment of GTS or tics is to decide if pharmacologic treatment is indicated. If the patient is not severely disabled, then reassure the patient and family that symptoms may improve and the prognosis is good. For patients with significant disability, guanfacine is a good initial choice due to lack of long-term AEs, especially in patients with coexisting ADHD
- In patients with severe ADHD, stimulants are more effective
- Clonidine, another alpha-2 adrenergic agonist, is often used for GTS or tics. Compared to guanfacine, more studies support its use but there was more somnolence. Rebound hypertension is greater and usually starts sooner after discontinuation compared to guanfacine
- Not a imidazoline ligand, which explains the lower incidence of somnolence compared to clonidine and tizanidine
- In children, case reports exist of guanfacine-related behavioral changes, including mania and aggression

 Suggested Reading

Jiménez-Jiménez FJ, García-Ruiz PJ. Pharmacological options for the treatment of Tourette's disorder. Drugs 2001;61(15):2207–20.

Sandor P. Pharmacological management of tics in patients with TS. J Psychosom Res 2003; 55(1):41–8.

Smith H, Elliott J. Alpha(2) receptors and agonists in pain management. Curr Opin Anaesthesiol 2001;14(5):513–8.

GUANIDINE HYDROCHLORIDE

THERAPEUTICS

Brands
• None

Generic?
Yes

Class
• Neuromuscular drug, cholinergic agonist

Commonly Prescribed for
(FDA approved in bold)
• Lambert-Eaton myasthenic syndrome (LEMS)
• Congenital myasthenia gravis (CMG)

How the Drug Works
• Exact mechanism of action unknown. Enhances release of acetylcholine following a nerve impulse and slows the rates of depolarization and repolarization of muscle cell membranes

How Long Until It Works
• Hours

If It Works
• Continue to use to reduce symptoms of LEMS or CMG at lowest required dose. Disease-modifying treatments, such as plasma exchange, intravenous immune globulin, corticosteroids, or immunosuppressives are helpful and identifying malignancy such as small-cell lung cancer is essential

If It Doesn't Work
• Treat with immunologic therapy
• Removal of neoplasm may improve symptoms
• Change to 3,4-Diaminopyridine

Best Augmenting Combos for Partial Response or Treatment-Resistance
• May be combined with pyridostigmine, which increases the available amount of acetylcholine for receptor binding which may allow reduction of dose and toxicity

Tests
• Obtain baseline CBC and monitor frequently during treatment. Monitor renal function and urinalysis

ADVERSE EFFECTS (AEs)

How Drug Causes AEs
• Most are related to cholinergic agonism

Notable AEs
• Paresthesias, nervousness, lightheadedness, tremor, ataxia
• Diarrhea, anorexia, increased peristalsis
• Rash, sweating, itching and skin eruptions
• Elevated hepatic transaminases, sore throat, fever
• Hypotension, palpitations, tachycardia
• Emotional lability, psychosis, hallucinations

Life-Threatening or Dangerous AEs
• Bone marrow suppression (anemia, leukopenia, thrombocytopenia) – often dose-related
• Atrial fibrillation
• Renal failure, interstitial nephritis

Weight Gain
• Unusual

Sedation
• Unusual

What to Do About AEs
• Lower to tolerable dose, supplement with pyridostigmine and discontinue for serious AEs

Best Augmenting Agents for AEs
• Atropine is helpful for reducing GI AEs

DOSING AND USE

Usual Dosage Range
• LEMS – up to 1000 mg/day

Dosage Forms
- Tablets: 125 mg

How to Dose
- Start at 1 tablet 3 times a day and increase as tolerated
- Increase up to 1000 mg per day in 3–4 divided doses
- Higher doses (up to 35 mg/kg/day) have been used but are associated with severe AEs

 Dosing Tips
- Dose requirements are highly variable and require careful titration

Overdose
- Early symptoms are gastrointestinal. Serious intoxication may produce tremor, convulsions, salivation, vomiting, hypoglycemia, and arrhythmias. Intravenous calcium may improve symptoms

Long-Term Use
- Requires frequent monitoring for hematologic and renal complications

Habit Forming
- No

How to Stop
- No need to taper but LEMS symptoms may worsen

Pharmacokinetics
- Rapidly absorbed with half-life of 7–8 hours. Not metabolized

 Drug Interactions
- No significant drug interactions due to lack of metabolism
- Do not combine with acetylcholinesterase inhibitors other than pyridostigmine

Do Not Use
- Hypersensitivity to drug

Renal Impairment
- Avoid using due to potential for worsening disease

Hepatic Impairment
- No known effects

Cardiac Impairment
- Avoid using in patients with tachyarrhythmias, hypotension

Elderly
- Unknown

 Children and Adolescents
- Unknown

 Pregnancy
- Unknown. Use only if benefits of medication outweigh risks

Breast Feeding
- Excreted in breast milk. Do not use

Potential Advantages
- First effective symptomatic treatment for LEMS

Potential Disadvantages
- Rarely used due to serious AEs

Primary Target Symptoms
- To improve weakness associated with LEMS

 Pearls
- Unlike MG, LEMS is a presynaptic disorder of neuromuscular transmission. LEMS is an autoimmune disease with antibodies directed against the voltage-gated calcium channels. LEMS is usually associated with small-cell lung cancer
- Pyridostigmine or other acetylcholinesterase inhibitors alone are not effective in LEMS
- A Lambert-Eaton-like CMG has been described and may respond to guanidine

Suggested Reading

Harper CM. Congenital myasthenic syndromes. Semin Neurol 2004;24(1):111–23.

Oh SJ, Kim DS, Head TC, Claussen GC. Low-dose guanidine and pyridostigmine: relatively safe and effective long-term symptomatic therapy in Lambert-Eaton myasthenic syndrome. Muscle Nerve 1997;20(9):1146–52.

Parr JR, Jayawant S. Childhood myasthenia: clinical subtypes and practical management. Dev Med Child Neurol. 2007;49(8):629–35.

Verschuuren JJ, Wirtz PW, Titulaer MJ, Willems LN, van Gerven J. Available treatment options for the management of Lambert-Eaton myasthenic syndrome. Expert Opin Pharmacother 2006;7(10):1323–36.

HALOPERIDOL

THERAPEUTICS

Brands
• Haldol, Dozic, Serenace

Generic?
Yes

 ### Class
• Antipsychotic

Commonly Prescribed for
(FDA approved in bold)
• **Tics in Gilles de la Tourette syndrome (GTS)**
• **Psychotic disorders**
• **Short-term treatment of severe behavior problems in children**
• Severe behavioral problems in children (second-line)
• Short-term treatment of hyperactivity in children (second-line)
• Schizophrenia (long-term parenteral therapy)
• Bipolar disorder
• Nausea and vomiting
• Headache
• Behavioral disturbances in dementias

 ### How the Drug Works
• Dopamine receptor antagonist with greater action at D2 receptors. Also blocks alpha-2 adrenergic receptors

How Long Until It Works
• Psychosis – usually within a week
• GTS – weeks to months

If It Works
• Use at lowest effective dose
• Monitor QT corrected (QTc) interval
• Continue to assess effect of the medication and if it is still needed

If It Doesn't Work
• Psychosis: increase dose or change to another agent
• GTS: discontinue or change to another agent

 ### Best Augmenting Combos for Partial Response or Treatment-Resistance
• Tics and GTS symptoms may change over time. Many patients improve with age. Behavioral and psychological therapy are useful. Education and reassurance are all that is needed in mild cases
• Identify and treat comorbid conditions, such as ADHD or obsessive compulsive disorder
• In GTS, alpha-2 adrenergic agonists such as clonidine and guanfacine, reserpine, and other neuroleptics are also useful
• For intractable migraine, often combined with NSAIDs or dihydroergotamine
• In general, avoid combining with other conventional antipsychotics

Tests
• Monitor weight, blood pressure, lipids, and fasting glucose with chronic use. Obtain blood pressure and pulse before initial IV use and monitor QTc with ECG

ADVERSE EFFECTS (AEs)

How Drug Causes AEs
• Motor AEs and prolactinemia – blocking of D2 receptors
• Hypotension – blocking of alpha-1 adrenergic receptors

Notable AEs
• Most common: Dizziness, sedation, dry mouth, constipation, weight gain
• Tachycardia, hypotension or hypertension
• Akathisia, parkinsonism

 ### Life-Threatening or Dangerous AEs
• Tardive dyskinesias
• Neuroleptic malignant syndrome
• Rare neurotoxicity in patients with thyrotoxicosis

Weight Gain
• Not unusual

unusual   not unusual   common   problematic

Sedation
• Common

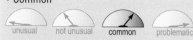

What to Do About AEs
• Take at night to avoid sedation. For severe AEs, change to another agent
• Rarely causes ECG changes. Use with caution in patients if QTc is above 450 (females) or 440 (males) and do not administer with QTc greater than 500
• If excessive sedation, use only as a rescue agent for intractable migraine in hospitalized patients or when patients can lie down or sleep

Best Augmenting Agents for AEs
• Give fluids to avoid hypotension, tachycardia and dizziness
• Give anticholinergics (diphenhydramine, trihexyphenidyl or benztropine) or benzodiazepines for motor AEs including extrapyramidal reactions and akathisia

DOSING AND USE

Usual Dosage Range
• GTS: 0.25–4 mg/day
• Migraine: 2–5 mg up to 3 times daily

Dosage Forms
• Tablets: 0.5 mg, 1 mg, 2 mg, 5 mg, 10 mg, 20 mg
• Concentrate: 2 mg/mL
• Solution: 1 mg/mL
• Injection: 5 mg/mL
• Decanoate Injection: 50 or 100 mg

How to Dose
• GTS: Start at 0.25–0.5 mg/day and increase slowly as needed to 3–4 mg/day if tolerated, depending on symptom relief
• Migraine: Give IV/IM or oral. Up to 5 mg 3–4 times daily for acute headache

 Dosing Tips
• Low doses are often effective in GTS and can be given as a once-daily dose at night
• For migraine, use often in hospitalized patients while monitoring blood pressure, pulse, and daily ECG

Overdose
• CNS depression, hypotension, and extrapyramidal reactions are most common. Respiratory suppression or death is rare

Long-Term Use
• Safe for long-term use but may cause irreversible AEs (tardive dyskinesias)

Habit Forming
• No

How to Stop
• No need to taper, but GTS/tics often recur

Pharmacokinetics
• Half-life 18 hours orally, 92% protein bound. Decanoate half-life is about 3 weeks

 Drug Interactions
• Use with CNS depressants (barbiturates, opiates, general anesthetics) potentiates CNS AEs
• Rifampin and carbamazepine may lower levels
• Fluoxetine may increase levels
• Haloperidol and lithium together may produce encephalopathy similar to neuroleptic malignant syndrome
• May enhance effects of antihypertensives
• Use with alcohol or diuretics may increase hypotension
• May decrease effectiveness of dopaminergic agents
• Reduces effectiveness of anticoagulants

 Other Warnings/ Precautions
• Use cautiously in patients with Parkinson's disease or dementia with Lewy bodies
• Neuroleptic malignant syndrome is characterized by fever, rigidity, confusion and autonomic instability, and is more common with typical neuroleptics, such as haloperidol, given IV

Do Not Use
• Hypersensitivity to drug, CNS depression/coma, or QTc greater than 500

SPECIAL POPULATIONS

Renal Impairment
• No dose adjustment needed

Hepatic Impairment
• Use with caution

Cardiac Impairment
• May worsen orthostatic hypotension

Elderly
• Start with lower doses and monitor for hypotension

Children and Adolescents
• Efficacy and safety unknown for children under age 3. Start at 0.05 mg/mg/day for GTS. Not a first-line agent in migraine

Pregnancy
• Category C. Limb deformities have been reported. Use only if benefit outweighs risks

Breast Feeding
• Use while breast feeding is generally not recommended

THE ART OF NEUROPHARMACOLOGY

Potential Advantages
• Perhaps the most effective drug in the treatment of GTS and tics

Potential Disadvantages
• Potential for long-term AEs (tardive dyskinesias), unlike alpha-2 adrenergic agonists

Primary Target Symptoms
• Tics, headache, and nausea

 Pearls
• In acute migraine, greater risk of abnormal movement AEs than other antiemetics, but less sedation and hypotension than chlorpromazine
• Pretreat or combine with diphenhydramine, 25–50 mg, to reduce rate of akathisia and dystonic reactions. Benztropine is also useful and may be given orally or IM
• Avoid in patients with Parkinson's disease or Lewy body dementia, but can be used as a 1-time dose in patients with florid psychosis (i.e., in emergency room setting). Non-pharmacologic approaches, clozapine, or quetiapine are preferred for psychosis or hallucinations in these patients
• Low doses less likely to induce negative symptoms in patients with schizophrenia

Suggested Reading

Backonja M, Beinlich B, Dulli D, Schutta HS. Haloperidol and lorazepam for the treatment of nausea and vomiting associated with the treatment of intractable migraine headaches. Arch Neurol 1989;46(7):724.

Honkaniemi J, Liimatainen S, Rainesalo S, Sulavuori S. Haloperidol in the acute treatment of migraine: a randomized, double-blind, placebo-controlled study. Headache 2006;46(5):781–7.

Kossoff EH, Singer HS. Tourette syndrome: clinical characteristics and current management strategies. Paediatr Drugs 2001;3(5):355–63.

Kudo S, Ishizaki T. Pharmacokinetics of haloperidol: an update. Clin Pharmacokinet 1999;37(6):435–56.

Siow HC, Young WB, Silberstein SD. Neuroleptics in headache. Headache 2005;45(4):358–71.

HEPARIN

THERAPEUTICS

Brands
• Hep-lock, Hepflush

Generic?
Yes

Class
• Anticoagulant

Commonly Prescribed for
(FDA approved in bold)
• **Deep venous thrombosis (DVT)/pulmonary embolism (PE)**
• **Atrial fibrillation with embolization**
• **Prevention of evolving thrombosis in acute ischemic stroke (IS)**
• **Coagulopathies (acute and chronic)**
• **Prophylaxis against postoperative DVT/PE in at-risk patients**
• **Clotting prevention (i.e., during procedures)**
• Prophylaxis of left ventricular thrombi and cerebrovascular accidents post-myocardial infarction (MI)
• Unstable angina
• After thrombolysis in acute MI

How the Drug Works
• Inhibits multiple sites in the coagulation system, preventing normal clotting of blood and formation of fibrin clots. Heparin, in combination with antithrombin III, inactivates activated Factor X and prevents the conversion of prothrombin to thrombin
• Larger doses inhibit further coagulation by inactivating thrombin and preventing conversion of fibrinogen to fibrin and inhibiting the activation of fibrin stabilizing factor

How Long Until It Works
• IV bolus: anticoagulant effect is immediate but increases in proportion to dose and duration of use. SC: peak levels occur at 2–4 hours

If It Works
• Monitor for bleeding complications and check activated partial thromboplastin time (aPTT)

If It Doesn't Work
• Patients can still have DVT/PE or IS despite treatment. Check aPTT to determine effectiveness

Best Augmenting Combos for Partial Response or Treatment-Resistance
• Often used with aspirin adjunctively in the setting of acute MI and coronary occlusion
• Usually used in acute setting after cardioembolic IS. Warfarin is usually used for long-term prophylaxis

Tests
• Monitor prothrombin time (aPPT) and INR to determine effectiveness. Periodically monitor platelet counts and test for occult blood in stool

ADVERSE EFFECTS (AEs)

How Drug Causes AEs
• Anticoagulation increases bleeding risk, hypersensitivity accounts for most other AEs

Notable AEs
• Generalized hypersensitivity (chills, fever, urticaria, rhinitis, headache). Mild thrombocytopenia. Osteoporosis with extended use

Life-Threatening or Dangerous AEs
• Heparin can cause retroperitoneal, adrenal, ovarian, GI, urinary tract, or intracranial bleeding. Complications can be life-threatening. Patients at increased risk include those with liver or renal disease, severe hypertension, bacterial endocarditis, ulcerative colitis, and diverticulitis
• Delayed thrombocytopenia (usually starting 7–12 days after initiation) can be severe. This can lead to new thrombus formation from irreversible platelet aggregation, called "white-clot syndrome."
• Vasospasm in limbs, up to 6 hours, may occur 6–10 days after initiating therapy
• Hypersensitivity reactions, including asthma, shock, or anaphylaxis

Weight Gain
• Unusual

unusual | not unusual | common | problematic

Sedation
• Unusual

unusual | not unusual | common | problematic

What to Do About AEs
• Stop infusion for serious AEs. Thrombocytopenia is not necessarily dose-related. Stop if platelets are below 100,000/mm³ or if recurrent thrombosis develops. Consider alternative anticoagulants, if patients require them

Best Augmenting Agents for AEs
• Most AEs cannot be improved by an augmenting agent

DOSING AND USE

Usual Dosage Range
• 5,000–20,000 units (u)/m²/24 h (as continuous IV infusion)
• 8000 – 20,000 u every 8–12 hours (SC)

Dosage Forms
• *Injection*: 1000 u in 500 mL or 2000 u in 1000 mL with 0.9% sodium chloride. With 0.45% sodium chloride, 12,500 u in 250 mL or 25,000 units in 250 or 500 mL
• *Multiple-dose vials*: 1000, 2000, 2500, 5000, 10,000, 20,000, or 40,000 u per mL
• *Single-dose ampules and vials*: 1000, 5000, 10,000, 20,000, 40,000 u per mL or 1000, 2500, 5000, 7500, 10,000, or 20,000 u per dose
• *Lock flush*: 1, 10 or 100 u/mL in 1, 2, 5, or 10 mL syringes

How to Dose
IV Infusion: start at 800–1000 u/hour (low-dose) for prevention of cardioembolic IS. Goal aPTT is usually higher for treatment of acute DVT or PE (see below). Perform coagulation tests every 4–6 hours in initial stages and adjust dose based on results
  • aPTT < 45, increase by 250 u/hour
  • aPTT 45–64, increase by 150 u/hour
  • aPTT 65–85, no change

  • aPTT 86–110, decrease by 150 u/hour
  • aPTT > 110, decrease by 250 u/hour
SC injection for DVT prevention: 5000 u every 8–12 hours for 7 days or until ambulatory

 Dosing Tips
• Note that heparin may increase prothrombin time as well as aPTT. This can cause confusion when starting oral anticoagulation. To ensure continuous anticoagulation, continue heparin for a few days after reaching therapeutic INR

Overdose
• Bleeding complications such as nosebleeds, hematuria, and GI bleeding are common. Protamine sulfate can reverse heparin effect

Long-Term Use
• Usually warfarin is preferred

Habit Forming
• No

How to Stop
• No need to taper, but patients will be at increased risk of thromboembolic complications after discontinuation

Pharmacokinetics
• Average half-life is 30–180 minutes but is non-linear and highly dose-dependent: increased with higher doses. Heparin is partially metabolized by the liver and reticuloendothelial system, but up to 50% is excreted unchanged in urine

 Drug Interactions
• Cephalosporins and penicillins may have additive effects and increase bleeding
• Platelet inhibitors including aspirin, NSAIDs, dipyridamole, hydroxychloraquine, dextran, and phenylbutazone interfere with platelet aggregation and may increase bleeding
• Digitalis, nicotine, tetracyclines, and antihistamines may partially counteract the anticoagulant effect of heparin
• Streptokinase administration before initiation may cause resistance to heparin
• May increase prothrombin time up to 5 hours after stopping drug. This may cause confusion when using with warfarin

Other Warnings/ Precautions

- May increase free fatty acid levels by induction of lipoprotein lipase
- Hyperkalemia, probably due to induced hypoaldosteronism, has been reported
- Elevation of hepatic transaminases is common but is unclear if these are related to heparin

Do Not Use

- Hypersensitivity to the drug, active bleeding, and severe thrombocytopenia

SPECIAL POPULATIONS

Renal Impairment

- Prolongs half-life, patients are more likely to experience bleeding complications. Use with caution

Hepatic Impairment

- Increased risk of bleeding complications due to increased half-life and decreased synthesis of clotting factors

Cardiac Impairment

- No known effects

Elderly

- Women over 60 have a higher rate of bleeding complications

Children and Adolescents

- Start with 50 u/kg bolus followed by 100 u/kg/dose every 4 hours or as continuous infusion 20,000 u/m^2/24 h. Safety in newborns is unknown. Low-birth-weight infants are at risk of germinal matrix hemorrhage

Pregnancy

- Category C. Stillbirths and prematurity may occur, but complications are fewer than with warfarin. Heparin (or low molecular weight heparin) is preferred in pregnant patients who require anticoagulation

Breast Feeding

- Not found in breast milk

THE ART OF NEUROPHARMACOLOGY

Potential Advantages

- Immediate effectiveness. Useful for prophylaxis of IS in patients with mechanical heart valves, cardiac thrombus, or atrial fibrillation

Potential Disadvantages

- Not a treatment for acute stroke. Generally used in hospital setting only. Serious bleeding and thrombocytopenia risks require frequent monitoring

Primary Target Symptoms

- Prevention of complications resulting from DVT, PE, or IS

 Pearls

- SC heparin 5000 units twice daily appeared to help prevent stroke recurrence with relatively low AEs after IS, but 6 month outcomes were not improved
- Higher doses of heparin are associated with greater AEs, including intracranial hemorrhage
- Delay anticoagulation in the setting of large IS or uncontrolled hypertension due to risk of hemorrhagic transformation
- Heparin does not have fibrinolytic activity; use alteplase for acute IS in the treatment window
- When using after cardioembolic IS, monitor patients for changes in exam that may indicate hemorrhagic conversion of stroke
- Large ventricular thrombus is a relative indication to begin heparin shortly after AIS
- Low weight molecular heparins, such as enoxaparin, are an alternative to SC heparin for DVT prophylaxis and can be used at higher weight-based doses for acute DVT or PE

Suggested Reading

Alberts MJ. Treatment of acute ischemic stroke. J Stroke Cerebrovasc Dis 2001; 10(2 Pt 2):10–7.

Cordonnier C, Leys D, Deplanque D, Hénon H. Antithrombotic agents' use in patients with atrial fibrillation and acute cerebral ischemia. J Neurol 2006;253(8):1076–82.

Hoffman JR. Cerebral venous thrombosis: hemorrhagic stroke requiring acute heparin anticoagulation. J Emerg Med 2006;31(1):111; author reply 111–3.

Moonis M, Fisher M. Considering the role of heparin and low-molecular-weight heparins in acute ischemic stroke. Stroke 2002;33(7):1927–33.

IMMUNE GLOBULIN INTRAVENOUS (IGIV)

Brands
• Gamunex, Polygam, Gammagard, Iveegam, Octagam, Flebogamma, Carimune, Panglobulin, Privigen

Generic?
No

Class
• Immune globulin, immunomodulator

Commonly Prescribed for
(FDA approved in bold)
• **Chronic inflammatory demyelinating polyneuropathy (CIDP)**
• **Primary humoral immunodeficiency**
• **Idiopathic thrombocytopenic purpura**
• **B-cell chronic lymphocytic leukemia**
• **Kawasaki syndrome**
• **Kidney transplant with a high antibody recipient or with an ABO incompatible donor**
• **Human immunodeficiency virus infection (pediatric only)**
• Guillain Barre syndrome (GBS)
• Myasthenia gravis (MG)
• Multifocal motor neuropathy (MMN)
• Inflammatory myopathies: dermatomyositis (DM) and polymyositis (PM)
• Stiff-person syndrome
• Adrenoleukodystrophy
• Paraneoplastic syndromes
• Paraproteinemic immunoglobulin M demyelinating polyneuropathy
• Intractable childhood epilepsy including West syndrome, Lennox-Gastaut and Rasmussen syndrome
• Acute demyelinating encephalomyelitis (ADEM)
• Optic neuritis and multiple sclerosis (MS)
• Central pontine myelinolysis
• Diabetic amyotrophy
• Peripheral polyneuropathy
• Myelopathy associated with human T-cell lymphotropic virus-1 infection (HTLV-1)
• Wegener's granulomatosis
• Churg-Strauss syndrome
• Amyotrophic lateral sclerosis (ALS)
• Alzheimer dementia

How the Drug Works
• IGIV preparations are derived from a pool of at least 1000 donors. They contain anti-idiotypic antibodies that bind to and neutralize pathogenic autoantibodies. The infused IG may downregulate production of endogenous IG. The IG from IGIV may block Fc receptors on immune cells
• IGIV contains high-affinity neutralizing antibodies against interleukin (IL)-1a, IL-6 and TNFα, which may downregulate synthesis of cytokines by T cells
• It forms complexes with products of complement activation, preventing the formation and deposition of attack complexes on target cells
• IGIV also causes transient lymphopenia and reduces the number of natural killer cells

How Long Until It Works
• Days. Usually there is some effect within a week

If It Works
• CIDP and GBS: Improves strength and sensory symptoms. In GBS improves prognosis and prevents residual disability
• MG: May allow improvement in symptoms and prevent acute deterioration. Often initiated at the time of a clinical flare, before starting long-term disease-modifying therapy
• MMN: Symptoms and conduction block improve, but GM1 antibody titers may remain elevated

If It Doesn't Work
• CIDP and GBS: Consider corticosteroids for CIDP. In GBS, plasma exchange is an alternative
• MG: Start or change disease-modifying therapies (usually at the same time as initiating IGIV)
• MMN: If no effect, reconsider the diagnosis, as treatment options for MMN are limited. If the effect of IGIV wears off, consider a short course of plasma exchange before repeating dose

Best Augmenting Combos for Partial Response or Treatment-Resistance
• CIDP and GBS: Most patients require corticosteroids for long-term treatment of

CIDP. There are small studies that suggest a combination with 500 mg methylprednisolone improves outcomes in GBS
- MG: Usually used with symptomatic treatment such as pyridostigmine. Often combined with other disease-modifying agents such as prednisone, azathioprine, cyclophosphamide, mycophenolate mofetil, or cyclosporine
- MMN: Cyclophosphamide may be useful in refractory cases

Tests
- Check renal function, CBC before starting treatment and monitor renal function periodically during therapy

- Change to an alternative formulation of IGIV (individuals have variable AEs to different formulations)

Best Augmenting Agents for AEs
- NSAIDs are generally effective for headache
- Hydrate and give aspirin before administration in patients with vascular disease or diabetes
- Antihistamines may help prevent hypersensitivity reactions
- Epinephrine should be available to treat anaphylaxis or severe hypotension

ADVERSE EFFECTS (AEs)

How Drug Causes AEs
- The cause of most AEs, except for hypersensitivity in patients with IgA deficiency, is unknown

Notable AEs
- Headache is the most common AE
- Chest tightness, edema, chills, fever, myalgia, nausea
- Hypotension

 Life-Threatening or Dangerous AEs
- Renal failure
- Congestive heart failure, thrombotic events and myocardial infarction, aseptic meningitis
- Anaphylaxis (especially in patients with IgA deficiency)

Weight Gain
- Unusual

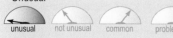

Sedation
- Unusual

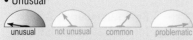

What to Do About AEs
- Administer at a slower rate

DOSING AND USE

Usual Dosage Range
- 1–2 g/kg each dose

Dosage Forms
- Carimune: Powder for solution in 1, 3, 6, and 12 g vials
- Flebogamma: 5% (50 mg/mL) in 10, 50, 100 and 200 mL vials
- Gamimune: 5% in 10% maltose
- Gammagard: 10% in 1, 2.5, 5, 10 and 20 g vials
- Iveegam: 5 g freeze dried powder for solution
- Privigen: 10% (100 mg/mL) in 5, 10, and 20 g vials
- Octagam: 5% (50 mg/mL) in 10, 50, 100, and 200 mL vials
- Polygam: 90% (50 mg/mL) in 2.5, 5 and 10 g single-use bottles
- Sandoglobulin: powder for injection

How to Dose
- The rate of infusion is based on the formulation. Start at a slow rate and increase after 30 minutes if tolerated and vital signs are normal. The infusions are generally given over 2–5 days for the 2 g dose. Occasionally 1 g doses can be given in 1–2 days in relatively healthy patients with previous exposure

 Dosing Tips
- Administer more slowly in chronically ill patients or those with renal insufficiency

- IGIV brands differ in their sodium and glucose content

Overdose
- Fluid overload and edema are most common

Long-Term Use
- Appears safe for long-term use

Habit Forming
- No

How to Stop
- No need to taper but monitor for recurrence of neurological disorder

Pharmacokinetics
- Peak action in a few days and half-life of about 3 weeks. 100% bioavailability after administration. IgG levels decline to about 40% of peak after 1 week

 Drug Interactions
- Do not give live vaccines within 3 months of IGIV administration

Do Not Use
- Known hypersensitivity to drug or its components, severe renal insufficiency, IgA deficiency, or presence of anti-immunoglobulin antibodies

SPECIAL POPULATIONS

Renal Impairment
- Use an iso-osmolar brand of IGIV to avoid worsening of renal function

Hepatic Impairment
- No known effects

Cardiac Impairment
- Use with caution in patients with diabetes or known vascular disease

Elderly
- May be more likely to experience complications. Use a low sodium and glucose brand

 Children and Adolescents
- Appears safe and effective in GBS, although experience is limited

 Pregnancy
- Category C. Probably safe in pregnancy

Breast Feeding
- Unknown if secreted in breast milk

THE ART OF NEUROPHARMACOLOGY

Potential Advantages
- Rapid onset of action in MG, CIDP, GBS, and many other neurologic disorders. Relatively well tolerated, with few long-term AEs

Potential Disadvantages
- Need for repeated IV administration and cost. Effectiveness varies depending on the disorder

Primary Target Symptoms
- Preventive treatment of complications from CIDP, MG, and GBS

 Pearls
- Often used as an alternative to plasma exchange (PE) for similar clinical situations (GBS, MG). In contrast to PE, does not require large-bore catheters or special equipment, and is safer in the setting of sepsis
- When compared to PE, outcomes in MG and GBS are similar with IGIV
- It is unclear if a second course of IGIV is beneficial in GBS for patients with suboptimal response to treatment
- Unlike GBS, CIDP requires long-term treatment. The use of monthly infusions (usually 1 g) for maintenance therapy may be beneficial, especially if corticosteroids are contraindicated
- MMN usually does not respond to corticosteroids or PE, so IGIV is the first-line treatment
- In a case series examining DM refractory to corticosteroids, IGIV was effective after multiple infusions
- Inclusion-body myositis does not typically respond to immunotherapy but open-label and controlled trials report functional improvement with IGIV in a minority of patients

- IGIV is a relatively rapid-acting disease-modifying treatment in MG. Small studies demonstrate effectiveness similar to PE. The role of maintenance infusions is unclear
- Paraproteinemic IgM demyelinating polyneuropathy (MGUS-associated neuropathy) patients showed modest benefit in open-label studies but antibody levels were unchanged
- Intractable childhood epilepsies may respond to treatment with IGIV, based on the assumption that seizures are related to postviral encephalitis. Rasmussen syndrome with glutamate receptor antibodies is one example and 8 of 9 IGIV-treated patients improved in 1 series
- Small series suggest IGIV is effective in stiff-person syndrome, producing clinical improvement and lower antibody titers
- Case reports suggest IGIV is useful for ADEM cases refractory to corticosteroids
- Clinical trials are underway to assess the effect of various IGIV regimens in relapsing-remitting MS
- IGIV appears ineffective in the treatment of ALS and adrenoleukodystrophy

Suggested Reading

Dalakas MC. The role of IVIg in the treatment of patients with stiff person syndrome and other neurological diseases associated with anti-GAD antibodies. J Neurol 2005;252 (Suppl 1):I19–25.

Dalakas MC. Role of IVIg in autoimmune, neuroinflammatory and neurodegenerative disorders of the central nervous system: present and future prospects. J Neurol 2006;253 (Suppl 5):V25–32.

Gajdos P, Chevret S, Toyka K. Intravenous immunoglobulin for myasthenia gravis. Cochrane Database Syst Rev 2008;(1): CD002277.

Granata T, Fusco L, Gobbi G, Freri E, Ragona F, Broggi G, Mantegazza R, Giordano L, Villani F, Capovilla G, Vigevano F, Bernardina BD, Spreafico R, Antozzi C. Experience with immunomodulatory treatments in Rasmussen's encephalitis. Neurology 2003;61(12):1807–10.

Koski CL, Patterson JV. Intravenous immunoglobulin use for neurologic diseases. J Infus Nurs 2006;29 (3 Suppl):S21–8.

Léger JM, Viala K, Cancalon F, Maisonobe T, Gruwez B, Waegemans T, Bouche P. Intravenous immunoglobulin as short- and long-term therapy of multifocal motor neuropathy: a retrospective study of response to IVIg and of its predictive criteria in 40 patients. J Neurol Neurosurg Psychiatry 2008;79(1):93–6.

Tasdemir HA, Dilber C, Kanber Y, Uysal S. Intravenous immunoglobulin for Guillain-Barré syndrome: how effective? J Child Neurol 2006;21(11):972–4.

INDOMETHACIN

THERAPEUTICS

Brands
- Indocin, Indocid, Indochron E-R, Indocin-SR

Generic?
Yes

Class
- Non-steroidal anti-inflammatory (NSAID)

Commonly Prescribed for
(FDA approved in bold)
- **Rheumatoid arthritis**
- **Ankylosing spondylitis**
- **Osteoarthritis**
- **Acute painful shoulder (bursitis, tendinitis)**
- **Acute gouty arthritis**
- Migraine, tension-type, and cluster headache
- Indomethacin-responsive headache disorders: Hemicrania continua (HC)
- Paroxysmal hemicrania, primary cough headache, primary exertional headache, preorgasmic headache, primary stabbing or "ice-pick" headache, hypnic headache
- Suppression of uterine activity to prevent premature labor

How the Drug Works
- Like other NSAIDs, inhibits cyclo-oxygenase (predominantly cox-1) thus inhibiting synthesis of prostaglandins, a mediator of inflammation
- The reason indomethacin is more effective than other NSAIDs for many headache disorders is unclear, but could be due to its structural similarities to serotonin, central vasoconstrictive and analgesic properties, or lowering of intracranial pressure. It also inhibits the metabolism of an active progesterone metabolite

How Long Until It Works
- Migraine: (acute) less than 2 hours
- Indomethacin-responsive headache disorders: (preventive) less than a week after starting a given daily dose

If It Works
- Continue to use

If It Doesn't Work
- Migraine: change to a triptan, dihydroergotamine, antiemetic or another NSAID
- Indomethacin-responsive headache disorders: reconsider the diagnosis

Best Augmenting Combos for Partial Response or Treatment-Resistance
- Migraine: combine with triptan or antiemetic

Tests
- None required

ADVERSE EFFECTS (AEs)

How Drug Causes AEs
- Effects on prostaglandins likely cause most GI and renal AEs

Notable AEs
- Dyspepsia, dizziness, nausea, diarrhea most common
- Inhibition of platelet aggregation is usually mild
- Elevation in hepatic transaminases (usually borderline)

Life-Threatening or Dangerous AEs
- GI ulcers and bleeding, increasing with duration of therapy
- May worsen depression, psychiatric disturbances, and parkinsonism
- May increase risk of fluid retention and edema, cardiovascular events, including myocardial infarction and stroke
- Renal insufficiency, proteinuria, and hyperkalemia
- Aseptic meningitis (rare)
- Hypersensitivity reactions – most common in patients with asthma

Weight Gain
- Unusual

unusual | not unusual | common | problematic

Sedation

• Not unusual

unusual / not unusual / common / problematic

What to Do About AEs

• For significant GI or intracranial bleeding, stop drug. Some AEs respond to lowering dose

Best Augmenting Agents for AEs

• Proton pump inhibitors may reduce risk of GI ulcers

DOSING AND USE

Usual Dosage Range

• Acute pain: 25–75 mg
• Preventive: 25–300 mg daily

Dosage Forms

• Capsules: 25 mg, 50 mg
• Sustained-release capsules: 75 mg
• Oral suspension: 25 mg/5 mL
• Suppository: 50 mg
• Injection: 100 mg

How to Dose

• Acute migraine: Give 25–50 mg orally or as suppository for acute pain
• HC and indomethacin-responsive headaches: Start at 75 mg/day (once daily sustained release or 25 mg 3 times daily with meals). If headache does not remit, increase dose in 3 days to 150 mg/day for another 3–10 days. Increase to 225 mg/day (75 mg 3 times daily) if no response, but if there is no benefit in less than 2 weeks discontinue drug. Occasional patients will require a higher dose (up to 300 mg/daily) or 4 weeks of treatment to improve

 Dosing Tips

• Taking with food decreases absorption and reduces GI AEs

Overdose

• GI distress, drowsiness, paresthesias, and numbness are most common. Severe overdose may cause hypertension, metabolic acidosis, hepatic or renal failure, and cardiac arrest. Consider multiple doses of activated charcoal or hemodialysis for severe cases

Long-Term Use

• Safe for long-term use. In patients with indomethacin-responsive headache disorders, periodically attempt to lower dose

Habit Forming

• No

How to Stop

• No need to taper

Pharmacokinetics

• Half-life is 4.5 hours, dose peak at 2 hours. Minimal hepatic metabolism. Renal excretion 60% and fecal 33%. 90% protein bound

 Drug Interactions

• Use with alcohol, bisphosphonates, corticosteroids, anticoagulants, and other NSAIDs increase GI bleeding risk
• Cyclosporine and NSAIDs increase risk of nephrotoxicity
• Cholestyramine may decrease absorption
• Aspirin use may decrease NSAID serum levels and increases risk of GI AEs
• May blunt effectiveness of beta-blockers and angiotensin-converting enzyme inhibitors
• May decrease effect of loop diuretics and spironolactone
• May increase drug levels and effects of digoxin, aminoglycosides, methotrexate, lithium, and phenytoin

 Other Warnings/ Precautions

• Risk factors for GI bleeding include smoking, alcoholism, older age, poor health status, and treatment with anticoagulants or corticosteroids
• May cause photosensitivity

Do Not Use

• Hypersensitivity to any NSAID, treatment with anticoagulants, renal or hepatic disease, age under 12, rectal bleeding or proctitis (suppositories)

Renal Impairment
• Use with caution in chronic renal insufficiency as may worsen renal function. Use low dose and monitor frequently

Hepatic Impairment
• Use with caution in patients with significant disease. May have increased risk of GI bleeding and toxicity

Cardiac Impairment
• May cause fluid retention and decompensation in patients with cardiac failure. May cause hypertension or lower effectiveness of antihypertensives

Elderly
• More likely to experience GI bleeding or CNS AEs

 Children and Adolescents
• Safety in children 14 and under is not established. Do not exceed 150–200 mg/day or 4 mg/kg/day

 Pregnancy
• Category B, except category D in 3rd trimester. May prolong pregnancy and increase risk of septal heart defects, incidence of dystocias, and delivery time. May cause premature closure of ductus arteriosus and pulmonary hypertension. Do not use, especially in 3rd trimester

Breast Feeding
• Most NSAIDs are excreted in breast milk. Do not breast feed due to effects on infant cardiovascular system

THE ART OF NEUROPHARMACOLOGY

Potential Advantages
• Fairly effective in many primary headache disorders and the drug of choice for many uncommon primary headache disorders

Potential Disadvantages
• More AEs than other NSAIDs. GI AEs increase with extended use

Primary Target Symptoms
• Headache pain severity with acute use, headache frequency and severity with chronic use

 Pearls
• Indomethacin suppositories are useful for severe migraine with nausea and vomiting
• HC is a continuous unilateral headache disorder, often with autonomic symptoms, that may be confused with migraine or cluster headache. HC responds absolutely to indomethacin, often at low doses (less than 100 mg/day). Patients with constant unilateral headache should receive a trial of indomethacin, which will usually improve HC in a few weeks. Because unilateral headache is common in migraine and other headache disorders, it may be difficult to diagnose HC without an appropriate trial
• Indomethacin injection, not available in the US, may be a more efficient way to diagnose indomethacin-responsive headaches. HC patients usually respond absolutely in a few hours
• Hypnic headache, a disorder of headache during sleep usually occurring later in life, may respond to a bedtime dose of indomethacin

Suggested Reading

Dodick DW. Indomethacin-responsive headache syndromes. Curr Pain Headache Rep 2004;8(1):19–26.

Dodick DW, Jones JM, Capobianco DJ. Hypnic headache: another indomethacin-responsive headache syndrome? Headache 2000;40(10):830–5.

Marmura MJ, Silberstein SD, Gupta M. Hemicrania continua: who responds to indomethacin? Cephalalgia 2009;29(3):300–7.

Peres MF, Silberstein SD, Nahmias S, Shechter AL, Youssef I, Rozen TD, Young WB. Hemicrania continua is not that rare. Neurology 2001;57(6):948–5

INTERFERON-BETA (1A AND 1B)

Brands
- Avonex (1a), Rebif (1a), CinnoVex (1a), Betaseron (1b), Extavia (1b)

Generic?
No

Class
- Immunomodulator

Commonly Prescribed for
(FDA approved in bold)
- **Reduction of relapses in patients with relapsing forms of multiple sclerosis (relapsing-remitting or secondary progressive with relapses)**
- Clinically isolated syndromes (CIS)

How the Drug Works
- By modifying the immune processes believed responsible in part for the development of MS. Interferon-beta has antiviral and immunomodulatory activities. Produces multiple gene products and markers, including beta-2 microglobulin, that affect immune function

How Long Until It Works
- At least 6 months

If It Works
- Continue to use

If It Doesn't Work
- Repeat brain MRI, check for neutralizing antibodies, change to glatiramer, reconsider the diagnosis of relapsing MS, and consider using natalizumab or mitoxantrone

Best Augmenting Combos for Partial Response or Treatment-Resistance
- Acute attacks are often treated with glucocorticoids, especially if there is functional impairment such as vision loss, weakness, or cerebellar symptoms
- Treat common clinical symptoms in MS with appropriate medication for spasticity (baclofen, tizanidine), neuropathic pain, and fatigue (modafinil)

- For patients with relapsing MS refractory to interferon-beta, as measured by clinical outcome and MRI accumulation of lesions, consider changing to glatiramer, natalizumab, or mitoxantrone. Other options, which are less proven, include monthly methylprednisolone, pulse cyclophosphamide, and other immunosuppressants
- Combination therapy may have a role, but has not been proven more effective than monotherapy. There is an ongoing clinical trial looking at combination treatment with interferon 1a (Avonex) and glatiramer acetate (Copaxone). Using interferon-beta with natalizumab may increase risk of progressive multifocal leukoencephalopathy

Tests
- None required

How Drug Causes AEs
- Except for injection site reactions, AEs from interferon component of drug

Notable AEs
- Flu-like symptoms, fatigue, weakness or myalgias, chest pain, and headache can occur within hours after starting drug. Long-term use may cause elevation of hepatic enzymes, leukopenia, photosensitivity, or injection site necrosis. Monitor for depression or worsening of existing psychiatric disorders

Life-Threatening or Dangerous AEs
- Hepatic injury, occasionally severe
- Rarely pancytopenia, thrombocytopenia, or autoimmune disorders, such as thyroid disease
- Rarely worsens existing cardiac disease such as angina, congestive heart failure, or arrhythmia

Weight Gain
- Unusual

unusual   not unusual   common   problematic

Sedation
• Not unusual

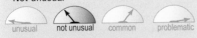

What to Do About AEs
• Most reactions are self-limiting and do not require any specific treatment but may cause some distress for the patient. Some patients have benefited from using anti-inflammatory medications (ibuprofen and naproxen) at the time of injection to decrease the AEs. If AEs are bothersome enough, change to another disease-modifying agent. For more serious AEs, discontinue drug

Best Augmenting Agents for AEs
• Most AEs cannot be improved with an augmenting agent

DOSING AND USE

Usual Dosage Range
• 8.8 mcg per 0.2 mL, 22 or 44 mcg per 0.5 mL (Rebif)
• 30 mcg per 0.5 mL as powder or prefilled syringe (Avonex)
• 0.25 mg in 1 mL (Betaseron)

Dosage Forms
1a: 8.8 mcg per 0.2 mL (titration only), 22 or 44 mcg per 0.5 mL (Rebif)
30 mcg per 0.5 mL as powder or prefilled syringe (Avonex)
1b: 0.25 mg in 1 mL (Betaseron)

How to Dose
• Interferon-beta 1a IM (Avonex): inject in the thigh or upper arm once weekly
• Interferon-beta 1a SC (Rebif): inject at different sites 3 times weekly, with more than 48 hours between doses. Start at 20% of final dose for 2 weeks, then increase to 50% of dose for 2 weeks. At week 5, start the maintenance dose (either 22 or 44 mcg)
• Interferon-beta 1b SC: (Betaseron): inject at different sites every other day. Start at 25% of initial dose for 2 weeks, then increase to 50% for 2 weeks, then 75% weeks 5–6. At week 7 start maintenance dose of 0.25 mg

 Dosing Tips
• Rebif and Betaseron are available as autoinjections
• Betaseron comes as a powder (no refrigeration needed) which must be reconstituted in saline before use

Overdose
• No information available

Long-Term Use
• Safe for long-term use

Habit Forming
• No

How to Stop
• No need to taper

Pharmacokinetics
• Biological response markers increase within 6–12 hours and stay elevated for 4–7 days. Peak levels of markers are at 48 hours

 Drug Interactions
• In general, do not combine with other immunosuppressant medications

 Other Warnings/ Precautions
• May worsen existing seizure disorders

Do Not Use
• Hypersensitivity to the drug or human albumin

SPECIAL POPULATIONS

Renal Impairment
• No known effects

Hepatic Impairment
• Use with caution in patients with significant disease

Cardiac Impairment
• No known effects

Elderly
• No known effects

Children and Adolescents

- Not studied in initial trials, but has been used since with AEs similar to those of adults. Disease-modifying therapy appears to have benefit in reducing long-term cognitive and physical disability from RRMS; it is reasonable to offer treatment early in the disease course

Pregnancy

- Category C. Use in pregnancy only if clearly needed. In most cases, it is discontinued and steroids are used for acute relapses during pregnancy

Breast Feeding

- Unknown if excreted in breast milk. Do not breast feed while on drug

---

THE ART OF NEUROPHARMACOLOGY

Potential Advantages

- Excellent treatment option for relapsing forms of MS. Multiple dosing schedule options. Least number of injection per year (Avonex). Less chest pain and fewer post-injection reactions than glatiramer

Potential Disadvantages

- Not effective for primary progressive MS. Many AEs, including some that are serious. Flu-like symptoms, depression, fever, myalgias, and liver function abnormalities are more common than with glatiramer. Risk of neutralizing antibodies

Primary Target Symptoms

- Decrease in relapse rates, delay/prevention of disability, and slower accumulation of lesions on MRI imaging

Pearls

- MRI studies and clinical experience demonstrate that relapsing MS usually changes over time into progressive MS, which has a more degenerative than inflammatory course. There is no evidence for using interferon-beta in non-relapsing forms of MS, but theoretically could be useful for some patients who have an inflammatory component
- May be more effective than glatiramer in preventing relapses
- Likely ineffective for primary progressive MS
- Disease-modifying therapy reduces MRI lesions but not brain atrophy
- Neutralizing antibodies are a subset of binding antibodies that can inhibit the activity of interferon-beta. The incidence of neutralizing antibodies with interferon-beta therapy varies widely in clinical trials. The prevalence is highest with interferon-beta 1b and lowest with IM interferon-1a
- Most patients develop antibodies within the first 3–18 months of treatment. Patients with proven neutralizing antibodies have about double the risk of relapses and have more new lesions on MRI. Check neutralizing antibodies in patients who experience clinical deterioration while being treated with interferon-beta. Because these antibodies are cross-reactive among the different forms, if patient has neutralizing antibodies, change to a disease-modifying agent that does not contain interferon-beta

Suggested Reading

Cohen JA, Calabresi PA, Chakraborty S, Edwards KR, Eickenhorst T, Felton WL 3rd, Fisher E, Fox RJ, Goodman AD, Hara-Cleaver C, Hutton GJ, Imrey PB, Ivancic DM, Mandell BF, Perryman JE, Scott TF, Skaramagas TT; ACT Investigators. Avonex Combination Trial in relapsing–remitting MS: rationale, design and baseline data. Mult Scler 2008;14(3):370–82.

Pachner AR, Cadavid D, Wolansky L, Skurnick J. Effect of anti-IFN{beta} antibodies on MRI lesions of MS patients in the BECOME study. Neurology 2009;73(18):1485–92.

Panitch H, Miller A, Paty D, Weinshenker B; North American Study Group on Interferon beta-1b in Secondary Progressive MS. Interferon beta-1b in secondary progressive MS: results from a 3-year controlled study. Neurology 2004;63 (10):1788–95.

Rudick RA, Stuart WH, Calabresi PA, Confavreux C, Galetta SL, Radue EW, Lublin FD, Weinstock-Guttman B, Wynn DR, Lynn F, Panzara MA, Sandrock AW; SENTINEL Investigators. Natalizumab plus interferon beta-1a for relapsing multiple sclerosis. N Engl J Med 2006;354(9):911–23.

Wingerchuk DM. Current evidence and therapeutic strategies for multiple sclerosis. Semin Neurol 2008;28(1):56–68.

LACOSAMIDE

THERAPEUTICS

Brands
• Vimpat

Generic?
No

Class
• Antiepileptic drug (AED)

Commonly Prescribed for
(FDA approved in bold)
• **Partial-onset seizures (adjunctive in ages 17 and older)**
• Neuropathic pain

How the Drug Works
• Lacosamide likely acts by enhancing slow inactivation of voltage-gated sodium channels, resulting in stabilization of hyperexcitable neuronal membranes and inhibition of repetitive neuronal firing
• It also binds to collapsin response mediator protein-2 (CRMP-2), which causes changes in axon outgrowth
• Unlike many AEDs, does not appear to affect AMPA, kainate, NMDA, or GABA receptors and does not block potassium or calcium currents

If It Works
• Seizures – goal is the remission of seizures. Continue as long as effective and well-tolerated. Consider tapering and slowly stopping after 2 years without seizures, depending on the type of epilepsy

If It Doesn't Work
• Increase to highest tolerated dose
• Epilepsy: consider changing to another agent, adding a second agent or referral for epilepsy surgery evaluation. When adding a second agent keep in mind the drug interactions that can occur

Best Augmenting Combos for Partial Response or Treatment-Resistance
• Epilepsy: Designed for use with other AEDs. No interactions with AEDs in terms of levels but risk of AEs and hepatic dysfunction increase with polytherapy

Tests
• No regular blood tests are recommended

ADVERSE EFFECTS (AEs)

How Drug Causes AEs
• CNS AEs are mostly related to changes in sodium channel function

Notable AEs
• Dizziness, ataxia, vomiting, diplopia, nausea, vertigo, blurry vision, and tremor are most common. Palpitations, dry mouth, tinnitus, paresthesias are less common. Injection site pain and erythema with intravenous administration
• Increase in hepatic transaminases in about 0.7% of patients. More common in patients on multiple AEDs

Life-Threatening or Dangerous AEs
• Hepatitis, neutropenia (both rare)
• Risk of behavioral or mood effects including depression, suicidal ideation
• Rare PR prolongation and first-degree AV block, atrial fibrillation or flutter. Does not affect QTc interval

Weight Gain
• Unusual

unusual   not unusual   common   problematic

Sedation
• Not unusual

unusual   not unusual   common   problematic

What to Do About AEs
• A small dose decrease may improve most AEs. Titrate more slowly

Best Augmenting Agents for AEs
• Most AEs cannot be improved by use of augmenting agents

DOSING AND USE

Usual Dosage Range
• Epilepsy: 200–400 mg/day

Dosage Forms
- Tablets: 50 mg, 100 mg, 150 mg, 200 mg
- Injection: 10 mg/mL

How to Dose
- Start at 100 mg/day (50 mg twice a day) for 1 week, then increase by 100 mg/day every week until reaching goal dose of 200–400 mg per day in 2 divided doses

 Dosing Tips
- The intravenous dose is equal to oral dose and only used in patients unable to take oral medications
- Food does not affect absorption

Overdose
- Little information is available. Hemodialysis would theoretically be useful

Long-Term Use
- Safe for long-term use

Habit Forming
- No physical dependence, but a small minority of patients (less than 1%) report euphoria with doses of 200 mg or more

How to Stop
- Taper slowly (over 1 week) in patients with epilepsy to prevent withdrawal seizures. No need to taper in patients with neuropathy without epilepsy

Pharmacokinetics
- Maximum concentrations at 1–4 hours, with steady state reached at 3 days of twice-daily dosing. Elimination half-life 13 hours. Metabolized by hepatic P450 system, primarily CYP2C19. Eliminated by renal excretion

 Drug Interactions
- Omeprazole, a CYP2C19 substrate and inhibitor, can theoretically decrease metabolism. Clinically this does not appear significant in studies. No significant interactions with other AEDs, oral contraceptives, or other commonly used medications

Do Not Use
- Patients with a proven allergy to lacosamide

Renal Impairment
- No adjustment is needed except in patients with severe or end-stage renal disease. In patients with severe disease, use maximum of 300 mg/day and give a supplemental 50% of daily dose after hemodialysis sessions

Hepatic Impairment
- Titrate with caution. Usual maximum dose 300 mg/day

Cardiac Impairment
- May cause arrhythmias, use with caution

Elderly
- Pharmacokinetics appear fairly similar to other adults with minor difference in drug levels. Monitor for AEs

 Children and Adolescents
- Not studied in children under age 17. The binding of drug to CRMP-2, a phosphoprotein important in neuronal differentiation and control of axonal outgrowth, is poorly understood. Its effect on CNS development is uncertain

 Pregnancy
- Risk category C. Relatively low rate of teratogenicity in animal studies compared to other AEDs. Patients taking for pain should generally stop before considering pregnancy
- Supplementation with 0.4 mg of folic acid before and during pregnancy is recommended

Breast Feeding
- Some drug is found in mother's breast milk
- Generally recommendations are to discontinue drug or bottle feed
- Monitor infant for sedation, poor feeding, or irritability

Potential Advantages
- Effective as an adjunctive agent with 2 new mechanisms of action and no significant interactions with other AEDs. Generally well-tolerated and available intravenously

Potential Disadvantages
- Less is known about usefulness in many common types of epilepsy

Primary Target Symptoms
- Seizure frequency and severity
- Pain

 Pearls
- AEs appear to be dose related. The 600 mg dose in clinical trials was associated with much higher rates of tremor, dizziness, fatigue, vomiting, and ataxia

- Potentially useful but not yet studied for treatment of partial-onset status epilepticus in humans
- In initial studies did not appear effective against clonic seizures
- Dizziness may be increased when combined with other sodium channel blockers
- Based on initial clinical trials, the effective dose for treatment of neuropathic pain may be higher – 400 mg per day or more

---

 Suggested Reading

Doty P, Rudd GD, Stoehr T, Thomas D. Lacosamide. Neurotherapeutics 2007;4(1):145–8.

Harris JA, Murphy JA. Lacosamide: an adjunctive agent for partial-onset seizures and potential therapy for neuropathic pain. Ann Pharmacother 2009;43(11):1809–17.

Kellinghaus C, Berning S, Besselmann M. Intravenous lacosamide as successful treatment for nonconvulsive status epilepticus after failure of first-line therapy. Epilepsy Behav 2009;14(2):429–31.

Shaibani A, Fares S, Selam JL, Arslanian A, Simpson J, Sen D, Bongardt S. Lacosamide in painful diabetic neuropathy: an 18-week double-blind placebo-controlled trial. J Pain 2009;10(8):818–28.

THERAPEUTICS

Brands
• Lamictal, Lamictin

Generic?
Yes

Class
• Antiepileptic drug (AED)

Commonly Prescribed for
(FDA approved in bold)
• **Complex partial seizures (adjunctive for age 16 or older)**
• **Conversion to monotherapy for partial seizures in adults 16 or older**
• **Lennox-Gastaut syndrome aged 2 and older**
• **Maintenance of bipolar disorder**
• Generalized tonic-clonic seizures including juvenile myoclonic epilepsy
• Absence seizures (children and adults)
• Temporal lobe epilepsy (children and adults)
• Migraine prophylaxis
• SUNCT (Short-lasting unilateral neuralgiform headache with conjunctival injection and tearing)
• Trigeminal neuralgia
• Bipolar depression or mania
• Psychosis/Schizophrenia (adjunctive)

How the Drug Works
• A use-dependent blocker of voltage-sensitive sodium channels, preventing release of excitatory neurotransmitters such as glutamate and aspartate
• May inhibit gamma-aminobutyric acid (GABA) release and interact with calcium channels
• Weakly inhibits serotonin-3 receptors

How Long Until It Works
• Seizures – should decrease by 2 weeks at a specific dose, but slow titration can delay time to effective dose
• Headaches – weeks to months
• Mania – may take weeks to months

If It Works
• Seizures – goal is the remission of seizures. Continue as long as effective and well-tolerated. Consider tapering and slowly stopping after 2 years without seizures, depending on the type of epilepsy
• Headache – goal is a 50% or greater decrease in frequency or severity of pain or aura

If It Doesn't Work
• Increase to highest tolerated dose
• Epilepsy: consider changing to another agent, adding a second agent or referral for epilepsy surgery evaluation. When adding a second agent keep in mind the drug interactions that can occur
• Headache: If not effective in 2 months, consider stopping or using another agent

Best Augmenting Combos for Partial Response or Treatment-Resistance
• Epilepsy: drug interactions complicate multi-drug therapy. Increase dose if using with enzyme-inducing drugs and lower when using with valproate. May be particularly effective in combination with valproate
• Headache: consider beta-blockers, antidepressants, natural products, other AEDs, and non-medication treatments such as biofeedback to improve headache control

Tests
• No regular blood tests are recommended

ADVERSE EFFECTS (AEs)

How Drug Causes AEs
• CNS AEs are probably caused by sodium channel blockade effects

Notable AEs
• Rash (usually benign) in about 10%
• Sedation, diplopia, ataxia, headache, tremor, insomnia
• Nausea, vomiting, abdominal pain, constipation
• In children, pharyngitis associated with flu syndrome

Life-Threatening or Dangerous AEs
• Severe dermatologic reactions include Stevens-Johnson syndrome, angioedema, toxic epidermal necrolysis, and

hypersensitivity. May include fever or multiorgan abnormalities
- Severe reaction in about 1/1000 adults but 8/1000 in children
- Rare blood dyscrasias

Weight Gain
- Unusual

unusual   not unusual   common   problematic

Sedation
- Unusual

unusual   not unusual   common   problematic

What to Do About AEs
- A small dose decrease may improve CNS AEs
- Rashes much more common with rapid dose increases, coadministration with valproic acid and in first 2–8 weeks after beginning therapy
- For mild rashes (non-tender, spotty, and non-confluent, peaks within a few days and improves by 2–3 weeks with no systemic features), evaluate and monitor closely. Stop drug or lower, do not increase dose. If rash does not worsen or quickly improves then can restart with slower titration
- For severe dermatologic reactions with systemic features or involvement of the eyes or mouth, stop the drug and investigate for any organ involvement (renal, hepatic, or hematologic). May require hospitalization

Best Augmenting Agents for AEs
- Topical corticosteroids or antihistamines for rash
- Initially dose at night to avoid sedation

DOSING AND USE

Usual Dosage Range
- Epilepsy: 100–500 mg/day. For patients on valproate, 100–150 mg/day
- Bipolar Maintenance: 100–200 mg/day, with lower dose for patients on valproate and higher if on enzyme-inducing AEDs

Dosage Forms
- Tablets: 25 mg, 100 mg, 150 mg, 200 mg
- Chewable dispersion tablets: 2 mg, 5 mg. 25 mg

- Oral disintegrating tablets: 25 mg, 50 mg, 100 mg, 200 mg
- Extended-release tablets: 25 mg, 50 mg, 100 mg, 200 mg

How to Dose
- Monotherapy: start at 25 mg/day (usually at night) for 2 weeks, then increase to 50 mg/day for 2 weeks, then 100 mg and continue to increase as needed by 100 mg/day every 2 weeks until goal dose. On lower dose (50 mg or less) administer qhs but on higher doses (over 100 mg) dose bid
- With valproate (DPX): start 25 mg every other day, week 3 increase to 25 mg/day, week 5 increase to 50 mg/day, week 6 increase to 100 mg/day if no side effects. If/when DPX dose is lowered then will need to increase dose of lamotrigine
- With enzyme-inducing AEDs (carbamazepine, phenytoin, primidone, phenobarbital): start at 50 mg/day (25 mg bid), week 3 increase to 100 mg/day, then increase by 100 mg/day every 1–2 weeks to usual dose of 300–500 mg/day

 ### Dosing Tips
- Slow increase will avoid complication of serious rash
- Patients may need to repeat slow titration when off lamotrigine for more than a few days
- For patients on both lamotrigine and DPX who are stopping DPX decrease DPX dose by 250/500 mg/day per week. This usually requires increasing lamotrigine dose by about 50%
- For patients on both lamotrigine and enzyme-inducing AEDs, decrease that AED dose slowly and only once the patient is on goal dose of lamotrigine

Overdose
- Coma, ataxia, nystagmus, dizziness in patients with overdoses > 4 grams. Intraventicular conduction delay. Supportive care and gastric lavage. Hemodialysis may help in severe cases

Long-Term Use
- Safe for long-term use

Habit Forming
- No

How to Stop

- Taper slowly over 2 weeks or more
- Abrupt withdrawal can lead to seizures in patients with epilepsy

Pharmacokinetics

- Metabolized by glucuronic acid conjugation, not via CYP450 system. Bioavailability is 98%. Half-life is 33 hours in adults on single-dose lamotrigine, but 59 hours in epilepsy patients on DPX and 14 hours when used with enzyme-inducing AEDs. May reduce folate by inhibiting dihydrofolate reductase. Renal excretion

 Drug Interactions

- DPX increases lamotrigine levels
- Enzyme-inducing AEDs (phenobarbital, phenytoin, carbamazepine) and rifampin decrease levels
- Oral contraceptives can decrease levels
- Does not interact with antidepressants, antipsychotics or lithium

 Other Warnings/ Precautions

- Rash is the most common serious reaction. Avoid starting lamotrigine at the same time as other medications and discontinue for serious rash. Risk of rash increases with rapid dose increases and in children
- CNS AEs increase when used with other CNS depressants
- Systemic symptoms such as fever, flu-like symptoms, swelling of eyelids along with any dermatologic changes require immediate evaluation
- May cause photosensitivity

Do Not Use

- Patients with a proven allergy to lamotrigine

Renal Impairment

- Renal excretion of drug requires lowering of dose. About 55% protein bound. Give supplemental doses after dialysis

Hepatic Impairment

- Patients with moderate-severe disease may need lower dose or slower titration

Cardiac Impairment

- No known effects

Elderly

- May need lower dose. More likely to experience AEs (except rash)

 Children and Adolescents

- Approved for use in children 16 and older or for children 2 or older with Lennox-Gastaut syndrome or partial seizures
- Children have an increased risk of rash
- With enzyme-inducing AEDs: start 2 mg/kg/day in 2 divided doses, week 3 increase to 5 mg/kg/day, then increase by 2–3 mg/kg/day every 1–2 weeks until at goal; usual therapeutic dose 5–15 mg/kg/day in 2 doses
- With VPX: start at 0.15 mg/kg/day, week 3 0.3 mg/kg/day, then increase by 0.3 mg/kg/day every 1–2 weeks until at goal, typically 1–14 mg/kg/day
- Monotherapy: 0.6 mg/kg/day, week 3 increase to 1.2 mg/kg/day, then increase by 1.2 mg/kg/day every 1–2 weeks until at goal, usually 5–15 mg/kg/day in 2 doses

 Pregnancy

- Risk category C. Relatively low rate of teratogenicity in animal studies compared to other AEDs. Patients taking for headache or pain should generally stop before considering pregnancy. For patients with bipolar disorder, risks of relapse may outweigh risks of drug
- Levels usually decrease during pregnancy. Check levels before and periodically during pregnancy to ensure therapeutic dose
- Supplementation with 0.4 mg of folic acid before and during pregnancy is recommended

Breast Feeding

- Some drug is found in mother's breast milk
- Generally recommendations are to discontinue drug or bottle feed
- Monitor infant for sedation, poor feeding or irritability

THE ART OF NEUROPHARMACOLOGY

Potential Advantages
- Effective for multiple types of epilepsy due to broad spectrum of action
- Treats generalized seizures as well as partial and useful in myoclonic epilepsies
- Useful for patients with more than 1 condition such as epilepsy and mania
- Less likely to cause weight changes than other agents

Potential Disadvantages
- Risk of rash requires a slow titration. Limited evidence for migraine

Primary Target Symptoms
- Seizure frequency and severity
- Pain
- Recurrent depression or mania in bipolar disorder

Pearls
- Effective for most patients with generalized and partial epilepsies and fairly well tolerated
- Effective in about 85% of patients with myoclonic epilepsy, but a minority may worsen
- Not superior to placebo in migraine trials, but multiple case series demonstrate utility for treating bothersome auras in patients with migraine. Consider as a prophylactic agent for migraine with aura in patients who don't respond or can't tolerate other agents
- Lamotrigine can help treat SUNCT (Short-lasting unilateral neuralgiform headache with conjunctival injection and tearing)
- Effective in maintaining bipolar depression patients, not proven for acute mania
- Most trials using lamotrigine for the treatment of neuropathic and central pain have been negative
- Rash is most common during titration phase, but can be delayed up to a year

Suggested Reading

Culy CR, Goa KL. Lamotrigine. A review of its use in childhood epilepsy. Paediatr Drugs 2000;2(4):299–330.

Goa KL, Ross SR, Chrisp P. Lamotrigine. A review of its pharmacological properties and clinical efficacy in epilepsy. Drugs 1993;46(1):152–76.

Gutierrez-Garcia JM. SUNCT syndrome responsive to lamotrigine. Headache 2002;42(8):823–5.

Harden CL, Pennell PB, Koppel BS, Hovinga CA, Gidal B, Meador KJ, Hopp J, Ting TY, Hauser WA, Thurman D, Kaplan PW, Robinson JN, French JA, Wiebe S, Wilner AN, Vazquez B, Holmes L, Krumholz A, Finnell R, Shafer PO, Le Guen C; American Academy of Neurology; American Epilepsy Society. Practice parameter update: management issues for women with epilepsy–focus on pregnancy (an evidence-based review): vitamin K, folic acid, blood levels, and breastfeeding: report of the Quality Standards Subcommittee and Therapeutics and Technology Assessment Subcommittee of the American Academy of Neurology and American Epilepsy Society. Neurology 2009;73(2):142–9.

Lampl C, Katsarava Z, Diener HC, Limmroth V. Lamotrigine reduces migraine aura and migraine attacks in patients with migraine with aura. J Neurol Neurosurg Psychiatry 2005;76(12):1730–2.

Sabers A, Petrenaite V. Seizure frequency in pregnant women treated with lamotrigine monotherapy. Epilepsia 2009;50(9):2163–6.

Silberstein SD. Preventive migraine treatment. Neurol Clin 2009;27(2):429–43.

LEVETIRACETAM

THERAPEUTICS

Brands
• Keppra, Kopodex, Keppra XR

Generic?
Yes

 Class
• Antiepileptic drug (AED)

Commonly Prescribed for
(FDA approved in bold)
• **Complex partial seizures (adjunctive in adults and children 4 and older)**
• **Primary generalized tonic-clonic seizures (adjunctive for patients 6 and older)**
• **Myoclonic seizures including juvenile myoclonic epilepsy (adjunctive for patients 12 and older)**
• Status epilepticus
• Neuropathic pain or headache
• Mania

 How the Drug Works
• Binds to synaptic vesicle protein isoform SV2A in the brain, a unique mechanism of action compared with other AEDs. SV2A is involved in synaptic vesicle exocytosis
• Does not appear to affect GABA transmission, sodium channel or calcium channel function
• Effective in rat kindling models

How Long Until It Works
• Seizures – effective within 48 hours at starting dose, and should reduce seizures by 2 weeks

If It Works
• Seizures – goal is the remission of seizures. Continue as long as effective and well-tolerated. Consider tapering and slowly stopping after 2 years without seizures, depending on the type of epilepsy
• Headache/Pain – goal is a 50% or greater decrease in frequency or severity

If It Doesn't Work
• Increase to highest tolerated dose
• Epilepsy: consider changing to another agent, adding a second agent or referral for epilepsy surgery evaluation

 Best Augmenting Combos for Partial Response or Treatment-Resistance
• Epilepsy: Commonly used in combination with other AEDs

Tests
• No regular blood tests are recommended

ADVERSE EFFECTS (AEs)

How Drug Causes AEs
• CNS AEs are probably caused by effects on SV2A synaptic vesicle proteins

Notable AEs
• Sedation, asthenia, nausea, dizziness, headache
• Behavioral symptoms: agitation, hostility, emotional liability, depression. More common when used in combination with other AEDs or history of a preexisting behavioral disorder

 Life-Threatening or Dangerous AEs
• Rare psychotic symptoms or suicidal ideation

Weight Gain
• Unusual

unusual   not unusual   common   problematic

Sedation
• Common

unusual   not unusual   common   problematic
• May wear off with time

What to Do About AEs
• A small dose decrease may improve CNS AEs
• Titrate slowly and start at low-dose (500 mg/day)
• Behavioral AEs resolve when medication stopped

Best Augmenting Agents for AEs
• No treatment for AEs other than lowering dose or stopping drug

DOSING AND USE

Usual Dosage Range
- Epilepsy: 1000–3000 mg/day
- Status Epilepticus: 500 – 1500 mg over 15 minutes

Dosage Forms
- Tablets: 250 mg, 500 mg, 750 mg, 1000 mg
- Oral solution: 100 mg/mL
- Injection: 500 mg/mL diluted in 100 mL. Give over 15 minutes
- Extended release: 500 mg, 750 mg

How to Dose
- Start at 1000 mg/day in twice-daily dosing. Titrate to effective dose by 500–1000 mg/day every 1–2 weeks
- Start at lower dose (250 mg twice a day or 500 mg extended release) in elderly or chronically ill patients
- For patients with myoclonic seizures, the 3000 mg/day dose is recommended

 Dosing Tips
- Increase PM dose first to avoid daytime sedation
- Effectiveness improves at higher doses up to 3000 mg/day

Overdose
- Somnolence. May worsen seizures at very high doses

Long-Term Use
- Safe for long-term use

Habit Forming
- No

How to Stop
- Taper slowly
- Abrupt withdrawal can lead to seizures in patients with epilepsy

Pharmacokinetics
- Some drug metabolized by enzymatic hydrolysis of acetamide group
- No P450 metabolism. Most drug is renally excreted unchanged
- Low protein binding (< 10%). Half-life is 6–8 hours in healthy patients

  Drug Interactions
- No major interactions with AEDs or other medications

 Other Warnings/ Precautions
- Uncommon minor but statistically significant decreases in WBC and neutrophils

Do Not Use
- Patients with a proven allergy to levetiracetam

SPECIAL POPULATIONS

Renal Impairment
- Renal excretion of drug requires lowering of dose
- Mild (creatinine clearance 50–80 mL/min) 500–1500 mg twice daily
- Moderate (30–50 mL/min) 500–1000 mg twice daily
- Severe (< 30 mL/min) 250–500 twice daily
- Dialysis patients 500–1000 mg once a day with 250–500 mg supplemental dose after dialysis

Hepatic Impairment
- No dose adjustment needed

Cardiac Impairment
- No known effects

Elderly
- May need lower dose. More likely to experience AE.

 Children and Adolescents
- Start at 20 mg/kg/day dose and increase every 2 weeks until at goal of 60 mg/kg/day in 2 divided doses
- The most common AEs in children are behavioral

 Pregnancy
- Risk category C. Teratogenicity in animal studies. Patients taking for pain should generally stop before considering pregnancy

- Levels often change during pregnancy. Check levels periodically during pregnancy to ensure therapeutic dose
- Supplementation with 0.4 mg of folic acid before and during pregnancy is recommended

Breast Feeding

- Some drug is found in mother's breast milk
- Generally recommendations are to discontinue drug or bottle feed
- Monitor infant for sedation, poor feeding or irritability

THE ART OF NEUROPHARMACOLOGY

Potential Advantages

- Broad-spectrum AED effective for multiple types of epilepsy. Unique mechanism of action. Safe, easy to combine with other AEDs, lack of significant drug interactions

Potential Disadvantages

- Limited evidence for pain or mood disorders. Rare but bothersome psychiatric symptoms

Primary Target Symptoms

- Seizure frequency and severity
- Pain

 Pearls

- For patients with excess sedation, or history of AEs on other AEDs, start at lower dose (250 mg twice a day)
- New intravenous form is potentially useful in refractory status epilepticus, especially in patients with contraindications to other agents
- Studies suggest particularly useful for photosensitive epilepsies and myoclonic seizures
- Unique mechanism of action suggests utility for patients with poor response to other AEDs (such as sodium channel modulators) or in combination with other agents
- Can treat post-myoclonic and post-encephalitic myoclonus
- Little evidence for use in migraine or neuropathic pain
- May be helpful in rapid cycling bipolar disorder

 Suggested Reading

Ben-Menachem E. Levetiracetam: treatment in epilepsy. Expert Opin Pharmacother 2003;4(11):2079–88.

Berning S, Boesebeck F, van Baalen A, Kellinghaus C. Intravenous levetiracetam as treatment for status epilepticus. J Neurol 2009;256(10):1634–42.

Krauss GL, Bergin A, Kramer RE, Cho YW, Reich SG. Suppression of post-hypoxic and post-encephalitic myoclonus with levetiracetam. Neurology 2001; 56(3):411–2.

Lynch BA, Lambeng N, Nocka K, Kensel-Hammes P, Bajjalieh SM, Matagne A, Fuks B. The synaptic vesicle protein SV2A is the binding site for the antiepileptic drug levetiracetam. Proc Natl Acad Sci U S A 2004;101(26):9861–6.

Pakalnis A, Kring D, Meier L. Levetiracetam prophylaxis in pediatric migraine–an open-label study. Headache 2007;47(3):427–30.

Wasterlain CG, Chen JW. Mechanistic and pharmacologic aspects of status epilepticus and its treatment with new antiepileptic drugs. Epilepsia 2008;49 (Suppl 9):63–73.

LITHIUM
(Carbonate or Citrate)

THERAPEUTICS

Brands
- Carbolith, Eskalith, Priadel, Litarex, Lithicarb, Lithotab, Camcolit, Quilonum

Generic?
Yes

Class
- Mood stabilizer

Commonly Prescribed for
(FDA approved in bold)
- **Manic episodes in bipolar disorder**
- **Maintenance treatment in bipolar disorder**
- Cluster headache prophylaxis
- Hypnic headache
- Major depressive disorder
- Bipolar depression

How the Drug Works
- Proposed mechanisms include effects on sodium or glutamate receptors similar to anticonvulsants such as valproate and lamotrigine, modulation of circadian rhythms by deactivation of the GSK-3B enzyme or interaction with nitric oxide. It appears to increase cytoprotective proteins, inhibit inositol monophosphatase and reduce protein kinase C activity. It is unclear which of these actions accounts for its efficacy

How Long Until It Works
- Cluster headache – usually effective in 2–3 weeks

If It Works
- Produces reduction in the severity or frequency of attacks. Consider tapering or stopping if headaches remit (more than 2 weeks in episodic cluster patients) or if considering pregnancy

If It Doesn't Work
- Increase to highest tolerated dose
- Migraine/cluster: address other issues, such as medication-overuse, other coexisting medical disorders, such as anxiety, and consider changing to another agent or adding a second agent

Best Augmenting Combos for Partial Response or Treatment-Resistance
- Cluster: At the start of the cycle can use a corticosteroid slam and taper. Verapamil is effective in cluster but may cause fluctuations in lithium levels. Valproate, topiramate, and methysergide are effective for many cluster patients

Tests
- Obtain baseline renal function, thyroid function, weight/BMI and ECG before starting
- Repeat renal function every 6–12 months, monitor lithium levels, thyroid function, and weight
- Trough lithium levels should be between 0.5–1.2 mEq/L for acute and chronic treatment

ADVERSE EFFECTS (AEs)

How Drug Causes AEs
- The cause of CNS AEs is unknown, but renal AEs are due to changes in ion transport

Notable AEs
- Bradycardia, hypotension
- Dizziness, vertigo, psychomotor retardation, tremor, restlessness, muscle hyperexcitability
- Anorexia, nausea, diarrhea, weight gain
- Polyuria, edema, metallic taste, fever, alopecia

Life-Threatening or Dangerous AEs
- Lithium toxicity, especially at levels above 1.5 mEq/L. Diarrhea, vomiting, drowsiness, weakness occur early. Ataxia, polyuria, tinnitus, blurred vision, seizures, cardiac arrhythmias, ECG changes, syncope, or hallucinations may be seen in severe cases
- Thyroid disease, including hypothyroidism with myxedema or hyperthyroidism
- Nephrogenic diabetes insipidus
- Movement disorders, such as chorea, rigidity, and acute dystonia
- Rarely intracranial hypertension

Weight Gain
• Common

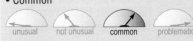

Sedation
• Common

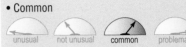

What to Do About AEs
• Check serum levels and reduce dose or stop drug for signs of toxicity
• Dose in the evening and take with food
• Maintain adequate hydration

Best Augmenting Agents for AEs
• For tremor, combine with propranolol. Most AEs cannot be improved with an augmenting agent

DOSING AND USE

Usual Dosage Range
• 600–1200 mg/day (for headache) in divided doses

Dosage Forms
• Tablets: 300 mg. Extended release 300 mg, 450 mg
• Capsules: 150 mg, 300 mg, 600 mg
• Syrup: 8 mEq (300 mg/5 mL) (citrate)

How to Dose
• Headache: start at 600 mg at night or 300 mg twice daily. Start 300 mg at night in sensitive or elderly patients. Increase dose after a few days until headaches improve. Usually effective at doses of 1200 mg/day or less

 Dosing Tips
• Dosing with extended-release tablets taken at night may reduce GI and other AEs

Overdose
• Tremor, dysarthria, delirium, coma, seizures, and death have been reported

Long-Term Use
• Safe for long-term use with monitoring

Habit Forming
• No

How to Stop
• Taper at 2 weeks after cessation of cluster attacks. Taper much more slowly in patients with bipolar disorder

Pharmacokinetics
• Elimination half-life about 24 hours. Mostly excreted unchanged in urine

 Drug Interactions
• Osmotic diuretics, theophyllines, urinary alkalinizers, and acetazolamide increase renal excretion and decrease levels
• Loop diuretics, angiotensin-converting enzyme inhibitors, and thiazide diuretics increase levels
• NSAIDs decrease renal clearance of lithium
• Topiramate decreases lithium levels
• Fluoxetine may increase levels
• Methyldopa, carbamazepine, phenytoin, haloperidol, and phenothiazines may increase neurotoxic effects, even with normal serum levels
• May increase effects of neuromuscular blocking drugs
• Verapamil may either reduce levels or cause toxicity
• Metronidazole may increase toxicity
• Use with SSRIs may cause diarrhea, tremor, dizziness, agitation (rare)

 Other Warnings/ Precautions
• Increases sodium excretion – maintain normal diet and consider salt supplementation
• Encephalopathy with irreversible brain damage may occur in patients taking lithium with haloperidol

Do Not Use
• Hypersensitivity to drug, cardiac arrhythmia, severe dehydration or hyponatremia, or severe kidney disease

Renal Impairment
- Chronic use is associated with glomerular and interstitial fibrosis. Avoid using in patients with significant disease or those developing abnormalities on treatment

Hepatic Impairment
- No known effects

Cardiac Impairment
- Do not use in patients with arrhythmias or heart failure

Elderly
- Require lower doses to achieve therapeutic levels and more likely to experience AEs

Children and Adolescents
- Appears safe in children over age 12. Monitor more closely

Pregnancy
- Category D. May increase cardiac abnormalities, such as Ebstein's anomaly. Do not use for headache disorders

Breast Feeding
- Not recommended. Lithium is found in breast milk and hypertonia, cyanosis, and ECG changes have been reported

THE ART OF NEUROPHARMACOLOGY

Potential Advantages
- Effective in cluster headache at levels below those needed for mood disorders

Potential Disadvantages
- Potential AEs with long-term therapy and narrow therapeutic window

Primary Target Symptoms
- Headache frequency and severity

Pearls
- Effective in cluster headache, even in patients with chronic cluster headache with no headache-free months. Most patients will require a relatively low dose (1200 mg/day or less) when compared with doses used for acute mania (often 1800 mg/day), but higher doses can be used if needed, with monitoring of serum levels
- For patients with episodic cycles of cluster headache, taper off starting 2 weeks after last attack. For chronic cluster, periodically taper medication every 6–12 months to detect remissions
- Patients with hypnic or "alarm-clock" headache may respond to doses of 300–600 mg at night. Hypnic headache is more common in elderly patients
- Limited if any efficacy in migraine
- CNS manifestations of lithium toxicity often persist for days after serum levels return to normal levels
- May work best in euphoric mania rather than mixed states or rapid cycling
- Lithium-related weight may be more common in women

Suggested Reading

Cohen AS, Matharu MS, Goadsby PJ. Trigeminal autonomic cephalalgias: current and future treatments. Headache 2007;47(6):969–80

Geddes JR, Burgess S, Hawton K, Jamison K, Goodwin GM. Long-term lithium therapy for bipolar disorder: systematic review and meta-analysis of randomized controlled trials. Am J Psychiatry 2004;161(2):217–22.

Karlovasitou A, Avdelidi E, Andriopoulou G, Baloyannis S. Transient hypnic headache syndrome in a patient with bipolar disorder after the withdrawal of long-term lithium treatment: a case report. Cephalalgia 2009;29(4):484–6.

Maj M. The effect of lithium in bipolar disorder: a review of recent research evidence. Bipolar Disord 2003;5(3):180–8.

Silberstein SD. Preventive migraine treatment. Neurol Clin 2009;27(2):429–43.

MANNITOL

THERAPEUTICS

Brands
- Osmitrol

Generic
- Yes

Class
- Osmotic diuretic

Commonly Prescribed for
(FDA approved in bold)
- **Reduction of elevated intracranial pressure (ICP)**
- **Reduction of elevated intraocular pressure**
- **Diuresis (prophylaxis in acute renal failure)**
- **Increased excretion of urinary toxins**
- **Urologic irrigation**

How the Drug Works
- Mannitol induces diuresis by elevating the osmolarity of the glomerular filtrate, which decreases tubular reabsorption of water

How Long Until It Works
- 15 minutes

If It Works
- Assess effectiveness and need for continued use. Usually used as a short-term measure before more definitive treatment

If It Doesn't Work
- Usually mannitol is a temporary measure for acute increases in ICP before more definitive treatment

Best Augmenting Combos for Partial Response or Treatment-Resistance
- Treatment of increased ICP depends on the etiology
- Causes of increased ICP due to general swelling include liver failure, hypertensive encephalopathy, and hypercarbia. Intervention should consist of treating the underlying medical problem
- In some cases, meningitis can cause increased production of CSF or obstruction of CSF flow
- Increased ICP due to mass effect from stroke (ischemic or hemorrhagic), may require neurosurgical intervention such as an intraventricular catheter, craniotomy, or craniectomy
- Permitting hypertension may increase perfusion and improve swelling, but calcium channel blockers may also be useful (especially in subarachnoid hemorrhage)
- Analgesia and sedation may be useful
- Hyperventilation, hypothermia, and barbiturate coma are occasionally used, usually in refractory cases
- Hypertonic saline is an alternative to mannitol for acutely increased ICP
- Corticosteroids are often used to reduce vasogenic edema, i.e., brain tumors

Tests
- Carefully monitor serum sodium, potassium, BUN, and urine output during therapy

ADVERSE EFFECTS (AEs)

How Drug Causes AEs
- Most are related to changes in electrolytes and diuresis

Notable AEs
- Pulmonary edema, hypo- or hypertension, tachycardia
- Headache, thirst, nausea, diarrhea, blurred vision, rhinitis, chills, fever

Life-Threatening or Dangerous AEs
- Severe hypernatremia or renal failure

Weight Gain
- Unusual

Sedation
- Unusual

What to Do About AEs
- Hold infusion for any significant AEs. Discontinue infusion if urine output is low

Best Augmenting Agents for AEs
- Most AEs cannot be improved by augmenting agents

DOSING AND USE

Usual Dosage Range
- 100–200 g/kg per day

Dosage Forms
- Infusion: 5% in 1000 mL, 10% in 500 or 1000 mL, 15% in 150 or 500 mL, 20% in 250 or 500 mL, 25% in 50 mL vials and 5 g/100 mL solution

How to Dose
- The 20% or 25% solution is the most efficient. Give 0.25 to 2 g/kg body weight over 30 to 60 minutes. Adjust to maintain a urine flow between 30 to 50 mL/hr

 Dosing Tips
- Effect of treatment should be apparent by 15 minutes, and peak effect occurs from 30–60 minutes

Overdose
- May result in increased renal excretion of sodium, potassium, or chloride. Risks include orthostatic tachycardia, hypotension, weakness, intestinal dilation, ileus, and pulmonary edema

Long-Term Use
- Unknown

Habit Forming
- No

How to Stop
- No need to taper. Monitor neurological status after discontinuation

Pharmacokinetics
- Only slightly metabolized. Excreted by kidney. About 80% of a dose renally excreted in 3 hours. Peak effect at 30–60 minutes

 Drug Interactions
- Many additives are incompatible with mannitol
- Do not give with blood products (may cause clumping of erythrocytes)

 Other Warnings/ Precautions
- May increase blood flow and the risk of postoperative neurosurgical bleeding

Do Not Use
- Anuria due to renal failure
- Pulmonary congestion or edema, congestive heart failure
- Active intracranial bleeding
- Progressive renal disease or dysfunction after mannitol
- Known hypersensitivity

SPECIAL POPULATIONS

Renal Impairment
- Do not use in anuric patients or worsening renal functioning after mannitol. In those with renal impairment, give a test dose of 0.2 g/kg body weight as a 15% to 25% solution over a period of 3 to 5 minutes. If urine output does not increase, give a second test dose. If no effect, discontinue use

Hepatic Impairment
- No known effects

Cardiac Impairment
- Do not use with severe congestive heart failure

Elderly
- No known effects

 Children and Adolescents
- As in adults, use 0.25 to 2 g/kg as a 15% to 20% solution. Give over a longer period – up to 6 hours

 Pregnancy
- Category B. Use only if clearly needed

Breast Feeding
- Unknown if excreted in breast milk

THE ART OF NEUROPHARMACOLOGY

Potential Advantages
- Rapid onset of action for treatment of increased ICP. No central line access needed for administration

Potential Disadvantages
- Does not address the cause of increased ICP and not always effective

Primary Target Symptoms
- Symptoms of increased ICP which may include nausea/vomiting, headache, papilledema, extraocular palsies, pupillary dilation, hypertension, bradycardia, or changes in breathing pattern (hyperventilation or Cheyne-Stokes respiration)

Pearls
- Long-standing first-line drug for increased ICP, but new available medical therapies have challenged this. Mannitol actually has little evidence for improving outcomes
- Recent studies suggest small boluses of hypertonic saline, 3–23.4%, may be superior to mannitol for acute ICP treatment, with greater reductions of ICP and more rapid effect. Prolonged use requires central line placement

Suggested Reading

Davis SM. Medical management of haemorrhagic stroke. Crit Care Resusc 2005;7(3):185–8.

Forsyth LL, Liu-DeRyke X, Parker D Jr, Rhoney DH. Role of hypertonic saline for the management of intracranial hypertension after stroke and traumatic brain injury. Pharmacotherapy 2008;28(4):469–84.

White H, Cook D, Venkatesh B. The use of hypertonic saline for treating intracranial hypertension after traumatic brain injury. Anesth Analg 2006;102(6):1836–46.

THERAPEUTICS

Brands
• Antivert, Bonine

Generic?
Yes

Class
• Antiemetic, vestibular suppressant, antihistamine

Commonly Prescribed for
(FDA approved in bold)
• **Motion sickness**
• **Vertigo**

 How the Drug Works
• Antihistamine and anticholinergic drug

How Long Until It Works
• 30 minutes

If It Works
• Continue to use as needed, especially in short-term disorders, such as viral labyrinthitis

If It Doesn't Work
• Treat the underlying disorder with appropriate agents for that disorder
• Benzodiazepines (valium) may be effective for vertigo; antiemetics, such as promethazine, help also treat motion sickness

 Best Augmenting Combos for Partial Response or Treatment-Resistance
• Benzodiazepines (valium) may be effective for vertigo
• Meniere's disease: diuretics, antiemetics, and low-salt diet
• Vestibular rehabilitation may be helpful

Tests
• None

ADVERSE EFFECTS (AEs)

How Drug Causes AEs
• Antihistamine and anticholinergic actions

Notable AEs
• Dry mouth, sedation are most common
• Paradoxical excitation (nervousness, agitation), blurred vision, rash, tinnitus
• Hypotension, tachycardia

 Life-Threatening or Dangerous AEs
• May precipitate narrow-angle glaucoma
• Risk of heat stroke, especially in elderly patients
• Can precipitate tachycardia, cardiac arrhythmias, and hypotension
• May cause urinary retention in patients with prostate hypertrophy

Weight Gain
• Common

unusual   not unusual   common   problematic

Sedation
• Common

unusual   not unusual   common   problematic

What to Do About AEs
• Sedation – give at night or lower dose
• Dry mouth – chewing gum or water

Best Augmenting Agents for AEs
• Most AEs cannot be improved with the use of an augmenting agent

DOSING AND USE

Usual Dosage Range
• Vertigo: 25–100 mg/day

Dosage Forms
• Tablets: 12.5 mg, 25 mg, 50 mg
• Chewable: 25 mg
• Capsules: 25 mg

How to Dose
• Motion sickness: 25–50 mg 1 hour before travel
• Vertigo: 25–50 mg 2–3 times daily (maximum 100 mg/day)

Dosing Tips
• Taking with meals may reduce AEs

Overdose
• Large overdoses may cause convulsions, hallucinations or respiratory depression

Long-Term Use
• Unknown, usually a short-term medication

Habit Forming
• No

How to Stop
• No need to taper

Pharmacokinetics
• Onset of action in 30–60 minutes, duration of action 4–24 hours depending on dose

 Drug Interactions
• Increases AEs of CNS depressants

 Other Warnings/ Precautions
• Use with caution in hot weather – may increase risk of heat stroke
• Tablets contain tartrazine, which may precipitate allergic-type reactions in asthmatic patients

Do Not Use
• Known hypersensitivity to the drug, severe asthma, glaucoma (especially angle-closure type), prostate hypertrophy or bladder neck obstructions, severe dyspnea

SPECIAL POPULATIONS

Renal Impairment
• No known effects

Hepatic Impairment
• Eliminated more slowly in patients with severe disease

Cardiac Impairment
• Use with caution in patients with orthostatic hypotension

Elderly
• Use with caution. More susceptible to AEs

 Children and Adolescents
• Appear safe in children over 12

 Pregnancy
• Category B. No known teratogenicity

Breast Feeding
• Use if benefits outweigh risk

THE ART OF NEUROPHARMACOLOGY

Potential Advantages
• Useful in the treatment of acute vertigo and motion sickness

Potential Disadvantages
• Often ineffective for long-term disorders associated with vertigo, such as migraine or Meniere's disease

Primary Target Symptoms
• Vertigo, nausea

 Pearls
• Usually used for the short-term management of viral labrynthitis
• Antihistamine and anticholinergic AEs often limit use

Suggested Reading

Baloh RW. Approach to the dizzy patient. Baillieres Clin Neurol 1994;3(3):453–65.

Horak FB, Jones-Rycewicz C, Black FO, Shumway-Cook A. Effects of vestibular rehabilitation on dizziness and imbalance. Otolaryngol Head Neck Surg 1992; 106(2):175–80.

Newman-Toker DE, Camargo CA Jr, Hsieh YH, Pelletier AJ, Edlow JA. Disconnect between charted vestibular diagnoses and emergency department management decisions: a cross-sectional analysis from a nationally representative sample. Acad Emerg Med 2009;16(10):970–7.

MEMANTINE

THERAPEUTICS

Brands
- Namenda, Ebixa

Generic?
No

Class
- NMDA receptor antagonist

Commonly Prescribed for
(FDA approved in bold)
- **Alzheimer dementia (AD) (moderate or severe)**
- Vascular dementia
- Parkinson's disease related dementia
- Dementia with Lewy bodies (DLB)
- HIV dementia
- Migraine prophylaxis
- Neuropathic pain
- Attention deficit hyperactivity disorder
- Binge-eating disorder

How the Drug Works
- Binds preferentially to NMDA receptors, preventing glutamate from activating these receptors. The excitatory effects of glutamate are postulated to contribute to the development of AD and lesions such as neurofibrillary tangles
- Although symptoms of AD can improve, memantine does not prevent disease progression

How Long Until It Works
- Weeks to months

If It Works
- Continue to use but symptoms of dementia usually continue to worsen

If It Doesn't Work
- Non-pharmacologic measures are the basis of dementia treatment. Maintain regular schedules and routines. Avoid prolonged travel, unnecessary medical procedures or emergency room visits, crowds, and large social gatherings
- Limit drugs with sedative properties such as opioids, hypnotics, antiepileptic drugs and tricyclic antidepressants

- Treat other disorders which can worsen symptoms such as hyperglycemia, or urinary difficulties

Best Augmenting Combos for Partial Response or Treatment-Resistance
- Addition of cholinesterase inhibitors may be beneficial. In one study donepezil plus memantine reduced the rate of progression compared to those taking donepezil alone
- Treat depression, if present, with SSRIs. Avoid tricyclic antidepressants in demented patients due to risk of confusion
- For significant confusion and agitation avoid neuroleptics (especially in Lewy body dementia) to avoid the risk of neuroleptic malignant syndrome. Atypical antipsychotics (risperidone, quetiapine, olanzapine, clozapine) can be used instead

Tests
- None required

ADVERSE EFFECTS (AEs)

How Drug Causes AEs
- Direct effect on NMDA receptors

Notable AEs
- Hypertension, dizziness, constipation, coughing, dyspnea, fatigue, pain, ataxia, vertigo, confusion

Life-Threatening or Dangerous AEs
- Syncope or cardiac arrhythmias can occur although it is unclear that these events are related to memantine

Weight Gain
- Unusual

Sedation
- Unusual

What to Do About AEs
- In patients with dementia, determining if AEs are related to medication or another medical

condition can be difficult. For CNS side effects, discontinuation of non-essential centrally acting medications may help. If a bothersome AE is clearly drug-related then discontinue memantine

Best Augmenting Agents for AEs

- Most AEs do not respond to adding other medications

DOSING AND USE

Usual Dosage Range

- 5–20 mg/daily

Dosage Forms

- Tablets: 5, 10 mg
- Oral Solution: 2 mg/mL

How to Dose

- Start at 5 mg in the evening. Increase by 5 mg per week until taking 10 mg twice daily or until reaching desired effect. Do not increase dose faster than intervals of 1 week. If AEs occur, titrate more slowly

 Dosing Tips

- Slow titration can reduce AEs. Food does not affect absorption

Overdose

- Symptoms may include restlessness, psychosis, hallucinations, and stupor. Treatment: acidification of urine will enhance urinary excretion of memantine

Long-Term Use

- Safe for long-term use. Effectiveness may decrease over time as the dementing illness progresses

Habit Forming

- No

How to Stop

- Abrupt discontinuation is unlikely to produce AEs except worsening of dementia symptoms

Pharmacokinetics

- Most drug is secreted in urine unchanged with an elimination half-life of 60–80 hours. Minimal inhibition of CYP p450 enzymes.

Metabolites have little clinical effect. Peak effect at 3–7 hours. Protein binding 45%

 Drug Interactions

- Use with caution with other drugs which are NMDA antagonists (amantadine, ketamine, dextromethorphan)
- Use with caution with drugs that also utilize renal mechanisms of excretion such as ranitidine, cimetidine, hydrochlorothiazide or nicotine
- Drugs that make urine alkaline (carbonic anhydrase inhibitors, sodium bicarbonate) reduce memantine clearance. Use with caution

Do Not Use

- Hypersensitivity to the drug

SPECIAL POPULATIONS

Renal Impairment

- Drug is renally excreted. Consider dose reduction with moderate impairment and do not use in patients with severe renal insufficiency

Hepatic Impairment

- No known effects

Cardiac Impairment

- No significant change in ECG observed in trials compared to placebo. No known effects

Elderly

- There is reduced drug clearance, but no dose adjustment needed as the dose used is the lowest that provides clinical improvement

 Children and Adolescents

- Not studied in children. AD does not occur in children

 Pregnancy

- Category B. Decreased birth weight in animal studies. Use only if benefits of medication outweigh risks

Breast Feeding

- Unknown if excreted in breast milk. Use with caution

THE ART OF NEUROPHARMACOLOGY

Potential Advantages
- Proven effectiveness for AD, even with severe dementia. Fewer cholinergic or GI AEs than cholinesterase inhibitors

Potential Disadvantages
- Cost and minimal effectiveness. Does not prevent progression of AD or other dementias. May be less effective for Lewy body dementia than cholinesterase inhibitors

Primary Target Symptoms
- Confusion, agitation, performing activities of daily living

Pearls
- May be used in combination with cholinesterase inhibitors with good effect
- Effective for migraine prophylaxis in open-label studies at doses of 10 mg/day or greater
- Structurally related to amantadine, a weak NMDA antagonist

Suggested Reading

Downey D. Pharmacologic management of Alzheimer disease. J Neurosci Nurs 2008;40(1):55–9.

Grossberg GT, Edwards KR, Zhao Q. Rationale for combination therapy with galantamine and memantine in Alzheimer's disease. J Clin Pharmacol. 2006;46 (7 Suppl 1):17S–26S

Krymchantowski A, Jevoux C. Memantine in the preventive treatment for migraine and refractory migraine. Headache 2009;49(3):481–2.

McKeage K. Memantine: a review of its use in moderate to severe Alzheimer's disease. CNS Drugs 2009;23(10):881–97.

Porsteinsson AP, Grossberg GT, Mintzer J, Olin JT; Memantine MEM-MD-12 Study Group. Memantine treatment in patients with mild to moderate Alzheimer's disease already receiving a cholinesterase inhibitor: a randomized, double-blind, placebo-controlled trial. Curr Alzheimer Res 2008;5(1):83–9.

Schmitt FA, van Dyck CH, Wichems CH, Olin JT; for the Memantine MEM-MD-02 Study Group. Cognitive response to memantine in moderate to severe Alzheimer disease patients already receiving donepezil: an exploratory reanalysis. Alzheimer Dis Assoc Disord 2006;20(4):255–62.

METAXALONE

THERAPEUTICS

Brands
- Skelaxin

Generic?
Yes

 Class
- Skeletal muscle relaxant, centrally acting

Commonly Prescribed for
(FDA approved in bold)
- **Musculoskeletal conditions. (Adjunct to rest and physical therapy for relief of acute pain.)**
- Spasticity

 How the Drug Works
- Unclear but might be related to general CNS depression effect

How Long Until It Works
- Pain – hours

If It Works
- Slowly titrate to most effective tolerated dose

If It Doesn't Work
- Increase to highest tolerated dose and consider alternative treatments

 Best Augmenting Combos for Partial Response or Treatment-Resistance
- Use other centrally acting muscle relaxants with caution due to potential CNS depressant effect
- Can combine with NSAIDs for acute pain

Tests
- None

ADVERSE EFFECTS (AEs)

How Drug Causes AEs
- CNS depression

Notable AEs
- Nausea, drowsiness, dizziness, headache, irritability, rash

 Life-Threatening or Dangerous AEs
- Hemolytic anemia or leukopenia have been reported

Weight Gain
- Unusual

unusual | not unusual | common | problematic

Sedation
- Common

unusual | not unusual | common | problematic

What to Do About AEs
- Lower the dose or discontinue drug

Best Augmenting Agents for AEs
- Most AEs cannot be improved by an augmenting agent

DOSING AND USE

Usual Dosage Range
- 800–3200 mg/day

Dosage Forms
- Tablets: 800 mg

How to Dose
- In children over 12 and adults, give 400–800 mg 3–4 times daily

 Dosing Tips
- Taking with food increases CNS depression

Overdose
- Overdose with alcohol can lead to death. Treat with gastric lavage and supportive therapy

Long-Term Use
- Not well studied

Habit Forming
- No

How to Stop
- Taper not required

Pharmacokinetics

- Peak effect at 3 hours and half-life 9 hours. Hepatic metabolism to metabolites excreted in urine

 Drug Interactions

- May enhance effect of other CNS depressants, such as alcohol, barbiturates, or benzodiazepines

 Other Warnings/ Precautions

- May impair mental or physical abilities when driving or performing hazardous tasks

Do Not Use

- Known hypersensitivity to the drug, hemolytic anemia, or severe renal or hepatic disease

SPECIAL POPULATIONS

Renal Impairment

- Not studied – use with caution

Hepatic Impairment

- Not studied – use with caution

Cardiac Impairment

- No known effects

Elderly

- Drug metabolism is slower in elderly patients. Use with caution

 Children and Adolescents

- Not studied in children under age 12

 Pregnancy

- Not categorized due to lack of data but likely category B. Use only if there is a clear need

Breast Feeding

- Unknown if excreted in breast milk but likely, due to drug structure

THE ART OF NEUROPHARMACOLOGY

Potential Advantages

- Relatively safe for the short-term treatment of pain with few drug interactions

Potential Disadvantages

- Not effective for most pain symptoms related to neurological disorders, such as spasticity due to multiple sclerosis, migraine, or neuropathic pain disorders

Primary Target Symptoms

- Spasticity, pain

Pearls

- Patients with spasticity due to multiple sclerosis or spinal cord disease are more likely to respond to baclofen or tizanidine

 Suggested Reading

Chou R, Peterson K, Helfand M. Comparative efficacy and safety of skeletal muscle relaxants for spasticity and musculoskeletal conditions: a systematic review. J Pain Symptom Manage 2004;28(2):140–75.

See S, Ginzburg R. Choosing a skeletal muscle relaxant. Am Fam Physician 2008;78(3):365–70.

Toth PP, Urtis J. Commonly used muscle relaxant therapies for acute low back pain: a review of carisoprodol, cyclobenzaprine hydrochloride, and metaxalone. Clin Ther 2004;26(9):1355–67. Review

METHOCARBAMOL

THERAPEUTICS

Brands
• Robaxin

Generic?
Yes

 Class
• Skeletal muscle relaxant, centrally acting

Commonly Prescribed for
(FDA approved in bold)
• **Musculoskeletal conditions. (Adjunct to rest and physical therapy for relief of acute pain.)**
• Muscle spasm

 How the Drug Works
• Unclear but might be related to general CNS depression effect

How Long Until It Works
• Pain – 30 minutes or less

If It Works
• Slowly titrate to most effective tolerated dose

If It Doesn't Work
• Increase to highest tolerated dose and consider alternative treatments

 Best Augmenting Combos for Partial Response or Treatment-Resistance
• Use other centrally acting muscle relaxants with caution due to potential additive CNS depressant effect
• Can combine with NSAIDs for acute pain

Tests
• None

ADVERSE EFFECTS (AEs)

How Drug Causes AEs
• Most AEs are due to CNS depression

Notable AEs
• Confusion, amnesia, dizziness, drowsiness, sedation, blurred vision, nystagmus, bradycardia, hypotension, pruritus, nasal congestion. Jaundice has been reported

 Life-Threatening or Dangerous AEs
• Leukopenia, seizures, and anaphylactic reactions have been reported

Weight Gain
• Unusual

unusual   not unusual   common   problematic

Sedation
• Common

unusual   not unusual   common   problematic

What to Do About AEs
• Lower the dose or discontinue drug

Best Augmenting Agents for AEs
• Most AEs cannot be improved by an augmenting agent

DOSING AND USE

Usual Dosage Range
• 4–8 grams per day in divided doses

Dosage Forms
• Tablets: 500 mg, 750 mg
• Injection: 100 mg/mL

How to Dose
• For acute muscle spasm, start 1500 mg 4 times daily (max 8 grams per day). Decrease dose to 1000 mg 4 times daily or 1500 mg 3 times daily after a few days

 Dosing Tips
• Initially give large doses at night if sedation is problematic

Overdose
• Overdose is most dangerous when combined with alcohol or other CNS depressants. Symptoms include nausea, drowsiness, hypotension, seizures, and

coma. Treat with gastric lavage and supportive therapy

Long-Term Use
• Not well studied

Habit Forming
• No

How to Stop
• Taper not required

Pharmacokinetics
• Peak effect at 2 hours and half-life 1–2 hours. Metabolized by dealkylation and hydroxylation to metabolites excreted in urine

 Drug Interactions
• May enhance effect of other CNS depressants such as alcohol, barbiturates or benzodiazepines
• Can inhibit the effect of pyridostigmine in myasthenia gravis
• Causes color interference in screening tests for 5-hydroxindoleacetic acid and urinary vanillylmandelic acid

 Other Warnings/ Precautions
• May impair mental or physical abilities when driving or performing hazardous tasks

Do Not Use
• Hypersensitivity to the drug, severe renal or hepatic disease

Renal Impairment
• Clearance reduced by 40% in end-stage renal disease. Use with caution

Hepatic Impairment
• Clearance reduced by about 70% in patients with alcoholic cirrhosis. Reduce dose and use with caution

Cardiac Impairment
• No known effects

Elderly
• Drug metabolism is slightly slower in elderly patients. Use with caution

 Children and Adolescents
• Not studied in children under age 16 except in tetanus. For the treatment of tetanus, give 15 mg/kg intravenously and repeat every 6 hours as needed

 Pregnancy
• Category C. Use only if there is a clear need

Breast Feeding
• Likely excreted in human milk, do not use

Potential Advantages
• Relatively safe for the short-term treatment of pain with few drug interactions. Useful in the treatment of tetanus

Potential Disadvantages
• Not effective for most pain symptoms related to neurological disorders such as spasticity due to multiple sclerosis, migraine, or neuropathic pain disorders

Primary Target Symptoms
• Spasticity, pain

 Pearls
• Most patients with spasticity due to multiple sclerosis or spinal cord diseases are more likely to respond to baclofen or tizanidine
• May be helpful as an injection in helping to control the neuromuscular manifestations of tetanus in addition to usual treatments

Suggested Reading

Chou R, Peterson K, Helfand M. Comparative efficacy and safety of skeletal muscle relaxants for spasticity and musculoskeletal conditions: a systematic review. J Pain Symptom Manage 2004;28(2):140–75.

See S, Ginzburg R. Choosing a skeletal muscle relaxant. Am Fam Physician 2008;78(3):365–70.

Valtonen EJ. A double-blind trial of methocarbamol versus placebo in painful muscle spasm. Curr Med Res Opin 1975;3(6):382–5.

METHOTREXATE

THERAPEUTICS

Brands
- Amethopterin, Emthexate, Ledertrexate, Maxtrex, Mexate, MTX, Trexall, Rheumatrex, Metoject

Generic?
Yes

Class
- Folic acid antagonist, immunomodulator

Commonly Prescribed for
(FDA approved in bold)
- **Treatment of malignancies, including non-Hodgkin lymphoma, gestational choriocarcinoma, head and neck epidermoid cancer, and lung and breast cancer**
- **Psoriasis**
- **Rheumatoid arthritis**
- Inflammatory myopathies: polymyositis (PM) and dermatomyositis (DM)
- Vasculitis, including Wegener's granulomatosis
- Relapsing-remitting or chronic progressive multiple sclerosis (MS)
- Ulcerative colitis or Crohn's disease
- Systemic lupus erythematosus
- Psoriatic arthritis

How the Drug Works
- Inhibits dihydrofolic acid reductase. Prevents synthesis of purine nucleotides and thymodylate. This interferes with DNA synthesis, repair, and replication

How Long Until It Works
- Within a week, but effect on neurological diseases may take months

If It Works
- DM/PM: improves strength, and may allow discontinuation or reduced dose of corticosteroids. Corticosteroids are tapered first. Taper slowly over 6 months if clinical remission occurs
- MS: May reduce relapses and new lesions on MRI
- Other disorders: Improves symptoms and clinical markers of the disease

If It Doesn't Work
- DM/PM: Question the diagnosis (inclusion-body myositis, hypothyroidism, muscular dystrophy), rule out corticosteroid-induced myopathy, and evaluate for undiagnosed malignancy (especially in DM). Change to azathioprine
- MS: If clearly not helpful, change to another agent

Best Augmenting Combos for Partial Response or Treatment-Resistance
- Usually used in combination with corticosteroids (to reduce corticosteroid dose) in DM and PM. Occasionally combined with other treatments for the treatment of MS

Tests
- Obtain CBC, liver and renal function tests, and chest x-ray at baseline and at dosage adjustments, or for any clinical symptoms. Use serum level and WBC to assess response to treatment

ADVERSE EFFECTS (AEs)

How Drug Causes AEs
- Folic acid antagonism

Notable AEs
- Ulcerative stomatitis, nausea, abdominal distress
- Malaise, fatigue, chills and fever, dizziness
- Headache, speech impairment, convulsions, encephalopathy
- Rash or photosensitivity
- Elevated liver function tests (up to 15%)

Life-Threatening or Dangerous AEs
- Leukopenia, anemia, aplastic anemia, thrombocytopenia
- Thrombotic events, such as cerebral thrombosis and pulmonary embolus
- Respiratory fibrosis and failure, renal failure
- Leukoencephalopathy, stroke-like symptoms (usually with high-doses IV only)

Weight Gain
- Unusual

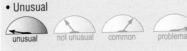

Sedation
- Unusual

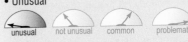

What to Do About AEs
- Renal failure – stop drug and ensure adequate hydration and urine alkalinization
- Hepatic failure – transient abnormalities are common. For persistently abnormal tests, perform liver biopsy and discontinue if moderate to severe changes. For significant disease, stop drug
- Pulmonary symptoms – cough or dyspnea could indicate significant disease. Stop drug and evaluate with chest x-ray

Best Augmenting Agents for AEs
- Leucovorin (a folate analog that is able to participate in reactions utilizing folates) is used after high-dose therapy as a rescue drug. Give 15 mg orally, IM, or IV every 6 hours for 10 doses

---

DOSING AND USE

Usual Dosage Range
- DM/PM – 7.5–30 mg/week
- Rheumatoid arthritis, MS – 7.5 mg/week

Dosage Forms
- Tablets: 2.5 mg, 5 mg, 7.5 mg, 10 mg, 15 mg
- Injection: 2.5 mg/mL or 25 mg/mL, powder for injection (20 mg, 50 mg, 100 mg, and 1 g)

How to Dose
- DM/PM – 2.5 mg 3 times a day, 1 day per week initially. Increase dose based on clinical response and creatine kinase levels as long as WBC is 3000/mm^3 or greater every 2 weeks or greater
- MS – 7.5 mg once weekly, or 2.5 mg 3 times a day, 1 day per week. Dose is generally not increased

---

Dosing Tips
- Food delays absorption and reduces peak concentration

Overdose
- GI bleeding or ulceration, mucositis, and oral ulceration are common
- Hematologic reactions are common. Rarely renal failure, aplastic anemia, sepsis, shock, or death. Often occurs as a consequence of daily dosing (instead of weekly)

Long-Term Use
- Usually used on a short-term basis for refractory disorders

Habit Forming
- No

How to Stop
- No need to taper but monitor for recurrence of neurological disorder

Pharmacokinetics
- Oral absorption is dose- and patient-dependent (lower percentage with higher dose). Peak serum levels in 1–2 hours. Terminal half-life is 3–10 hours at low doses but 8–15 hours with high doses. Mostly (about 90%) renal excretion

Drug Interactions
- NSAIDs or salicylates may elevate levels and increase GI and hematologic toxicity
- Salicylates, phenylbutazone, phenytoin, and sulfonamides may displace methotrexate from albumin and increase toxicity
- Probenecid reduces renal tubular transport and increases levels
- Oral antibiotics such as aminoglycosides, chloramphenicol may decrease absorption
- May increase hepatotoxicity when used with other hepatotoxic agents, such as azathioprine
- May decrease clearance of theophylline, increasing levels
- Folic acid vitamins may reduce response to methotrexate, and folate deficiency may increase toxicity

Do Not Use

- Known hypersensitivity, pregnancy or breast feeding, preexisting blood dyscrasias, chronic liver disease, or alcoholism

Renal Impairment

- At greater risk for toxicity and renal function may worsen. Use with caution

Hepatic Impairment

- Do not use. Alcoholism, obesity, advanced age, and diabetes are risk factors for hepatotoxicity

Cardiac Impairment

- No known effects

Elderly

- Monitor closely. Bone marrow suppression, thrombocytopenia, and pneumonitis are more common

 Children and Adolescents

- In the treatment of cancer and rheumatoid arthritis, AEs are similar to adults. Not well-studied in children with DM or MS

 Pregnancy

- Category X. Causes abortion, embryotoxicity, and fetal defects. Avoid pregnancy after use for 3 months in men and at least 1 ovulatory cycle in women

Breast Feeding

- Do not breast feed

Potential Advantages

- Useful corticosteroid-sparing agent in PM/DM. Once-weekly dosing

Potential Disadvantages

- Multiple AEs complicate use

Primary Target Symptoms

- Preventive treatment of complications from PM, DM or MS

 Pearls

- In DM or PM, use azathioprine instead of methotrexate as a corticosteroid-sparing agent in patients with interstitial lung disease, liver disease or in those that refuse to abstain from alcohol
- Improvement in muscle strength a better predictor of improvement in PM or DM than a decrease in creatine kinase
- Anti-Jo-1 antibodies are predictive of worsening response in PM and DM
- PM in general is less likely to respond to corticosteroids (about 50%) than DM (over 80%), but DM patients may have a more difficult time tapering corticosteroids
- In RRMS, clinical studies demonstrated preservation of upper extremity function with low-dose weekly methotrexate at a dose of 7.5 mg/day once weekly (2.5 mg 3 times a day for 1 day). One study showed effectiveness in reducing the rate of progression in chronic progressive MS

Suggested Reading

Gray OM, McDonnell GV, Forbes RB. A systematic review of oral methotrexate for multiple sclerosis. Mult Scler 2006;12(4):507–10.

Hengstman GJ, van den Hoogen FH, van Engelen BG. Treatment of the inflammatory myopathies: update and practical recommendations. Expert Opin Pharmacother 2009;10(7):1183–90.

Tsuji G, Maekawa S, Saigo K, Nobuhara Y, Nakamura T, Kawano S, Koshiba M, Asahara S, Chinzei T, Kumagai S. Dermatomyositis and myelodysplastic syndrome with myelofibrosis responding to methotrexate therapy. Am J Hematol 2003;74(3):175–8.

Vencovský J, Jarosová K, Machácek S, Studýnková J, Kafková J, Bartůnková J, Nemcová D, Charvát F. Cyclosporine A versus methotrexate in the treatment of polymyositis and dermatomyositis. Scand J Rheumatol 2000;29 (2):95–102.

White ES, Lynch JP. Pharmacological therapy for Wegener's granulomatosis. Drugs 2006;66 (9):1209–28.

THERAPEUTICS

Brands
• Methergine

Generic?
Yes

Class
• Ergot, migraine preventive

Commonly Prescribed for
(FDA approved in bold)
• **Uterine contractions/bleeding after delivery**
• Migraine prophylaxis
• Cluster headache

How the Drug Works
• 5-HT2$_{A/B/C}$ receptor antagonist and 5-HT1$_{B/D}$ agonist
• Used to prevent or control excessive bleeding following childbirth and spontaneous or elective abortion. Causes uterine contractions to aid in expulsion of retained products of conception after miscarriage and to help deliver the placenta after childbirth
• Migraine/cluster: Proposed mechanisms include vasoconstrictive actions or inhibition of the release of inflammatory neuropeptides, such as calcitonin gene-related peptide. Prevention of cortical spreading depression may be the mechanism of action for all migraine preventatives. An active metabolite of methysergide

How Long Until It Works
• Obstetrical: hours, or minutes as an injection
• Migraines – within 2 weeks, but can take up to 2 months on a stable dose to see full effect

If It Works
• In migraine, the goal is a 50% or greater decrease in migraine frequency or severity. Consider tapering or stopping if headaches remit for more than 6 months or if considering pregnancy

If It Doesn't Work
• Increase to highest tolerated dose
• Migraine: address other issues, such as medication-overuse, other coexisting

medical disorders, such as anxiety, and consider changing to another drug or adding a second drug

Best Augmenting Combos for Partial Response or Treatment-Resistance
• Migraine: Usually used in refractory cases of migraine and cluster headache, usually as an adjunctive agent. May use in combination with AEDs, antidepressants, natural products, and non-pharmacologic treatments, such as biofeedback, to improve headache control

Tests
• Monitor blood pressure. In patients on long-term continuous therapy, consider screening for fibrotic disorders

ADVERSE EFFECTS (AEs)

How Drug Causes AEs
• Actions on serotonin receptors, including vasoconstriction. Fibrotic complications are related to 5H-T2$_B$ actions

Notable AEs
• Muscle aching, claudication, nausea, vomiting, weight gain
• Dizziness, giddiness, drowsiness, paresthesias
• Hypertension
• Rarely hallucinations

Life-Threatening or Dangerous AEs
• Severe hypertension
• Ergots and related drugs are associated with the development of retroperitoneal, pulmonary, or endocardial fibrosis. Long-term continuous use appears to be the biggest risk factor

Weight Gain
• Not unusual

Sedation
• Unusual

What to Do About AEs
- Lower dose for nausea, stop for serious AEs

Best Augmenting Agents for AEs
- Most AEs cannot be treated with an augmenting agent

DOSING AND USE

Usual Dosage Range
- 0.4–1.2 mg/day

Dosage Forms
- Tablets: 0.2 mg
- Injection: 0.2 mg/mL

How to Dose
- Obstetrical: 1 tablet 3–4 times daily, or injection (IM or IV) 0.2 mg every 2–4 hours
- Migraine: One tablet twice a day, increase by 1–2 tablets every week in 2–3 divided doses to maximum of 6 tablets per day

 Dosing Tips
- Taper off slowly to avoid headache recurrence

Overdose
- Abdominal pain, nausea, numbness, vomiting, paresthesias, and hypertension are most common. Convulsions, coma, hypotension, and respiratory depression have been reported

Long-Term Use
- Long-term, continuous use of methysergide (methylergonovine is a metabolite) is associated with the development of retroperitoneal, pulmonary, or endocardial fibrosis

Habit Forming
- No

How to Stop
- In migraine prophylaxis, reduce/taper dose over 2–4 weeks, as stopping quickly may trigger headache

Pharmacokinetics
- Mean elimination half-life 3–4 hours. Bioavailability is 60%. Hepatic metabolism and excretion

 Drug Interactions
- Use with caution with other vasoconstrictive agents, ergot alkaloids, or triptans
- Do not administer with potent CYP3A4 inhibitors, including macrolide antibiotics (erythromycin, clarithromycin), HIV protease or reverse transcriptase inhibitors (delaviridine, ritonavir, nelfinavir, indinavir), or azole antifungals (ketoconazole, itraconazole, voriconazole). Less potent 3A4 inhibitors include saquinavir, nefazodone, fluconazole, fluoxetine, fluvoxamine, grapefruit juice, and clotrimazole

 Other Warnings/ Precautions
- Use with caution in the setting of sepsis

Do Not Use
- With CYP-450 3A4 inhibitors
- Hypertension, toxemia, pregnancy,
- Proven hypersensitivity to drug

SPECIAL POPULATIONS

Renal Impairment
- Safety and effect of significant disease on drug metabolism unknown. Use with caution

Hepatic Impairment
- Safety and effect of significant disease on drug metabolism unknown. Avoid using in patients with severe disease

Cardiac Impairment
- Do not use in patients with hypertension or significant vascular disease

Elderly
- Use with caution, especially in those with known hypertension

 Children and Adolescents
- Not studied in children. The pediatric dose is unknown

Pregnancy
- Category C, but contraindicated due to uterotonic effects

Breast Feeding
- A small amount is found in breast milk. Use with caution

THE ART OF NEUROPHARMACOLOGY

Potential Advantages
- Believed effective and well-tolerated prophylactic agent in refractory migraine

Potential Disadvantages
- Potential for serious AEs, including fibrosis. Limited clinical trial evidence

Primary Target Symptoms
- Migraine frequency and severity

 Pearls
- Not a first-line drug, but may be used as a rescue preventive for very frequent migraines. Well-tolerated but long-term AEs of ergots may raise concerns. Most frequently used in tertiary headache clinics
- A metabolite of methysergide, an FDA-approved migraine prophylactic agent no longer available in the US
- Safety with other potentially vasoconstrictive drugs (i.e., triptans) is unknown
- Because methylergonovine and methysergide are weak vasoconstrictors compared with oral ergots, they are occasionally used for patients using triptans for acute attacks. In early clinical studies of sumatriptan many patients were on 5-HT2 agonists, such as methysergide or pizotifen. Consider the risks and benefit of treatment
- Perhaps most effective in cluster headache
- Reportedly effective in post-dural puncture headache

 Suggested Reading

Dodick DW, Silberstein SD. Migraine prevention. Pract Neurol 2007;7(6):383–93.

Gaiser R. Postdural puncture headache. Curr Opin Anaesthesiol 2006;19(3):249–53.

Graff-Radford SB, Bittar GT. The use of methylergonovine (Methergine) in the initial control of drug induced refractory headache. Headache 1993;33(7):390–3.

Mueller L, Gallagher RM, Ciervo CA. Methylergonovine maleate as a cluster headache prophylactic: a study and review. Headache 1997;37(7):437–42.

Silberstein SD. Preventive migraine treatment. Neurol Clin 2009;27(2):429–43.

THERAPEUTICS

Brands
• Sansert, Deseril

Generic?
Yes

Class
• Ergot, migraine preventative

Commonly Prescribed for
(FDA approved in bold)
• Migraine prophylaxis
• Cluster headache prophylaxis
• Diarrhea associated with carcinoid syndrome

How the Drug Works
• 5-HT2 and 5-HT1$_{A/B/C}$ receptor antagonist and partial agonist of 5-HT1$_{B/D}$. It is unclear which action accounts for drug effectiveness
• Migraine/cluster: Proposed mechanisms include vasoconstrictive actions or inhibition of the release of inflammatory neuropeptides, such as calcitonin gene-related peptide. Prevention of cortical spreading depression may be the mechanism of action for all migraine preventatives

How Long Until It Works
• Migraines – within 2 weeks, but can take up to 2 months on a stable dose to see full effect

If It Works
• In migraine, the goal is a 50% or greater decrease in migraine frequency or severity. Consider tapering or stopping if headaches remit for more than 6 months or if considering pregnancy

If It Doesn't Work
• Increase to highest tolerated dose
• Migraine/cluster: address other issues such as medication-overuse, other coexisting medical disorders, such as anxiety, and consider changing to another drug or adding a second drug

Best Augmenting Combos for Partial Response or Treatment-Resistance
• Migraine/cluster: Usually used in refractory cases of migraine and cluster headache, usually as an adjunctive agent. May use in combination with AEDs, antidepressants, natural products, and non-pharmacologic treatments, such as biofeedback, to improve headache control

Tests
• Monitor blood pressure. In patients on long-term continuous therapy, consider screening for fibrotic disorders

ADVERSE EFFECTS (AEs)

How Drug Causes AEs
• Actions on serotonin receptors including vasoconstriction. Fibrotic complications are related to 5-HT2$_B$ actions

Notable AEs
• Muscle aching, claudication, nausea, vomiting, weight gain
• Dizziness, giddiness, drowsiness, paresthesias, insomnia
• Hypertension, postural hypertension, tachycardia
• Rarely hallucinations, seizures, blood dyscrasias, such as neutropenia, eosinophilia, or thrombocytopenia

Life-Threatening or Dangerous AEs
• Severe hypertension
• Ergots and related drugs are associated with the development of retroperitoneal, pulmonary, or endocardial fibrosis. Long-term continuous use appears to be the biggest risk factor

Weight Gain
• Not Unusual

Sedation
• Unusual

What to Do About AEs
• Lower dose for nausea, stop for serious AEs

Best Augmenting Agents for AEs
- Most AEs cannot be treated with an augmenting agent

DOSING AND USE

Usual Dosage Range
- 4–8 mg/day

Dosage Forms
- Tablets: 1 mg, 2 mg

 Dosing Tips
- Taper off slowly to avoid headache recurrence

How to Dose
- Start 1 mg at bedtime, increase gradually over 2 weeks to 1–2 mg 2 times daily with food

Overdose
- Peripheral vasospasm, with diminished pulses, coldness, mottling, and cyanosis, have been reported. In children, hyperactivity, euphoria, and tachycardia have been reported. Remove with emesis or gastric lavage if needed

Long-Term Use
- Long-term, continuous use of methysergide is associated with the development of retroperitoneal, pulmonary, or endocardial fibrosis

Habit Forming
- No

How to Stop
- In migraine prophylaxis, reduce/taper dose over 2–4 weeks, as stopping quickly may trigger headache

Pharmacokinetics
- Methysergide is likely a prodrug rapidly converted to methylergometrine. Half-life is 60 minutes, but half-life of methylergometrine is 220 minutes. Bioavailability is only 13% due to high first-pass metabolism

 Drug Interactions
- Use with caution with other vasoconstrictive agents, ergot alkaloids, or triptans
- Do not administer with potent CYP3A4 inhibitors, including macrolide antibiotics (erythromycin, clarithromycin), HIV protease or reverse transcriptase inhibitors (delaviridine, ritonavir, nelfinavir, indinavir), or azole antifungals (ketoconazole, itraconazole, voriconazole). Less potent 3A4 inhibitors include saquinavir, nefazodone, fluconazole, fluoxetine, fluvoxamine, grapefruit juice, and clotrimazole
- May reverse the effect of opioid analgesics

⚠ Other Warnings/ Precautions
- Use with caution in the setting of sepsis or infection

Do Not Use
- Proven hypersensitivity to the drug or its components, pregnancy, lactation, peripheral vascular disease, severe hypertension, coronary artery disease, phlebitis or cellulitis of the lower limbs, pulmonary disease, collagen diseases or fibrotic processes, valvular heart disease, debilitated states, and serious infections

SPECIAL POPULATIONS

Renal Impairment
- Safety and effect of significant disease on drug metabolism unknown. Use with caution

Hepatic Impairment
- Safety and effect of significant disease on drug metabolism unknown. Avoid using in patients with significant disease

Cardiac Impairment
- Do not use in patients with hypertension, significant vascular or valvular disease

Elderly
- Use with caution, especially in those with known hypertension

Children and Adolescents

• Not studied in children. The pediatric dose is unknown

 Pregnancy

• Category X. Contraindicated due to uterotonic effects

Breast Feeding

• Found in breast milk. Do not breast feed while taking drug

THE ART OF NEUROPHARMACOLOGY

Potential Advantages

• Effective and well-tolerated prophylactic agent in refractory headache

Potential Disadvantages

• Potential for serious AEs, including fibrosis

Primary Target Symptoms

• Headache frequency and severity

 Pearls

• Not a first-line drug, but may be used as a rescue preventive for very frequent migraines. Well-tolerated but long-term AEs of ergots may raise concerns. Most frequently used in tertiary headache centers
• Compared to its metabolite, methylergonovine, is about 6 times more potent in its serotonin antagonism
• Safety with other potentially vasoconstrictive drugs (i.e., triptans) is unknown
• Because methergine and methysergide are weak vasoconstrictors compared with oral ergots, they are occasionally used for patients using triptans for acute attacks. In early clinical studies of sumatriptan, many patients were on 5-HT2 antagonists, such as methysergide or pizotifen. Consider the risks and benefit of treatment
• Perhaps most effective in cluster headache

 Suggested Reading

Dodick DW, Silberstein SD. Migraine prevention. Pract Neurol 2007;7(6):383–93.

Dodick DW, Capobianco DJ. Treatment and management of cluster headache. Curr Pain Headache Rep 2001;5(1):83–91.

Kottra JJ, Dunnick NR. Retroperitoneal fibrosis. Radiol Clin North Am 1996;34(6):1259–75.

Silberstein SD. Methysergide. Cephalalgia 1998;18(7):421–35.

METOCLOPRAMIDE

THERAPEUTICS

Brands
• Reglan, Maxolon

Generic?
Yes

Class
• Antiemetic, GI stimulant, antipsychotic

Commonly Prescribed for
(FDA approved in bold)
• **Diabetic gastroparesis**
• **Nausea and vomiting (postoperative, chemotherapy)**
• **Small bowel intubation**
• Symptomatic gastroesophageal reflux
• Migraine
• Tics in Gilles de la Tourette syndrome (GTS)

How the Drug Works
• Dopamine receptor antagonism (specifically D2) decreases nausea. It may also increase absorption of coadministered drugs. May stimulate GI motility by sensitizing tissues to the actions of acetylcholine or from 5-HT$_4$ receptor agonism

How Long Until It Works
• 30–60 minutes with oral dose for nausea. Gastroparesis improves maximally by 3 weeks

If It Works
• Use at lowest effective dose
• Continue to assess effect of the medication and if it is still needed

If It Doesn't Work
• Increase dose, or discontinue and change to another agent
• Migraine: change to another antiemetic (prochlorperazine, droperidol, chlorpromazine) or combine with other agents
• Gastroparesis: domperidone (where available) is an alternative. Smaller, more frequent meals with low fat and fiber might improve symptoms

Best Augmenting Combos for Partial Response or Treatment-Resistance
• Migraine: often combined with NSAIDs and triptans or ergots. Usually not used as monotherapy
• Gastroparesis: may be combined with erythromycin, Botulinum toxin, electrical gastric stimulation

Tests
• None required

ADVERSE EFFECTS (AEs)

How Drug Causes AEs
• Motor AEs and prolactinemia – blocking of D2 receptors

Notable AEs
• Most common: Sedation, CNS depression
• Fluid retention, bradycardia or superventricular tachycardia, hypo- or hypertension, rash, galactorrhea, urinary frequency or incontinence
• Akathisia, parkinsonism (bradykinesia, tremor, rigidity), acute dystonic reactions

Life-Threatening or Dangerous AEs
• Tardive dyskinesias
• Neuroleptic malignant syndrome (rare)
• Hepatotoxicity (rare)

Weight Gain
• Unusual

unusual / not unusual / common / problematic

Sedation
• Not unusual

unusual / not unusual / common / problematic

What to Do About AEs
• Excessive sedation: lower dose or use only as a rescue agent when patient can lie down or sleep
• Movement disorders: lower dose or stop

Best Augmenting Agents for AEs

- Give fluids to avoid hypotension, tachycardia, and dizziness
- Give anticholinergics (diphenhydramine or benztropine) or benzodiazepines for extrapyramidal reactions

DOSING AND USE

Usual Dosage Range

- Migraine: 5–30 mg/dose
- Gastroparesis: 10–15 mg 3–4 times daily before meals

Dosage Forms

- Tablets: 5 mg, 10 mg
- Syrup: 5 mg/5 mL
- Injection: 5 mg/mL

How to Dose

- Migraine/vertigo: IV, IM or oral. Non-oral routes are useful for severe vomiting. IV/IM: 10–30 mg 3–4 times daily. Oral: 10–20 mg, usually as adjunctive treatment

 Dosing Tips

- Give before meals for gastroparesis, and 10–20 minutes (oral or IM) before other medications for migraine. To reduce risk of motor AEs including akathisia, administer IV formulation more slowly (over 10–15 minutes)

Overdose

- Drowsiness, confusion, and extrapyramidal reactions may occur

Long-Term Use

- Risk of movement AEs (tardive dyskinesias, parkinsonism) with frequent use

Habit Forming

- No

How to Stop

- No need to taper

Pharmacokinetics

- Half-life 5–6 hours. Peak effect 1–2 hours

 Drug Interactions

- Increases bioavailability of levodopa due to increased absorption, which in turn decreases metoclopramide effect of gastric emptying
- Anticholinergics and opioids decrease effects on GI motility
- Releases catecholamines and may increase effect of MAO inhibitors
- May increase absorption and enhance effects of alcohol and cyclosporine
- May decrease effectiveness of cimetidine and digoxin due to decreased absorption due to faster transit time
- Increases the neuromuscular blocking effects of succinylcholine

 Other Warnings/ Precautions

- May precipitate hypertensive crisis in patients with pheochromocytoma
- Parkinsonism may occur, usually within 6 months of starting, and may persist for 2–3 months after discontinuation

Do Not Use

- Hypersensitivity to drug, known pheochromocytoma, or any condition where GI stimulation could be dangerous (bowel obstruction, hemorrhage, or perforation)

SPECIAL POPULATIONS

Renal Impairment

- Clearance decreased. Use lower doses

Hepatic Impairment

- Use with caution

Cardiac Impairment

- May alter blood pressure or cause fluid retention in patients with heart failure

Elderly

- More likely to experience movement AEs

 Children and Adolescents

- Efficacy and safety unknown. Poorly studied, but a dose of 0.15 mg/kg in acute migraine has been studied. In GTS, give 10–60 mg/daily in divided doses

Pregnancy
- Category B. Use for significant migraine or nausea during pregnancy if needed

Breast Feeding
- Found in breast milk. Monitor infant for sedation

THE ART OF NEUROPHARMACOLOGY

Potential Advantages
- Effective medication for intractable migraine, vomiting, or vertigo. Less sedation and orthostasis than most antiemetics and no risk of ECG changes

Potential Disadvantages
- Usually not effective as monotherapy in oral form. Potential for movement disorders, especially with long-term use

Primary Target Symptoms
- Headache, vertigo, and nausea

 Pearls
- In the treatment of status migrainosus, combining metoclopramide and dihydroergotamine for up to 1 week is usually effective. Give the metoclopramide first
- Pretreat or combine with diphenhydramine, 25–50 mg, to reduce rate of akathisia and dystonic reactions. Benztropine is also useful and may be given orally or IM
- In outpatients with severe or daily headache, may be used daily for short periods of time (3–10 days) as a bridge treatment in conjunction with NSAIDs before preventive medication becomes effective
- Appears safe for migraine treatment during pregnancy
- Originally thought to be peripherally acting, but CNS AEs including parkinsonism, tardive dyskinesias or dystonias are common with prolonged use
- In GTS, less weight gain or sedation compared to neuroleptics, but less evidence of effectiveness

 Suggested Reading

Friedman BW, Esses D, Solorzano C, Dua N, Greenwald P, Radulescu R, Chang E, Hochberg M, Campbell C, Aghera A, Valentin T, Paternoster J, Bijur P, Lipton RB, Gallagher EJ. A randomized controlled trial of prochlorperazine versus metoclopramide for treatment of acute migraine. Ann Emerg Med 2008;52(4):399–406.

Marmura MJ. Silberstein SD. Migraine: essentials of patient evaluation and acute treatment. Pract Neurol 2009;8(3):12–7.

Raskin NH. Repetitive intravenous dihydroergotamine as therapy for intractable migraine. Neurology 1986;36(7):995–7.

Regan LA, Hoffman RS, Nelson LS. Slower infusion of metoclopramide decreases the rate of akathisia. Am J Emerg Med 2009;27(4):475–80.

Silberstein SD, Ruoff G. Combination therapy in acute migraine treatment: the rationale behind the current treatment options. Postgrad Med 2006;Spec No:20–6.

Skidmore F, Reich SG. Tardive dystonia. Curr Treat Options Neurol 2005;7(3):231–6.

MEXILETINE

THERAPEUTICS

Brands
• Mexitil

Generic?
Yes

Class
• Antiarrhythmic

Commonly Prescribed for
(FDA approved in bold)
• **Cardiac arrhythmias**
• Symptomatic myotonia (myotonia congenita, myotonic dystrophy)
• Pain in peripheral neuropathy
• Intractable headache

How the Drug Works
• Class 1B antiarrhythmic agent that depresses phase 0 (reduces the rate of rise of the action potential). An oral analogue of lidocaine. It has actions on surfaces and membranes of skeletal muscle and neuronal sodium-channel blocking properties. It also reduces the effective refractory period in Purkinje fibers

How Long Until It Works
• Antiarrhythmic effect will occur within hours, although it may take time to find optimal dose. May take more time (days or weeks) to see relief and determine most effective dose in myotonia or pain disorders

If It Works
• Continue to use with appropriate monitoring

If It Doesn't Work
• Check serum levels and if not effective change to an alternative agent

Best Augmenting Combos for Partial Response or Treatment-Resistance
• Myotonia: Quinine and other anticonvulsants are occasionally used. Phenytoin is also effective but has similar antiarrhythmic properties and may interact with mexiletine
• Neuropathic pain: other anticonvulsants and antidepressants can be used

Tests
• Monitor hepatic enzymes and CBC during therapy. Obtain ECG at baseline and for any new symptoms. Check a serum mexiletine level to guide therapy and for any AEs

ADVERSE EFFECTS (AEs)

How Drug Causes AEs
• Drug effect blocking sodium channels

Notable AEs
• GI AEs (nausea, vomiting, heartburn) are most common. CNS AEs (tremor, nervousness, coordination difficulties, blurred vision, confusion) are much more common when serum levels exceed 2 mcg/mL

Life-Threatening or Dangerous AEs
• New or worsening cardiac arrhythmias
• Acute hepatic injury (usually in the first few weeks of therapy)
• Blood dyscrasias, including leukopenia (rare)

Weight Gain
• Unusual

unusual | not unusual | common | problematic

Sedation
• Not unusual

unusual | not unusual | common | problematic

What to Do About AEs
• Check serum level and ECG. For serious AEs, discontinue drug

Best Augmenting Agents for AEs
• Most AEs cannot be improved by an augmenting agent

DOSING AND USE

Usual Dosage Range
• 400–1200 mg/day in divided doses

Dosage Forms
• Tablets: 150, 200, 250 mg

How to Dose

- In patients on lidocaine infusion, stop lidocaine before starting mexiletine. Start at 200 mg every 8 hours. Adjust daily dose by 50–100 mg based on clinical effect every 3 or more days. Base dose on serum levels. Consider changing patients on a stable dose to twice-daily dosing

Dosing Tips

- Take with food to reduce AEs

Overdose

- Nausea, hypotension, sinus bradycardia, paresthesia, seizures, AV heart block, and ventricular tachycardias

Long-Term Use

- Safe for long-term use with appropriate monitoring

Habit Forming

- No

How to Stop

- No need to taper for the treatment of neurological disorders

Pharmacokinetics

- Hepatic metabolism via CYP2D6 and 1A2 to less potent metabolites. Half-life 10–12 hours. Protein binding 50–60%

Drug Interactions

- Mexiletine may decrease clearance and increase levels of caffeine and theophylline
- Cimetidine may affect (increase or decrease) mexiletine levels
- Atropine, opioids, aluminum-magnesium hydroxide may slow absorption and decrease effect
- Metaclopramide increases absorption and increases levels
- CYP1A2 inhibitors, such as fluvoxamine, decrease mexiletine clearance and increase levels
- CYP2D6 inhibitors, such as propafenone, paroxetine, fluoxetine and duloxetine, may increase levels

- Enzyme inducers, such as hydantoins and rifampin, increase drug clearance and lower levels
- Urinary pH affects renal clearance of mexiletine. Acidifiers increase clearance and lower levels and alkalinizers decrease clearance

 ### Other Warnings/ Precautions

- All antiarrhythmic agents can worsen or cause new arrhythmias. These may include increase in premature ventricular arrhythmias to life-threatening tachycardias

Do Not Use

- Known hypersensitivity to the drug, cardiogenic shock, or preexisting second or third degree AV block (without pacemaker)

Renal Impairment

- Likely no effect on dose

Hepatic Impairment

- Use with caution. Patients with severe disease may need a lower dose

Cardiac Impairment

- Right-sided congestive heart failure can reduce hepatic metabolism and increase blood level, and patients may require a reduced dose. Cardiac patients with existing disease are more prone to life-threatening arrhythmias

Elderly

- No known effects

 ### Children and Adolescents

- Not studied in children

 ### Pregnancy

- Category C but not studied. Only use in pregnancy if clearly needed

Breast Feeding

- Excreted in breast milk. Do not use

THE ART OF NEUROPHARMACOLOGY

Potential Advantages

- Useful treatment for myotonia and refractory pain disorders

Potential Disadvantages

- Multiple AEs and need for monitoring complicate use

Primary Target Symptoms

- Symptoms of myotonia (muscle pain, stiffness, weakness, dysphagia), pain

 Pearls

- Many patients with myotonia (delayed relaxation of muscles after activity) do not require pharmacologic treatment of their symptoms
- Weakness in myotonia is usually in the arms or hands
- Other medications of putative usefulness in myotonia include other sodium channel blockers, such as phenytoin, procainamide, tricyclic antidepressants, benzodiazepines, calcium channel blockers, taurine, and prednisone. There are no large controlled drug trials for myotonia treatment
- Physical therapy may be of some benefit in myotonia
- Mexiletine is occasionally used for refractory neuropathic pain disorders and headache. Successful treatment with intravenous lidocaine, if practical, may predict response to mexiletine

 Suggested Reading

Cruccu G. Treatment of painful neuropathy. Curr Opin Neurol 2007;20(5):531–5.

Marmura MJ, Passero FC Jr, Young WB. Mexiletine for refractory chronic daily headache: a report of nine cases. Headache 2008; 48(10):1506–10.

Trip J, Drost G, van Engelen BG, Faber CG. Drug treatment for myotonia. Cochrane Database Syst Rev 2006;(1):CD004762.

Wright JM, Oki JC, Graves L 3rd. Mexiletine in the symptomatic treatment of diabetic peripheral neuropathy. Ann Pharmacother 1997;31(1):29–34.

MITOXANTRONE

THERAPEUTICS

Brands
- Novantrone

Generic?
Yes

Class
- Antineoplastic agent, immunomodulator

Commonly Prescribed for
(FDA approved in bold)
- **Reducing neurologic disability or relapses in patients with secondary progressive, progressive relapsing, or worsening relapsing-remitting multiple sclerosis (MS)**
- **Acute nonlymphoblastic leukemia**
- Prostate cancer
- Breast cancer
- Non-Hodgkin's lymphoma

How the Drug Works
- A DNA-reactive agent that causes crosslinks and strand breaks, interferes with DNA uncoiling and repair, and has a cytocidal effect on cells. In MS, it appears to blunt the immune processes believed to be responsible in part for the disease
- It suppresses B-cell, T-cell, and macrophage function, impairs antigen proliferation, and decreases the secretion of inflammatory cytokines, including TNFα, IL-2, and interferon gamma, that mediate demyelination
- Due to its slow release from sequestered tissue into blood it is a long-acting immunosuppressant

How Long Until It Works
- MS: Months-years. In trials treated patients had fewer relapses at 1 and 2 years

If It Works
- MS: Continue to use for up to 2–3 years or a total of 140 mg/m^2 then discontinue because of cardiotoxicity risk

If It Doesn't Work
- For patients failing first-line agents in MS (interferons, glatiramer) and mitoxantrone with frequent relapses (measured by clinical outcome and MRI accumulation of lesions)

consider using natalizumab, monthly methylprednisolone, or pulse cyclophosphamide

Best Augmenting Combos for Partial Response or Treatment-Resistance
- Acute attacks in MS are often treated with glucocorticoids, especially if there is functional impairment due to vision loss, weakness, or cerebellar symptoms
- Treat common clinical symptoms with appropriate medication for spasticity (baclofen, tizanidine), neuropathic pain, and fatigue (modafinil)
- Generally not combined with most other MS disease-modifying treatments (natalizumab, interferons, glatiramer) but 1 study showed that adding monthly mitoxantrone to monthly doses of 1 gram methylprednisolone improved outcomes

Tests
- Assess cardiac left ventricular function using echocardiogram or MUGA (multi gated acquisition scan) at baseline and before each dose of mitoxantrone. Obtain a baseline blood count and recheck if symptoms of infection occur

ADVERSE EFFECTS (AEs)

How Drug Causes AEs
- Most AEs are likely related to affect on DNA synthesis and function and its immunosuppressive effect

Notable AEs
- Arrhythmias or ECG changes, leukopenia, anemia, thrombocytopenia, hepatic enzyme elevations, amenorrhea, nausea, urinary tract infections, anorexia, malaise/fatigue, alopecia, weakness, pharyngitis, extravasation at IV sites, peripheral edema, dyspnea, chills, infection. Urine may turn blue-green color

Life-Threatening or Dangerous AEs
- Suppression of left ventricular (LV) ejection fraction can lead to heart failure and death
- Serious infections have occurred in patients developing neutropenia on mitoxantrone

Weight Gain
• Unusual

Sedation
• Common

What to Do About AEs
• Discontinue if LV fraction changes significantly or < 50%
• Discontinue for significant neutropenia (< 1500 cells/mm^3)

Best Augmenting Agents for AEs
• Pretreat to prevent nausea before first infusion. Topical corticosteroids for IV extravasation

Pharmacokinetics
• Drug has a wide distribution into tissue, exceeding the concentrations in the blood. The drug is slowly released into the bloodstream from tissue. The elimination half-life is 23–215 hours (mean 75). 78% of drug is protein bound. Excreted in urine or feces as unchanged or inactive metabolites

 Drug Interactions
• No known drug interactions

 Other Warnings/ Precautions
• Risk of acute myeloblastic leukemia even years after stopping the medication

Do Not Use
• Known hypersensitivity to the drug. Known liver or heart failure

---

DOSING AND USE

Usual Dosage Range
• 12 mg/m^2 is the standard dose in MS

Dosage Forms
• Injection: 2 mg/mL in 10, 12.5, and 15 mL vials

Dosing Tips
• Should be given in specialty infusion center

How to Dose
• Give 12 mg/m^2 every 3 months as an infusion. Infusing slowly (over 30 minutes) may reduce risk of cardiotoxicity

Overdose
• Some patients died as a result of leukopenia and infection

Long-Term Use
• Use is limited to 2–3 years (a total of 140 mg/ body surface area in m^2) due to cardiac toxicity

Habit Forming
• No

How to Stop
• No need to taper

SPECIAL POPULATIONS

Renal Impairment
• No known effects

Hepatic Impairment
• Do not use for treatment of MS

Cardiac Impairment
• Do not use in patients with LV ejection fraction of 50% or less, or in patients experiencing significant decrease after starting treatment

Elderly
• Clearance of drug might be slower

 Children and Adolescents
• Safety and efficacy are not established

 Pregnancy
• Category D. Considered teratogenic based on mechanism of action. Do not use, and do a pregnancy test in women with MS of childbearing potential before starting treatment

Breast Feeding
• Drug is excreted in breast milk. Do not breast feed on drug

THE ART OF NEUROPHARMACOLOGY
Potential Advantages
• Effective treatment for some of the most disabled MS patients including those failing first-line agents and those with secondary progressive or relapsing progressive MS. Effective in preserving ambulation in patients with progressive MS

Potential Disadvantages
• Potential for multiple AEs, including irreversible heart failure, limits use. Not effective for primary progressive MS. Needs to be infused by physicians familiar with chemotherapeutic agents. Risk of acute myeloblastic leukemia, even years after stopping the medication

Primary Target Symptoms
• Decrease in relapse rate, prevention of disability, and slower accumulation of lesions on MRI imaging

Pearls
• An effective treatment but toxicity requires appropriate patient selection
• Appropriate patient selection is important. Patients with an aggressive form of RRMS with a need to preserve ambulation and independence. Effective in decreasing disability for 2–3 years while on the medication
• In clinical trials, decreased disability based on expanded disability status scores by about 60% or more compared to placebo. Increase in T2 MRI lesions was 80% less than placebo
• Hematologic effects are more common at the higher doses used in leukemia treatment
• Some suggest a minority (about 25%) of MS patients have subclinical ventricular dysfunction, making monitoring of LV ejection fraction even more essential

Suggested Reading

Cohen BA, Mikol DD. Mitoxantrone treatment of multiple sclerosis: safety considerations. Neurology 2004;63 (12 Suppl 6):S28–32.

Krapf H, Morrissey SP, Zenker O, Zwingers T, Gonsette R, Hartung HP; MIMS Study Group. Effect of mitoxantrone on MRI in progressive MS: results of the MIMS trial. Neurology 2005; 65(5):690–5.

Le Page E, Leray E, Taurin G, Coustans M, Chaperon J, Morrissey SP, Edan G. Mitoxantrone as induction treatment in aggressive relapsing remitting multiple sclerosis: treatment response factors in a 5 year follow-up observational study of 100 consecutive patients. J Neurol Neurosurg Psychiatry 2008;79(1):52–6.

Zipoli V, Portaccio E, Hakiki B, Siracusa G, Sorbi S, Amato MP. Intravenous mitoxantrone and cyclophosphamide as second-line therapy in multiple sclerosis: an open-label comparative study of efficacy and safety. J Neurol Sci 2008;266(1–2):25–30.

THERAPEUTICS

Brands
- Provigil, Alertec, Modiodal

Generic?
No

Class
- Wake-promoting agent

Commonly Prescribed for
(FDA approved in bold)
- **Reducing excessive sleepiness in patients with narcolepsy or shift-work related sleep disorder**
- **Reducing excessive sleepiness in patients with obstructive sleep apnea (OSA)/ hypopnea syndrome**
- Treatment of fatigue in multiple sclerosis (MS)
- Fatigue in depression
- Attention deficit hyperactivity disorder
- Fatigue in cancer, HIV, or post-stroke patients

How the Drug Works
- Unlike traditional stimulants which act directly via dopaminergic pathways, it may also act in the hypothalamus by stimulating wake-promoting areas, or inhibiting sleep-promoting areas
- It may also have effects on dopamine transporter pathways similar to other stimulants, hypothetically inhibiting the dopamine transporter
- Increases neuronal activity selectively in the hypothalamus and activates tuberomammillary nucleus neurons that release histamine
- It also activates hypothalamic neurons that release orexin/hypocretin

How Long Until It Works
- Typically 1–2 hours, although maximal benefit may take days-weeks

If It Works
- Continue to use indefinitely as long as symptoms persist. Complete resolution of symptoms is unusual. Does not cause insomnia when dosed correctly

If It Doesn't Work
- Change to most effective dose or alternative agent. Re-evaluate treatment of underlying cause (i.e., OSA) of fatigue. Consider other causes of fatigue (i.e., anemia, heart disease) as appropriate. Screen for use of CNS depressants that can interfere with sleep, i.e., opioids or alcohol

Best Augmenting Combos for Partial Response or Treatment-Resistance
- In treating OSA, modafinil is an adjunct to standard treatments such as continuous positive airway pressure (CPAP), weight loss and treatment of obstruction when possible
- In MS change drug regimen, i.e., antispasticity or disease-modifying agents when possible if they are significantly contributing to fatigue. Amantadine is an alternative treatment for MS-related fatigue
- Treat coexisting medical illnesses such as HIV, depression, or chronic pain disorders with appropriate agents

Tests
- None required

ADVERSE EFFECTS (AEs)

How Drug Causes AEs
- Unknown but most AEs are likely related to drug actions on CNS neurotransmitters

Notable AEs
- Nervousness, insomnia, headache, nausea, anorexia, palpitations, dry mouth, diarrhea, hypertension

Life-Threatening or Dangerous AEs
- Transient ECG changes have been reported in patients with preexisting heart disease
- Rare psychiatric reactions (activation of mania, anxiety)
- Rare severe dermatologic reactions

Weight Gain
- Unusual

unusual   not unusual   common   problematic

Sedation

- Unusual

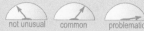

What to Do About AEs

- Try lowering the dose or dividing doses. If insomnia, do not take later in the day

Best Augmenting Agents for AEs

- Most AEs do not respond to adding other medications

DOSING AND USE

Usual Dosage Range

- 100–400 mg daily

Dosage Forms

- Tablets: 100, 200 mg (scored)

How to Dose

- Start at 200 mg in the morning
- In patients sensitive to medications, start at 100 mg in the morning
- When dividing dose, give the first dose in the morning, the second 4–6 hours later (i.e., at noon)
- If sleepiness does not improve on 200 mg/day dose, increase to 400 mg if no AEs

 Dosing Tips

- Dose requirements can escalate over time due to autoinduction. A drug holiday may restore effectiveness of lower dose
- In general, patients with sleepiness do better with higher doses (200 mg or more) and patients with fatigue or inability to concentrate may do well at lower doses
- In patients with shift-work related sleep disorder, take 1 hour prior to beginning a shift

Overdose

- No reported deaths. Agitation, anxiety and hypertension are common

Long-Term Use

- Although most initial trials were only a few months, appears safe. Periodically re-evaluate need for use

Habit Forming

- Class IV medication, but rarely abused in clinical practice

How to Stop

- Withdrawal is not problematic, unlike traditional stimulants. Symptoms of sleepiness may recur

Pharmacokinetics

- Metabolized by CYP450 system including isoenzymes 2C19, 3A4, among others. Peak concentrations at 2 hours and elimination half-life is 10–12 hours. About 10% of drug is excreted unchanged in urine. Mild CYP3A4 induction

 Drug Interactions

- Can increase plasma levels and effect of many drugs metabolized by 2C19 or 2D6 including phenytoin, diazepam, propranolol, tricyclic antidepressants, and SSRIs
- Can induce CYP450 3A4 reducing plasma levels of triazolam, and many steroidal contraceptives
- Carbamazepine can lower modafinil plasma levels and fluvoxamine and fluoxetine can increase levels
- Modafinil can affect warfarin effectiveness requiring closer monitoring of prothrombin times
- May interact with MAO inhibitors

 Other Warnings/ Precautions

- May adversely affect mood. Can cause activation of psychosis or mania

Do Not Use

- Known hypersensitivity to the drug, severe hypertension or cardiac arrhythmias

SPECIAL POPULATIONS

Renal Impairment

- No known effects. May require lower dose

Hepatic Impairment

- Reduce dose in patients with severe impairment

Cardiac Impairment
- Do not use in patients with ischemic ECG changes, chest pain, left ventricular hypertrophy or recent myocardial infarction

Elderly
- No known effects

Children and Adolescents
- Not studied in children under 16. Not a first-line agent in ADHD

Pregnancy
- Category C. Generally not used in pregnancy

Breast Feeding
- Unknown if excreted in breast milk. Do not use

THE ART OF NEUROPHARMACOLOGY

Potential Advantages
- Less risk of addiction, withdrawal and abuse compared to other stimulants

Potential Disadvantages
- Cost. May be less effective than other stimulants

Primary Target Symptoms
- Sleepiness, fatigue, concentration difficulties

Pearls
- The Epworth sleepiness scale is a reliable way to measure daytime sleepiness and response to treatment. It is a self-administered 8 item questionnaire with scores of 0–24. A score of 10 or greater indicates excessive daytime sleepiness. A reduction of 4 or more points on the Epworth is considered a good response to treatment
- Narcolepsy is characterized by excessive daytime sleepiness, uncontrollable sleep and observed cataplexy. Hypnagogic or hypnopompic hallucinations or sleep paralysis suggest the diagnosis. In sleep studies, a sleep latency of 8 minutes or less and quick onset of REM sleep confirms the diagnosis. The maintenance of wakefulness test can monitor response to treatment or be used to document safety in patients in which wakefulness is important for public safety (e.g., pilots). An increase of 1–2 minutes in maintenance of wakefulness is considered a good response to treatment
- Dividing doses and giving a second dose at noon does not appear to affect sleep architecture
- For MS-related fatigue, amantadine is another commonly used treatment. Modafinil is usually most effective at the 200 mg/day dose
- May be effective in treating excessive sleepiness in Parkinson's disease (at 200 mg/day dose) but does not usually improve motor scores
- Technically not a psychostimulant and minimal abuse potential

Suggested Reading

Gerrard P, Malcolm R. Mechanisms of modafinil: a review of current research. Neuropsychiatr Dis Treat 2007;3(3):349–64.

Keating GM, Raffin MJ. Modafinil: a review of its use in excessive sleepiness associated with obstructive sleep apnoea/hypopnoea syndrome and shift work sleep disorder. CNS Drugs 2005;19(9):785–803.

Kumar R. Approved and investigational uses of modafinil: an evidence-based review. Drugs 2008;68(13):1803–39.

Parmentier R, Anaclet C, Guhennec C, Brousseau E, Bricout D, Giboulot T, Bozyczko-Coyne D, Spiegel K, Ohtsu H, Williams M, Lin JS. The brain H3-receptor as a novel therapeutic target for vigilance and sleep-wake disorders. Biochem Pharmacol 2007;73(8):1157–71.

Stankoff B, Waubant E, Confavreux C, Edan G, Debouverie M, Rumbach L, Moreau T, Pelletier J, Lubetzki C, Clanet M; French Modafinil Study Group. Modafinil for fatigue in MS: a randomized placebo-controlled double-blind study. Neurology 2005;64(7):1139–43.

MYCOPHENOLATE MOFETIL

THERAPEUTICS

Brands
• CellCept, Myfortic

Generic?
Yes

Class
• Immunosuppressive agent, immunomodulator

Commonly Prescribed for
(FDA approved in bold)
• **Prophylaxis of organ rejection in patients with allogenic renal, cardiac or hepatic transplants**
• Myasthenia gravis (MG)
• Refractory uveitis
• Churg-Straus syndrome
• Diffuse proliferative lupus nephritis
• Psoriasis

How the Drug Works
• Prodrug that is actively metabolized to mycophenolic acid, a selective inhibitor of inosine monophosphate dehydrogenase, an important enzyme in de nova synthesis of guanine nucleotide. This alters purine metabolism, which preferentially affects T and B lymphocytes that depend on this pathway
• Inhibits proliferation of T and B lymphocytes and suppresses antibody formation
• May inhibit recruitment of leukocytes into sites of inflammation and graft rejection
• Does not affect production of interleukins

How Long Until It Works
• In as little as 2–3 weeks, and usually within 2 months

If It Works
• Usually used as a steroid-sparing agent. May allow reduction in dose or discontinuation of corticosteroids. Most MG patients require long-term treatment, but occasionally may remit allowing careful discontinuation

If It Doesn't Work
• Usually used as an adjunctive agent in conjunction with corticosteroids in MG. Azathioprine, cyclosporine, cyclophosphamide, plasma exchange, and intravenous immune globulin are alternative long-term treatments. Thymectomy may also be effective for selected patients

 Best Augmenting Combos for Partial Response or Treatment-Resistance
• Generally combined with prednisone or other corticosteroids for treatment of MG, allowing eventual decrease in dose, and occasionally combined with other immunosuppressive agents

Tests
• Obtain a CBC when initiating treatment, then weekly in the first month, twice monthly in months 2–3, and monthly through the first year

ADVERSE EFFECTS (AEs)

How Drug Causes AEs
• Serious AEs are related to immunosuppression and neutropenia

Notable AEs
• Diarrhea is most common. Other frequent AEs include abdominal pain, insomnia, nausea, peripheral edema, anxiety, back pain or headache, cough, and mild leukopenia. GI bleeding can also occur

 Life-Threatening or Dangerous AEs
• Increased risk of lymphomas or other malignancies, including skin cancers. Increased risk of infection or sepsis, severe neutropenia

Weight Gain
• Unusual

unusual not unusual common problematic

Sedation
• Unusual

unusual not unusual common problematic

What to Do About AEs
• Decrease dose or change to another agent. Diarrhea may decrease if taken with food or

use lower doses taken more frequently
(3 times daily)

Best Augmenting Agents for AEs

- Diarrhea: loperamide or diphenoxylate
  hydrochloride-atropine. Most other
  AEs do not respond to augmenting
  agents

DOSING AND USE

Usual Dosage Range

- MG – 1–3 g/day in 2 divided doses

Dosage Forms

- Capsules: 250 mg
- Tablets: 500 mg
- Powder for oral suspension: 200 mg/mL
- Powder for injection: 500 mg in 20 mL vials

How to Dose

- Start at 500 mg twice a day for 1–2 weeks
- Increase by 1 gram a day if CBC stable up to
  1500 mg twice daily

Dosing Tips

- Take with food to reduce GI AEs

Overdose

- Little clinical experience, but GI AEs are
  more common at higher doses.
  Bile acid sequestrants, such as
  cholestyramine, may increase excretion
  of drug

Long-Term Use

- Safe for long-term use with appropriate
  monitoring

Habit Forming

- No

How to Stop

- No need to taper but monitor for recurrence
  of MG complications

Pharmacokinetics

- Rapidly metabolized to active
  metabolite mycophenolic acid.
  97% protein bound. Tmax less than 1 hour
  in healthy patients. Oral doses are 94%
  of intravenous. Metabolites are excreted in
  urine

Drug Interactions

- Decreases protein binding and
  increases free levels of phenytoin and
  theophylline
- Decreases levels of oral contraceptives
- Competes for tubular secretion when used
  with acyclovir or ganciclovir, resulting in
  increased levels of both drugs
- Iron, antacids, and cholestyramine decrease
  levels of mycophenolate
- Probenecid increases levels of
  mycophenolate and salicylates can increase
  free drug level
- Calcium supplements inhibit absorption of
  mycophenolate. Take calcium supplements
  1 hour before or 2 hours after
  mycophenolate

Other Warnings/
Precautions

- Oral suspension contains aspartame and
  should not be given to phenylketonurics
- Live attenuated vaccines may be less
  effective and should be avoided
- Patients with hereditary defects in purine
  metabolism, such as Lesch-Nyhan
  syndrome, should avoid

Do Not Use

- Known hypersensitivity to the drug or its
  components

SPECIAL POPULATIONS

Renal Impairment

- Concentration of metabolites can be
  dramatically increased in renal
  insufficiency. Monitor closely and use with
  caution. In renal transplant patients, a daily
  dose of 2 g/day is recommended, unlike liver
  or cardiac transplant patients, who usually
  take 3 g/day

Hepatic Impairment

- Appears safe in many disorders, including
  alcoholic cirrhosis. Its safety in patients with
  hepatic failure related to primary biliary
  cirrhosis is unknown

Cardiac Impairment

- No known effects

Elderly
• Use with caution, may be more prone to AEs

Children and Adolescents
• Mostly used in transplant patients. Dose based on surface area, usually 600 mg/m^2 twice a day, up to a maximum of 2 g/daily

Pregnancy
• Category D. Do not use within 6 weeks of considering pregnancy. High rate of 1st trimester pregnancy loss and congenital malformations. Women with childbearing potential must have a negative pregnancy test before starting drug. Use 2 forms of contraception while on drug if sexually active

Breast Feeding
• Excreted in breast milk. Choose between discontinuing breast feeding or the drug

THE ART OF NEUROPHARMACOLOGY

Potential Advantages
• Relatively fewer AEs than many other immunosuppressive agents and relatively rapid onset of effect compared to other treatments, such as azathioprine

Potential Disadvantages
• May be less effective than other treatments. Diarrhea

Primary Target Symptoms
• Long-term preventive treatment of MG complications, such as weakness, visual problems, respiratory difficulties

Pearls
• An attractive treatment based on tolerability and rapid effect, but not always effective in MG
• Avoid using telithromycin, aminoglycosides, interferon alpha, penicillamine, intravenous magnesium, and intravenous lidocaine in MG patients
• Use beta-blockers, fluroquinolones, and CNS depressants such as opioids or muscle relaxants with caution in MG
• Recent phase III placebo-controlled studies of 2g/day mycophenolate do not demonstrate superiority to placebo in allowing MG patients to taper off steroids, or in the initial treatment of MG when combined with prednisone 20 mg

Suggested Reading

Benatar M, Rowland LP. The muddle of mycophenolate mofetil in myasthenia. Neurology 2008;71(6):390–1.

Hanisch F, Wendt M, Zierz S. Mycophenolate mofetil as second line immunosuppressant in Myasthenia gravis – a long-term prospective open-label study. Eur J Med Res 2009r; 14(8):364–6.

Heatwole C, Ciafaloni E. Mycophenolate mofetil for myasthenia gravis: a clear and present controversy. Neuropsychiatr Dis Treat 2008;4(6):1203–9.

Sanders DB, Hart IK, Mantegazza R, Shukla SS, Siddiqi ZA, De Baets MH, Melms A, Nicolle MW, Solomons N, Richman DP. An international, phase III, randomized trial of mycophenolate mofetil in myasthenia gravis. Neurology 2008; 71(6):400–6.

Villarroel MC, Hidalgo M, Jimeno A. Mycophenolate mofetil: An update. Drugs Today (Barc) 2009;45(7):521–32

NARATRIPTAN

THERAPEUTICS

Brands
- Amerge, Naramig

Generic?
No

 Class
- Triptan

Commonly Prescribed for
(FDA approved in bold)
- **Migraine**

 How the Drug Works
- Selective 5-HT1 receptor agonist, working predominantly at the D receptor subtype. Effectiveness may be due to blocking the transmission of pain signals from the trigeminal nerve to the trigeminal nucleus caudalis and preventing release of inflammatory neuropeptides rather than just causing vasoconstriction

How Long Until It Works
- 2 hours or less

If It Works
- Continue to take as needed. Patients taking acute treatment more than 2 days/ week are at risk for medication-overuse headache, especially if they have migraine

If It Doesn't Work
- Treat early in the attack – triptans are less likely to work after the development of cutaneous allodynia, a marker of central sensitization
- For patients with partial response or reoccurrence, add an NSAID
- Change to another agent

 Best Augmenting Combos for Partial Response or Treatment-Resistance
- NSAIDs or neuroleptics are often used to augment response

Tests
- None required

ADVERSE EFFECTS (AEs)

How Drug Causes AEs
- Direct effect on serotonin receptors

Notable AEs
- Tingling, flushing, warm/cold temperature sensations, palpitations, sensation of burning, vertigo, sensation of pressure, nausea

 Life-Threatening or Dangerous AEs
- Rare cardiac events including acute MI, cardiac arrhythmias, and coronary artery vasospasm have been reported with naratriptan

Weight Gain
- Unusual

unusual   not unusual   common   problematic

Sedation
- Unusual

unusual   not unusual   common   problematic

What to Do About AEs
- In most cases, only reassurance is needed. Lower dose, change to another triptan or use an alternative headache treatment

Best Augmenting Agents for AEs
- Treatment of nausea with antiemetics is acceptable. Other AEs improve with time

DOSING AND USE

Usual Dosage Range
- 1–2.5 mg

Dosage Forms
- Tablets: 1 and 2.5 mg

How to Dose
- Tablets: Most patients respond best with 2.5 mg oral dose. Give 1 pill at the onset of an attack and repeat in 4 hours for a partial response or the headache returns. Maximum 5 mg/day. Limit 10 days per month

Dosing Tips
- Treat early in attack

Overdose
- May cause hypertension, cardiovascular symptoms. Other possible symptoms include seizure, tremor, extremity erythema, cyanosis or ataxia. For patients with angina, perform ECG and monitor for ischemia for at least 24 hours

Long-Term Use
- Monitor for cardiac risk factors with continued use

Habit Forming
- No

How to Stop
- No need to taper. Patients who overuse triptans often experience withdrawal headaches up to several days

Pharmacokinetics
- Half-life 5.5 hours. Tmax 2 hours. Bioavailability is 74%. Metabolized by cytochrome P450 enzymes. 28% protein binding

 Drug Interactions
- Theoretical interactions with SSRI/SNRI. It is unclear that triptans pose any risk for the development of serotonin syndrome in clinical practice
- Use with sibutramine, a weight loss drug, can cause a serotonin syndrome including weakness, irritability, myoclonus and confusion

Do Not Use
- Within 24 hours of ergot-containing medications such as dihydroergotamine
- Patients with proven hypersensitivity to naratriptan, known cardiovascular disease, uncontrolled hypertension, or Prinzmetal's angina
- Almotriptan was not studied in patients with hemiplegic and basilar migraine
- May worsen symptoms in ischemic bowel disease

Renal Impairment
- Concentration increases in those with moderate-severe renal impairment (creatinine clearance less than 39 mL/min) and half-life doubles. Use with caution. May be at increased cardiovascular risk

Hepatic Impairment
- Drug metabolism is decreased with moderate disease. Do not use with severe hepatic impairment

Cardiac Impairment
- Do not use in patients with known cardiovascular or peripheral vascular disease

Elderly
- May be at increased cardiovascular risk

 Children and Adolescents
- Safety and efficacy have not been established
- Triptan trials in children were negative, due to higher placebo response

 Pregnancy
- Category C. Use only if potential benefit outweighs risk to the fetus. Pregnancy registries are ongoing. Migraine often improves in pregnancy, and other acute agents (opioids, neuroleptics, prednisone) have more proven safety

Breast Feeding
- Naratriptan is found in breast milk. Use with caution

Potential Advantages:
- Excellent tolerability and less recurrence, even compared to other oral triptans. Less risk of abuse than opioids or barbiturate-containing treatments

Potential Disadvantages:
- Cost, potential for medication-overuse headache. Not as effective as other triptans

Primary Target Symptoms
- Headache pain, nausea, photo- and phonophobia

Pearls
- Early treatment of migraine is most effective
- Fewer AEs and longer half-life than most triptans but less effective
- May not be effective when taken during aura, before headache begins
- In patients with "status migrainosus" (migraine lasting more than 72 hours)

neuroleptics and DHE are more effective
- Triptans were not originally studied for use in the treatment of basilar or hemiplegic migraine
- Patients taking triptans more than 10 days/month are at increased risk of medication-overuse headache which is less responsive to treatment
- Chest and throat tightness are usually benign and may be related to esophageal spasm rather than cardiac ischemia. These symptoms occur more commonly in patients without cardiac risk factors

Suggested Reading

Ferrari MD, Roon KI, Lipton RB, Goadsby PJ. Oral triptans (serotonin 5-HT(1B/1D) agonists) in acute migraine treatment: a meta-analysis of 53 trials. Lancet 2001;358(9294):1668–75.

Gladstone JP, Gawel M. Newer formulations of the triptans: advances in migraine management. Drugs 2003;63(21):2285–305.

Mannix LK, Savani N, Landy S, Valade D, Shackelford S, Ames MH, Jones MW. Efficacy and tolerability of naratriptan for short-term prevention of menstrually related migraine: data from two randomized, double-blind, placebo-controlled studies. Headache 2007; 47(7):1037–49.

Pringsheim T, Davenport WJ, Dodick D. Acute treatment and prevention of menstrually related migraine headache: evidence-based review. Neurology 2008;70(17):1555–63.

Silberstein SD, Berner T, Tobin J, Xiang Q, Campbell JC. Scheduled short-term prevention with frovatriptan for migraine occurring exclusively in association with menstruation. Headache 2009;49(9):1283–97.

Wenzel RG, Tepper S, Korab WE, Freitag F. Serotonin syndrome risks when combining SSRI/SNRI drugs and triptans: is the FDA's alert warranted? Ann Pharmacother 2008; 42(11):1692–6.

NATALIZUMAB

THERAPEUTICS

Brands
• Tysabri, Antegren

Generic?
No

Class
• Immunosuppressive agent, immunomodulator

Commonly Prescribed for
(FDA approved in bold)
• **Reducing neurologic disability or relapses in patients with progressive relapsing, or worsening relapsing-remitting multiple sclerosis. (MS)**
• Crohn's disease (adults)

How the Drug Works
• Natalizumab is a monoclonal antibody that binds to the alpha-4 integrin chain of the very late activation antigen (VLA)-4 adhesion molecule and blocks mononuclear cell migration and costimulatory activating signals. These receptors include vascular cell adhesion molecule -1 (VCAM-1), which is expressed on activated vascular endothelium
• Disruption of these interactions prevents migration of leukocytes across the blood-brain barrier and reduces plaque formation as measured by MRI. It does not affect the absolute neutrophil count

How Long Until It Works
• Months-years. In trials treated patients had fewer relapses up to 2 years

If It Works
• Continue to use with appropriate monitoring

If It Doesn't Work
• For patients failing first-line agents (interferons, glatiramer) and with frequent relapses (measured by clinical outcome and MRI accumulation of lesions), consider using mitoxantrone, monthly methylprednisolone, or pulse cyclophosphamide

Best Augmenting Combos for Partial Response or Treatment-Resistance
• Acute attacks are often treated with glucocorticoids, especially if there is functional impairment due to vision loss, weakness, or cerebellar symptoms
• Treat common clinical symptoms with appropriate medication for spasticity (baclofen, tizanidine), neuropathic pain, and fatigue (modafinil)
• The SENTINEL study showed that adding natalizumab to Interferon 1β-1a decreases clinical relapses, MRI measures of disease severity and disability compared to Interferon 1β alone, but did not compare this combination to natalizumab alone. Given that combination therapy may increase risk of adverse events, combination therapy is not recommended at this time

Tests
• Progressive multifocal leukoencephalopathy (PML) is a rare complication of treatment with natalizumab. For suspected cases, stop drug and evaluate with MRI with gadolinium and cerebrospinal fluid analysis for JC virus DNA

ADVERSE EFFECTS (AEs)

How Drug Causes AEs
• Most AEs are likely related to immunosuppression or hypersensitivity

Notable AEs
• Headache, fatigue, abdominal discomfort, depression, dermatitis, rash, pruritus, menstrual irregularities, weight changes, urinary tract infection, and vaginitis

Life-Threatening or Dangerous AEs
• PML is a neurologic infection seen in immunosuppressed patients related to activation of the JC virus. PML can cause weakness (usually unilateral), clumsiness, or changes in cognition, personality, and memory. This can progress to severe disability or death over a period of weeks-months. Occurs in 1/1000 patients receiving natalizumab

- Opportunistic infections are also uncommon, but there have been cases of acute cytomegalovirus infection, pulmonary aspergillosis, and *Pneumocystis carinii* pneumonia in patients treated, with natalizumab. It is unclear if drug increases the risk of infection in patients receiving short courses of steroids for acute attacks

Weight Gain
- Unusual

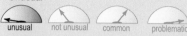

Sedation
- Common

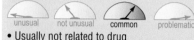

- Usually not related to drug

What to Do About AEs
- For milder infections, such as upper respiratory or urinary tract infection, treat with appropriate agents. In cases of PML or opportunistic infection, discontinue drug

Best Augmenting Agents for AEs
- Most AEs will not respond to augmenting agents

evaluating patients no less than every 6 months, and determining the effectiveness of treatment. Treatment must be authorized every 6 months

Habit Forming
- No

How to Stop
- No need to taper. There is no evidence to date of "rebound" from stopping drug

Pharmacokinetics
- Approximate time to steady state is about 24 weeks after q4 week dosing. The mean half-life is 11 days and mean clearance 16 days

 Drug Interactions
- Increases risk of serious infection when used with other immunosuppressants, especially in those on concomitant immunosuppressants (such as azathioprine, cyclosporine, methotrexate, and 6-mercaptopurine) or inhibitors of TNFα

Do Not Use
- Hypersensitivity to drug. Patients who have or have had PML. Patients treated with other immunosuppressants

DOSING AND USE

Usual Dosage Range
- 300 mg is the standard dose

Dosage Forms
- Injection: 300 mg in 15 mL single-use vial

 Dosing Tips
- Not applicable

How to Dose
- Give 300 mg over 1 hour every 4 weeks

Overdose
- Unknown

Long-Term Use
- Drug is available only under a restricted distribution program called the TOUCH prescribing program. These centers are responsible for reporting serious infections,

SPECIAL POPULATIONS

Renal Impairment
- No known effects

Hepatic Impairment
- No known effects

Cardiac Impairment
- No known effects

Elderly
- No known effects

 Children and Adolescents
- Safety and efficacy are not established

Pregnancy

- Category C. Pregnancy registry is ongoing. Use only if benefit of preventing MS relapse outweighs risk

Breast Feeding

- Unknown if excreted in breast milk. Do not breast feed on drug

THE ART OF NEUROPHARMACOLOGY

Potential Advantages

- Effective treatment for some of the most disabled MS patients including those failing first-line agents. Efficacy may be superior to other disease-modifying agents. Once a month treatment

Potential Disadvantages

- Rare but potentially fatal AE of PML or opportunistic infection. Only available through specific infusion centers as IV infusion

Primary Target Symptoms

- Decrease in relapse rate, prevention of disability, and slower accumulation of lesions on MRI imaging

Pearls

- After initial launch, three cases of PML resulted in the drug being pulled from the market. Four subsequent cases have been reported in the approximately ten thousand patients treated for 18 months since drug approval
- In theory, because natalizumab blocks immune cells from entering the CNS, there could be rebound progression with drug discontinuation. It is unknown if the immune cells die or remain sequestered in blood. A preliminary study showed no serious AEs in the year after discontinuation
- Patients who do not respond to other disease-modifying agents or with a particularly aggressive disease course are candidates for natalizumab. In studies there was a reduction in mean attack rate of 68%

Suggested Reading

Gold R. Combination therapies in multiple sclerosis. J Neurol 2008;255 (Suppl 1):51–60.

Kappos L, Bates D, Hartung HP, Havrdova E, Miller D, Polman CH, Ravnborg M, Hauser SL, Rudick RA, Weiner HL, O'Connor PW, King J, Radue EW, Yousry T, Major EO, Clifford DB. Natalizumab treatment for multiple sclerosis: recommendations for patient selection and monitoring. Lancet Neurol 2007;6(5):431–41.

Lindå H, von Heijne A, Major EO, Ryschkewitsch C, Berg J, Olsson T, Martin C. Progressive multifocal leukoencephalopathy after natalizumab monotherapy. N Engl J Med 2009;361(11):1081–7.

Stuart WH. Combination therapy for the treatment of multiple sclerosis: challenges and opportunities. Curr Med Res Opin 2007; 23(6):1199–208.

NIMODIPINE

THERAPEUTICS

Brands
- Nimotop

Generic?
Yes

Class
- Calcium channel blocker

Commonly Prescribed for
(FDA approved in bold)
- **Prevention of vasospasm in subarachnoid hemorrhage (SAH)**
- Hypertension
- Traumatic brain injury
- Reversible cerebral vasoconstrictive syndromes

How the Drug Works
- Cardiac and vascular smooth muscle contraction depends on movement of calcium through L-type calcium channels into cells, which is inhibited by nimodipine. In animals, nimodipine has a greater effect on cerebral arteries compared with other calcium channel blockers, probably because it is more lipophilic. There is no angiographic evidence that this is correct

How Long Until It Works
- Within hours for both SAH vasospasm and hypertension

If It Works
- Prevents delayed ischemic complications after SAH caused by vasospasm, improves recovery time and reduces disability
- Typically used for 3 weeks

If It Doesn't Work
- Continue supportive care. Alternative but unproven treatments include statins and magnesium sulfate

Best Augmenting Combos for Partial Response or Treatment-Resistance
- Treatment of SAH should take place in a medical center with experience and 24-hour physician availability

- Occlude the aneurysm in SAH by surgery or coiling
- Do not treat hypertension aggressively
- Normovolemia is preferred
- Treat hyperglycemia and use measures to avoid deep vein thrombosis

Tests
- Monitor blood pressure and heart rate

ADVERSE EFFECTS (AEs)

How Drug Causes AEs
- Direct effects of L-type calcium receptor antagonism on cardiac and smooth muscle

Notable AEs
- Hypotension, bradycardia
- Flushing, headache, constipation, nausea, myalgia, edema

Life-Threatening or Dangerous AEs
- Rare elevation of hepatic transaminases or thrombocytopenia
- May slow AV conduction or worsen symptoms of heart failure

Weight Gain
- Unusual

unusual   not unusual   common   problematic

Sedation
- Unusual

unusual   not unusual   common   problematic

What to Do About AEs
- Complications of SAH are more serious than significant AEs due to nimodipine. Continue or lower dose

Best Augmenting Agents for AEs
- Constipation can be treated by usual agents such as magnesium

Usual Dosage Range
• 360 mg/day

Dosage Forms
• Tablets: 30 mg

How to Dose
• Start within 4 days of SAH. Give 2 tablets (60 mg) every 4 hours for 21 days

Dosing Tips
• If patients are unable to take orally, give the contents of the tablet via nasogastric tube and flush with saline. Food decreases absorption. Doses should be not less than 1 hour before or 2 hours after meals

Overdose
• There are no reports of overdose. Bradycardia, hypotension, and low-output heart failure are among the risks with calcium channel blocker overdose

Long-Term Use
• Unknown

Habit Forming
• No

How to Stop
• No need to taper. Less risk of rebound tachycardia than beta-blockers

Pharmacokinetics
• Hepatic metabolism by CYP450 system. Elimination half-life 8–9 h. Tmax 1 h. Oral bioavailability 13% with > 95% protein binding

Drug Interactions
• Use with caution with other antihypertensives, especially other calcium channel blockers
• H2 antagonists (cimetidine, ranitidine) increase nimodipine levels
• Use with beta-blockers can be synergistic or additive, use with caution
• Potent CYP3A4 inhibitors, such as ketoconazole, may increase levels

Do Not Use
• Proven hypersensitivity to nimodipine or other calcium-channel blockers

Renal Impairment
• Unknown. Use with caution

Hepatic Impairment
• Decrease dose to 30 mg every 4 hours in patients with cirrhosis

Cardiac Impairment
• Do not use in acute shock. Use with caution in severe CHF, hypotension, and greater than first-degree heart block

Elderly
• Use with caution

Children and Adolescents
• Little is known about efficacy or safety

Pregnancy
• Category C (all calcium channel blockers.). Use only if potential benefit outweighs risk to the fetus

Breast Feeding
• Not recommended. Nimodipine is probably excreted in breast milk

THE ART OF NEUROPHARMACOLOGY

Potential Advantages
• Multiple studies show efficacy for the treatment of vasospasm after SAH

Potential Disadvantages
• Limited evidence of efficacy. Outcomes are still often poor in SAH

Primary Target Symptoms
• Prevention of delayed ischemic complications from vasospasm after SAH

Pearls

- No longer available in intravenous form. Studies failed to show that intravenous administration was superior and serious AEs including cardiac events were greater

- In one study, nimodipine showed potential usefulness in severe traumatic brain injury. Reduces jugular lactate and intracranial pressure
- May be useful in the treatment of cerebral vasoconstrictive syndromes, a potential cause of "thunderclap headache." The best dose and duration of use is unknown

Suggested Reading

Aslan A, Gurelik M, Cemek M, Goksel HM, Buyukokuroglu ME. Nimodipine can improve cerebral metabolism and outcome in patients with severe head trauma. Pharmacol Res 2009;59(2):120–4.

Deshaies EM, Boulos AS, Drazin D, Popp AJ. Evidence-based pharmacotherapy for cerebral vasospasm. Neurol Res 2009;31(6):615–20.

Dorhout Mees SM, Rinkel GJ, Feigin VL, Algra A, van den Bergh WM, Vermeulen M, van Gijn J. Calcium antagonists for aneurysmal subarachnoid haemorrhage. Cochrane Database Syst Rev 2007;(3):CD000277.

Ducros A, Bousser MG. Reversible cerebral vasoconstriction syndrome. Pract Neurol 2009;9(5):256–67.

NORTRIPTYLINE

THERAPEUTICS

Brands
- Sensoval, Aventyl, Pamelor, Norpress, Allegron, Nortrilen

Generic?
Yes

Class
- Tricyclic antidepressant (TCA)

Commonly Prescribed for
(FDA approved in bold)
- **Depression**
- Migraine prophylaxis
- Tension-type headache prophylaxis
- Diabetic neuropathy
- Post-herpetic neuralgia
- Other painful peripheral neuropathies
- Back or neck pain
- Phantom limb pain
- Fibromyalgia
- Bulimia nervosa
- Insomnia
- Anxiety
- Nocturnal enuresis
- ADHD
- Smoking cessation

How the Drug Works
- Blocks serotonin and norepinephrine reuptake pumps, increasing their levels within hours, but antidepressant effect takes weeks. Effect is more likely related to adaptive changes in serotonin and norepinephrine receptor systems over time
- It also has antihistamine properties, which most likely causes the sedation treating insomnia

How Long Until It Works
- Migraines – effective in as little as 2 weeks, but can take up to 3 months on a stable dose to see full effect
- Neuropathic pain – usually some effect within 4 weeks
- Depression – 2 weeks but up to 2 months for full effect
- Insomnia, anxiety, depression – may be effective immediately, but effects often delayed 2 to 4 weeks

If It Works
- Migraine – goal is a 50% or greater decrease in migraine frequency or severity. Consider tapering or stopping if headaches remit for more than 6 months or if considering pregnancy
- Neuropathic pain – the goal is to reduce pain intensity and symptoms, but usually does not produce remission
- Insomnia – continue to use if tolerated and encourage good sleep hygiene
- Depression – continue to use and monitor for AEs. Usually not first-line treatment for depression

If It Doesn't Work
- Increase to highest tolerated dose
- Migraine: address other issues, such as medication overuse, other coexisting medical disorders, such as anxiety, and consider changing to another agent or adding a second agent
- Chronic pain: either change to another agent or add a second agent
- Insomnia: if no sedation occurs despite adequate dosing, stop and change to another agent

Best Augmenting Combos for Partial Response or Treatment-Resistance
- Migraine: For some patients, low-dose polytherapy with 2 or more drugs may be better tolerated and more effective than high-dose monotherapy. May use in combination with AEDs, antihypertensives, natural products, and non-medication treatments, such as biofeedback, to improve headache control
- Chronic pain: AEDs such as gabapentin, pregabalin, carbamazepine, and capsaicin, mexiletine are agents used for neuropathic pain. Opioids are appropriate for long-term use in some cases but require careful monitoring

Tests
- Consider checking ECG for QTc prolongation at baseline and when increasing dose, especially in those with a personal or family history of QTc prolongation, cardiac arrhythmia, heart failure or recent myocardial infarction. In patients on diuretics, measure potassium and magnesium at baseline and periodically

ADVERSE EFFECTS (AEs)

How Drug Causes AEs

- Anticholinergic and antihistaminic properties are causes of most common AEs. Blockade of alpha-1 adrenergic receptors may cause orthostasis and sedation

Notable AEs

- Constipation, dry mouth, blurry vision, increased appetite, nausea, diarrhea, heartburn, weight gain, urinary retention, sexual dysfunction, sweating, itching, rash, fatigue, weakness, sedation, nervousness, restlessness

 Life-Threatening or Dangerous AEs

- Orthostatic hypotension, tachycardia, QTc prolongation, and rarely death
- Increased intraocular pressure
- Paralytic ileus, hyperthermia
- Rare activation of mania or suicidal ideation
- Rare worsening of existing seizure disorders

Weight Gain

- Common

Sedation

- Common

What to Do About AEs

- For minor AEs, lower dose or switch to another agent. If tiredness/sedation are bothersome, lower dose or consider desipramine or protriptyline. For serious AEs, lower dose and consider stopping

Best Augmenting Agents for AEs

- Try magnesium for constipation. For migraine, consider using with agents that cause weight loss as an AE (e.g., topiramate)

DOSING AND USE

Usual Dosage Range

- Migraine/pain: 10–100 mg/day
- Depression, anxiety: 75–150 mg/day

Dosage Forms

- Capsules: 10, 25, 50, 75 mg
- Liquid solution: 10 mg/5 mL

How to Dose

- Initial dose 10–25 mg/day taken about 1 hour before retiring. Effective range from 10–150 mg but typically 100 mg or less

 Dosing Tips

- Start at a low dose, usually 10 mg, and titrate up every few days as tolerated. Low doses are often effective for pain even though they are below the usual effective antidepressant dose. At doses of 100 mg or greater, monitor plasma levels of drug. Patients may choose to divide doses to 3–4 times daily dosing

Overdose

- Cardiac arrhythmias and ECG changes; death can occur. CNS depression, convulsions, severe hypotension, and coma are not rare. Patients should be hospitalized. Sodium bicarbonate can treat dysrhythmias and hypotension. Treat shock with vasopressors, oxygen, or corticosteroids

Long-Term Use

- Safe for long-term use

Habit Forming

- No

How to Stop

- Taper slowly to avoid withdrawal, including rebound insomnia. Withdrawal usually lasts less than 2 weeks. For patients with well-controlled pain disorders, taper very slowly (over months) and monitor for recurrence of symptoms

Pharmacokinetics

- Metabolized by CYP450 system, especially CYP2D6, 1A2. Half-life 18–44 h and time to reach steady-state 4–19 days

 Drug Interactions

- CYP2D6 inhibitors (duloxetine, paroxetine, fluoxetine, bupropion), cimetidine, and valproic acid can increase drug concentration
- Phenothiazines increase tricyclic levels

- Enzyme inducers such as rifamycin, smoking, phenobarbital can lower levels. Carbamazepine use can also lower TCA levels
- Use with clonidine has been associated with increases in blood pressure and hypertensive crisis
- Tramadol increases risk of seizures in patients taking TCAs
- May reduce absorption and bioavailability of levodopa
- May alter effects of antihypertensive medications, and prolongation of QTc, especially problematic in patients taking drugs that induce bradycardia
- Quinolones, such as grepafloxacin and sparfloxacin, increase risk of cardiac arrhythmias when used with TCAs
- Use together with anticholinergics can increase AEs (e.g., risk of ileus)
- Methylphenidate may inhibit metabolism and increase AEs
- Use within 2 weeks of monoamine oxidase (MAO) inhibitors may risk serotonin syndrome

 Other Warnings/ Precautions

- May increase risk of seizure

Do Not Use
- Proven hypersensitivity to drug or other TCAs
- In acute recovery after myocardial infarction or uncompensated heart failure
- In conjunction with antiarrhythmics that prolong QTc interval
- In conjunction with medications that inhibit CYP2D6

Renal Impairment
- Use with caution. May need to lower dose

Hepatic Impairment
- Use with caution. May need to lower dose

Cardiac Impairment
- Do not use in patients with recent myocardial infarction, severe heart failure, with a history of QTc prolongation or orthostatic hypotension

Elderly
- More sensitive to AEs such as sedation, hypotension. Start with lower doses

 Children and Adolescents

- Not as well studied but similar effectiveness compared with amitriptyline in children. In children less than 12, most commonly used at low dose for treatment of enuresis

 Pregnancy

- Category D. Crosses the placenta and may cause fetal malformations or withdrawal. Generally not recommended for the treatment of pain or insomnia during pregnancy. For patients with depression or anxiety, selective serotonin-reuptake inhibitors (SSRIs) may be safer than TCAs

Breast Feeding
- Some drug is found in breast milk and use while breast feeding is not recommended

Potential Advantages
- Very effective in the treatment of multiple pain disorders. Useful for treatment of depression, anxiety, and insomnia, which are common in chronic pain disorders. Less sedation than tertiary amine TCAs (e.g., amitriptyline)

Potential Disadvantages
- AEs are often greater than SSRIs or SNRIs and many AEDs. Less effective for insomnia than tertiary amine TCAs (e.g., amitriptyline)

Primary Target Symptoms
- Headache frequency and severity
- Neuropathic pain

 Pearls

- In patients with chronic pain, offers relief at doses below usual antidepressant doses
- For patients with significant anxiety or depressive disorders, as effective as newer drugs but much more AEs. Consider treatment of depression or anxiety with

another agent and using a low dose of nortriptyline or other TCA for pain
- TCAs can often precipitate mania in patients with bipolar disorder. Use with caution
- Despite interactions, expert psychiatrists may use with MAO inhibitors for refractory depression. Combination with atypical neuroleptics is another option
- For post-stroke depression, may be superior to SSRIs and may even increase survival
- Many patients do not improve. The number needed to treat for moderate pain relief in neuropathic pain is 2–3
- Increases non-REM sleep time and decreases sleep latency. When starting, there is often an activating effect,

and insomnia may temporarily worsen
- Nortriptyline and other secondary amines (amoxapine, desipramine, protriptyline) have lower rates of sedation and orthostatic hypotension than tertiary amines (amitriptyline, clomipramine, doxepin, imipramine, trimipramine) and relatively more norepinephrine than serotonin blocking activity
- Previously used for ADHD before new treatments became available. May be useful as an adjunct for patients with pain and co-existing ADHD
- TCAs may increase risk of metabolic syndrome

 Suggested Reading

Heymann RE, Helfenstein M, Feldman D. A double-blind, randomized, controlled study of amitriptyline, nortriptyline and placebo in patients with fibromyalgia. An analysis of outcome measures. Clin Exp Rheumatol 2001; 19(6):697–702.

Silberstein SD, Goadsby PJ. Migraine: preventive treatment. Cephalalgia 2002;22(7):491–512.

Verdu B, Decosterd I, Buclin T, Stiefel F, Berney A. Antidepressants for the treatment of chronic pain. Drugs 2008;68(18):2611–32.

Wilens TE, Biederman J, Mick E, Spencer TJ. A systematic assessment of tricyclic antidepressants in the treatment of adult attention-deficit hyperactivity disorder. J Nerv Ment Dis 1995;183(1):48–50.

Zin CS, Nissen LM, Smith MT, O'Callaghan JP, Moore BJ. An update on the pharmacological management of post-herpetic neuralgia and painful diabetic neuropathy. CNS Drugs 2008; 22(5):417–42

OXCARBAZEPINE

Brands
- Trileptal

Generic?
Yes

Class
- Antiepileptic drug (AED)

Commonly Prescribed for
(FDA approved in bold)
- **Complex partial seizures with or without secondary generalization (adults and children), monotherapy (ages 4 and up) and adjunctive(ages 2 and up)**
- Generalized tonic-clonic seizures
- Mixed seizure patterns
- Trigeminal neuralgia
- Temporal lobe epilepsy (children and adults)
- Neuropathic pain
- Alcohol withdrawal
- Bipolar I Disorder (acute manic and mixed episodes)

How the Drug Works
- Inhibits voltage-dependent sodium channel conductance
- Modulates calcium channels, potassium conductance, glutamate release and NMDA receptors

How Long Until It Works
- Seizures –2 weeks or less
- Trigeminal neuralgia or neuropathic pain – hours to weeks

If It Works
- Seizures – goal is the remission of seizures. Continue as long as effective and well-tolerated. Consider tapering and slowly stopping after 2 years without seizures, depending on the type of epilepsy
- Trigeminal neuralgia – should dramatically reduce or eliminate attacks. Periodically attempt to reduce to lowest effective dose or discontinue

If It Doesn't Work
- Increase to highest tolerated dose
- Epilepsy: consider changing to another agent, adding a second agent or referral for epilepsy surgery evaluation. When adding a second agent, keep drug interactions in mind
- Trigeminal neuralgia: Try an alternative agent. For truly refractory patients referral to tertiary headache center, consider surgical or other procedures

 Best Augmenting Combos for Partial Response or Treatment-Resistance
- Epilepsy: drug interactions can complicate multi-drug therapy
- Pain: Can combine with other AEDs (gabapentin or pregabalin) or tricyclic antidepressants

Tests
- Check sodium levels for symptoms of hyponatremia or in patients susceptible to hyponatremia

How Drug Causes AEs
- CNS AEs are probably caused by sodium channel blockade effects

Notable AEs
- Sedation, dizziness, ataxia, headache, tremor, emotional lability
- Nausea, vomiting, anorexia, dyspepsia
- Blurry or double vision, upper respiratory tract infection, rhinitis

 Life-Threatening or Dangerous AEs
- Rare blood dyscrasias: leukopenia, thrombocytopenia
- Dermatologic reactions uncommon and rarely severe but include erythema multiforme, toxic epidermal necrolysis, and Stevens-Johnson syndrome
- Hyponatremia/SIADH (syndrome of inappropiate antidiuretic hormone secretion)

Weight Gain
- Not unusual

unusual — not unusual — common — problematic

Sedation
• Common

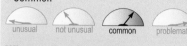

What to Do About AEs
• Use with caution in patients with low sodium at baseline, or those on medications that can lower sodium such as diuretics

Best Augmenting Agents for AEs
• Most AEs cannot be improved with an augmenting agent

DOSING AND USE

Usual Dosage Range
• Epilepsy: 900–2400 mg/day
• Pain: Often a low dose is effective. Usually 1200 mg/day or less

Dosage Forms
• Tablets: 150 mg, 300 mg, 600 mg
• Oral suspension: 300 mg/5 mL

How to Dose
• Epilepsy: start at 600 mg/day in 2 divided doses
• Increase by up to 600 mg/day every week to goal dose
• Some increased effectiveness but also more side effects above 1200 mg/day dose
• Trigeminal neuralgia/pain: Start at 150–300 mg/day and increase every 3 days by 150–300 mg/day until pain relief
• Adjust dose as needed when using with AEDs or other drugs that affect levels

 Dosing Tips
• Can dose twice daily or 3 times daily in sensitive patients, titrate slowly
• Levels typically need to be 1/3 higher than carbamazepine dose for a similar effect

Overdose
• Sedation, ataxia. No reported deaths

Long-Term Use
• Safe for long-term use

Habit Forming
• No

How to Stop
• Taper slowly
• Abrupt withdrawal can lead to seizures in patients with epilepsy

Pharmacokinetics
• Most of the pharmacologic activity is through the 10-monohydroxy metabolite of oxcarbazepine. Half-life is 2 hours, but its metabolite is 9 hours
• Hepatic metabolism converts to metabolite. About 40% protein bound, mostly renally excreted. Bioavailability is over 95%

 Drug Interactions
• Inhibitor of CYP2C19 and mild inducer of CYP3A4/5, but not other P450 enzymes
• Oxcarbazepine increases levels of phenytoin and phenobarbital and lowers levels of lamotrigine
• Phenytoin, primidone, phenobarbital, carbamazepine, and other CYP450 3A4 inducers decrease levels of oxcarbazepine metabolite
• Valproate and verapamil lower levels
• Can decrease concentration of hormonal contraceptives

 Other Warnings/ Precautions
• CNS AEs increase when used with other CNS depressants
• Rare systemic disorders: Systemic lupus erythematosus
• May affect bone metabolism with long-term treatment
• Risk of hyponatremia is highest in the first 3 months. Check sodium level for symptoms of hyponatremia (nausea, headache, lethargy, or worsening headache)

Do Not Use
• Patients with a proven allergy to oxcarbazepine. Patients with carbamazepine allergies have a 30% chance of allergy to oxcarbazepine

Renal Impairment

- Lower dose for patients with renal insufficiency (creatinine clearance < 30 mL/min). Reduce initial dose by half and titrate slowly

Hepatic Impairment

- Safe for patients with mild-moderate disease at usual doses. Use with caution in patients with severe disease

Cardiac Impairment

- No known effects

Elderly

- May need lower dose, especially when creatinine clearance is reduced

 ### Children and Adolescents

- Start at 8–10 mg/kg/day and increase every 1–2 weeks as tolerated to goal dose, usually 30 mg/kg/day. Maximum 46 mg/kg/day
- Side effects similar to adults

 ### Pregnancy

- Risk category C. Teratogenicity in animal studies
- Risks of stopping medication must outweigh risk to fetus for patients with epilepsy. Seizures and potential status epilepticus place the woman and fetus at risk and can cause reduced oxygen and blood supply to the womb
- Patients taking for headache, pain, or bipolar disorder should generally stop before considering pregnancy
- Levels may change during pregnancy. Checking levels may ensure therapeutic dose
- Supplementation with 0.4 mg of folic acid before and during pregnancy is recommended

Breast Feeding

- Some drug is found in mother's breast milk
- Generally recommendations are to discontinue drug or bottle feed
- Monitor infant for sedation, poor feeding or irritability

Potential Advantages

- Proven effectiveness as monotherapy and adjunctive for partial seizures. Generally fewer AEs than carbamazepine and no autoinduction

Potential Disadvantages

- Ineffective for absence, atypical absence and myoclonic seizures. Similar or greater rate of hyponatremia than carbamazepine

Primary Target Symptoms

- Seizure frequency and severity
- Pain

 ### Pearls

- Effective for partial epilepsies but not absence or myoclonic seizures, infantile spasms
- May worsen or improve generalized tonic-clonic seizure control
- To measure levels, check levels of monohydroxy derivative (the metabolite)
- Hyponatremia (less than 125) occurs in about 2.5% of patients
- Consider as an alternative for the treatment of trigeminal neuralgia, often effective in hours or days. Better tolerated than, carbamazepine. Benefit may not be sustained
- Recent studies suggest ineffective in migraine
- May be helpful for neuropathic pain, such as painful diabetic neuropathy
- May be helpful as adjunctive agent in bipolar disorder, or for acute mania

Suggested Reading

Ettinger AB, Argoff CE. Use of antiepileptic drugs for nonepileptic conditions: psychiatric disorders and chronic pain. Neurotherapeutics 2007; 4(1):75–83.

Gomez-Arguelles JM, Dorado R, Sepulveda JM, Herrera A, Arrojo FG, Aragón E, Huete CR, Terrón C, Anciones B. Oxcarbazepine monotherapy in carbamazepine-unresponsive trigeminal neuralgia. J Clin Neurosci 2008;15(5):516–9.

Harden CL, Pennell PB, Koppel BS, Hovinga CA, Gidal B, Meador KJ, Hopp J, Ting TY, Hauser WA, Thurman D, Kaplan PW, Robinson JN, French JA, Wiebe S, Wilner AN, Vazquez B, Holmes L, Krumholz A, Finnell R, Shafer PO, Le Guen C; American Academy of Neurology; American Epilepsy Society. Practice parameter update: management issues for women with epilepsy– focus on pregnancy (an evidence-based review): vitamin K, folic acid, blood levels, and breastfeeding: report of the Quality Standards Subcommittee and Therapeutics and Technology Assessment Subcommittee of the American Academy of Neurology and American Epilepsy Society. Neurology 2009;73(2):142–9.

Koch MW, Polman SK. Oxcarbazepine versus carbamazepine monotherapy for partial onset seizures. Cochrane Database Syst Rev 2009;(4): CD006453.

Muller M, Marson AG, Williamson PR. Oxcarbazepine versus phenytoin monotherapy for epilepsy. Cochrane Database Syst Rev 2006; (2):CD003615.

Silberstein S, Saper J, Berenson F, Somogyi M, McCague K, D'Souza J. Oxcarbazepine in migraine headache: a double-blind, randomized, placebo-controlled study. Neurology 2008; 70(7):548–55.

PENICILLAMINE

THERAPEUTICS

Brands
• Cuprimine, Depen

Generic?
Yes

 ### Class
• Cystine-depleting agent, chelating agent

Commonly Prescribed for
(FDA approved in bold)
• **Wilson's disease (WD)**
• **Cystinuria**
• **Rheumatoid arthritis (severe, active)**

 ### How the Drug Works
• In WD, copper accumulates in body tissues, causing neurological/psychiatric problems and/or liver failure. Penicillamine is cysteine, doubly substituted with methyl groups. Penicillamine binds to (chelates) copper, allowing it to be excreted in the urine

How Long Until It Works
• Urinary excretion of copper will increase in less than 24 hours. Clinical improvement usually takes 6 months or more; many patients may experience paradoxical worsening after starting treatment

If It Works
• Continue treatment, if tolerated, and aim for 24-hour urine copper excretion of 2 mg. Most patients remain on drug for the rest of their life but if all results return to normal (serum copper < 10 μg/dL), consider changing to zinc. Monitor for recurrence of symptoms or changes in urinary copper excretion

If It Doesn't Work
• Increase to as much as 2 g daily. Intolerance is more common than ineffectiveness. Change to trientine, and for liver failure or truly refractory patients, liver transplantation is curative

 ### Best Augmenting Combos for Partial Response or Treatment-Resistance
• Change to trientine if ineffective or poorly tolerated. A diet low in copper-containing foods, such as nuts, chocolate, liver, and dried fruit, is recommended

Tests
• Patients with WD have low serum ceruloplasmin and serum copper, but increased urinary excretion of copper is diagnostic. In pediatric patients, a 24-hour urinary copper excretion more than 1600 μg after 500 mg dose of penicillamine is considered diagnostic of WD. While on treatment, check blood counts and urinalysis, and monitor for skin changes and fever twice weekly for 1 month, then every 2 weeks for the next 5 months, and monthly for the remainder of treatment

ADVERSE EFFECTS (AEs)

How Drug Causes AEs
• Unknown

Notable AEs
• Fever, pruritus, changes in taste perception, tinnitus, optic neuritis, neuropathies, abdominal pain, anorexia, pancreatitis, proteinuria/hematuria, oral ulcerations, alopecia

 ### Life-Threatening or Dangerous AEs
• Myasthenic syndrome, usually starting with ptosis and diplopia, that can lead to generalized myasthenia if penicillamine is not stopped. Hematological AEs, such as leukopenia, thrombocytopenia. Nephrotic syndrome/renal failure. Drug fever, often with a macular cutaneous eruption and often in 2–3 weeks after starting treatment. Rarely obliterative bronchiolitis, with unexplained cough or wheezing

Weight Gain
• Unusual

unusual | not unusual | common | problematic

Sedation
• Unusual

unusual | not unusual | common | problematic

What to Do About AEs

- Leukopenia, neutropenia – discontinue drug
- Patients with moderate proteinuria can continue drug cautiously at lower dose but if renal function worsens or urinary protein is more than 1 g in 24 hours, discontinue drug. Urinary proteinuria can take up to a year to improve
- Give vitamin B6 (pyridoxine) 25 mg weekly, or 50 mg weekly to children, pregnant women, and patients with malnutrition or an intercurrent illness
- For drug fever, temporarily discontinue drug, give corticosteroid therapy, and restart drug at lower dose with a slower titration
- Pulmonary symptoms: check pulmonary function tests
- Patients with significant AEs: change to trientine

Best Augmenting Agents for AEs

- Most AEs cannot be improved with the use of an augmenting agent

DOSING AND USE

Usual Dosage Range

- 0.75 g–2g/day

Dosage Forms

- Tablets: 125, 250 mg

How to Dose

- Start at 250 mg/day and increase gradually over the next 1–2 weeks to target dose. The usual dose is between 0.75 to 1.5 g daily, although patients will occasionally require as much as 2 g/day. The goal is to achieve a 24-hour copper excretion over 2 mg/day for the first 3 months. After the first few months, the urinary copper excretion decreases to less than 0.5 mg/day and eventually less than 150 μg per day, with a serum copper less than 10 mcg/dL. Usually the dose will not require adjustment after the first 2 weeks

 Dosing Tips

- Give at least 1 hour before or 2 hours after meals to ensure absorption

Overdose

- Symptoms unknown

Long-Term Use

- Many AEs, such as nephrotoxicity (a lupus-like syndrome), bone marrow suppression/thrombocytopenia, can develop after extended use. Can cause skin complications, such as elastosis perforans serpiginosa, and aphthous stomatitis and can affect pyridoxine metabolism

Habit Forming

- No

How to Stop

- No need to taper

Pharmacokinetics

- Bioavailability is 40–70%, and drug is 80% protein bound with peak plasma levels 1–3 hours after ingestion. When stopping, after prolonged usage, there is a slow elimination phase for 4–6 days

 Drug Interactions

- Decreases levels of digoxin
- Increases effects and toxicity of gold therapy, antimalarial or cytotoxic drugs, phenylbutazone, and oxyphenbutazone
- Iron salts and antacids decrease absorption of penicillamine

 Other Warnings/ Precautions

- May cause a positive anti-nuclear antibody (ANA) test and lupus erythematous-like syndrome. Some patients allergic to penicillin may have cross-sensitivity to penicillamine

Do Not Use

- Patients with known hypersensitivity to the drug, history of penicillamine-related aplastic anemia, or agranulocytosis

SPECIAL POPULATIONS

Renal Impairment

- Use with caution in WD due to lack of alternatives. In rheumatoid arthritis, use another agent

Hepatic Impairment

- Usually improves hepatic disease in WD, even if severe

Cardiac Impairment
- No known effects

Elderly
- Use with caution

 Children and Adolescents
- WD can occur in children, usually ages 5 or older. Start with lower dose penicillamine, and adjust based on urinary copper excretion

Pregnancy
- Category C. Use only for WD or cystinuria (not rheumatoid arthritis). Reduce dose to 750 mg daily, and reduce to 250 mg/daily for a planned cesarean section 6 weeks before the planned birth date

Breast Feeding
- Patients taking penicillamine should not breast feed

Potential Advantages
- Proven, long-standing treatment for WD, usually effective

Potential Disadvantages
- Multiple AEs, including paradoxical worsening in 20–50% of patients

Primary Target Symptoms
- Monitor urinary copper to determine effectiveness. Treatment should improve neurological symptoms, such as parkinsonism, dystonia, ataxia, depression, and psychosis, over time

 Pearls
- The high incidence of paradoxical worsening and multiple AEs seen with penicillamine have led many to suggest that trientine should be the first-line agent in WD
- Other agents with known effects in WD include tetrathiomolybdate and intramuscular dimercaprol
- In asymptomatic individuals diagnosed by abnormal test results or family screening, it is uncertain if zinc or penicillamine is the most appropriate initial treatment

 Suggested Reading

Brewer GJ. Novel therapeutic approaches to the treatment of Wilson's disease. Expert Opin Pharmacother 2006;7(3):317–24.

Brewer GJ. The risks of free copper in the body and the development of useful anticopper drugs. Curr Opin Clin Nutr Metab Care 2008;11(6):727–32.

Das SK, Ray K. Wilson's disease: an update. Nat Clin Pract Neurol 2006;2(9):482–93.

Wiggelinkhuizen M, Tilanus ME, Bollen CW, Houwen RH. Systematic review: clinical efficacy of chelator agents and zinc in the initial treatment of Wilson disease. Aliment Pharmacol The 2009;29(9):947–58.

PHENOBARBITAL

THERAPEUTICS

Brands
- Luminal, Alkabel

Generic?
Yes

 Class
- Antiepileptic drug (AED), barbiturate

Commonly Prescribed for
(FDA approved in bold)
- **Generalized tonic-clonic, psychomotor, and partial seizures (monotherapy and adjunctive, children and adults)**
- Status epilepticus
- Seizures resulting from cerebral malaria
- Sedation
- Anxiety
- Alcohol or barbiturate withdrawal

 How the Drug Works
- Phenobarbital raises seizure thresholds or alters seizure patterns in animal models
- The exact mechanism of action is unknown but likely enhances GABA-A receptor activity
- Depresses glutamate excitability, alters sodium, calcium, and potassium channel conductance

How Long Until It Works
- Seizures – should decrease by 2 weeks

If It Works
- Seizures – goal is the remission of seizures. Continue as long as effective and well-tolerated. Consider tapering and slowly stopping after 2 years without seizures, depending on the type of epilepsy

If It Doesn't Work
- Increase to highest tolerated dose
- Epilepsy: consider changing to another agent, adding a second agent or referral for epilepsy surgery evaluation. When adding a second agent, keep in mind drug interactions

 Best Augmenting Combos for Partial Response or Treatment-Resistance
- Epilepsy: drug interactions complicate multi-drug therapy. Phenobarbital is a second-line agent in developed countries due to AE profile

Tests
- CBC, hepatic and kidney function panels at baseline and every 6 months

ADVERSE EFFECTS (AEs)

How Drug Causes AEs
- CNS AEs are probably caused by effects of increased GABA activity and alteration of ion channel function
- Vitamin D deficiency is caused by induction of metabolism

Notable AEs
- Sedation, ataxia, vertigo, cognitive dulling, depression, nystagmus, irritability, emotional disturbances
- Nausea, vomiting, hypotension
- Rash, uncommonly Stevens-Johnson syndrome

 Life-Threatening or Dangerous AEs
- Megaloblastic anemia, rarely agranulocytosis
- Respiratory depression: use with caution in patients with asthma or pulmonary disease

Weight Gain
- Common

unusual not unusual common problematic

Sedation
- Problematic

unusual not unusual common problematic

What to Do About AEs
- A dose decrease may improve CNS AEs
- For megaloblastic anemia, treat with folate

Best Augmenting Agents for AEs
- No treatment for most AEs other than lowering dose or stopping drug

DOSING AND USE

Usual Dosage Range

- Epilepsy: 30–180 mg/day (as monotherapy)

Dosage Forms

- Tablets: 15, 16, 30, 32, 60, 65, and 100 mg
- Capsules: 16 mg
- Elixir 15 or 20 mg/5 mL
- Intravenous solution: 30, 60 or 65 or 130 mg/mL

How to Dose

- Epilepsy as monotherapy: start at 30–50 mg at bedtime. Increase in 5–30 mg increments every week until goal dose (usually 90–180 mg/day)
- Status epilepticus: Give 20 mg/kg at rate no greater than 100 mg/min. Do not substitute oral or intramuscular
- When adding to other AEDs start at 30 mg at bedtime and titrate more slowly
- When changing from another AED, the transition should take at least 2 weeks

 Dosing Tips

- May induce its own metabolism
- Most patients can take once daily
- Check a serum level (usual goal 10–40 µg/mL) for optimal dosage. Required dose may be higher for the control of simple and complex partial, compared with tonic-clonic, seizures

Overdose

- Similar to barbiturates. Respiratory depression, ataxia, nystagmus, tachycardia, hypotension, hypothermia can all occur

Long-Term Use

- Safe for long-term use with periodic laboratory monitoring

Habit Forming

- Tolerance, psychological and physical dependence can occur, especially with long-term use at high doses. Use with caution in patients with depression or history of substance abuse

How to Stop

- Abrupt withdrawal can lead to seizures in patients with epilepsy
- Often requires prolonged taper compared to other AEDs

Pharmacokinetics

- Hepatic metabolism. Potent hepatic P450 CYP3A4 inducer. Mean half-life in adults is 100 hours, in children mean is 65 hours. Peak drug levels at 1–3 hours. 25% of drug is excreted renally. Bioavailability is 100%. May reduce folate by inhibiting dihydrofolate reductase. About 50% protein bound

 Drug Interactions

- Potent inducer of hepatic P450 metabolism. Lowers levels of many medications including warfarin, lamotrigine, tricyclic antidepressants, corticosteroids, methadone, cyclosporine, ACTH, vitamin D, verapamil, and nifedipine, among many others
- Variable effect on phenytoin metabolism
- Many AEDs inhibit CYP2C9 or CYP2C19 and can increase serum levels of phenobarbital, including phenytoin, valproic acid, carbamazepine, and felbamate
- Acetazolamide, ethosuximide, and antacids can lower levels

 Other Warnings/ Precautions

- CNS AEs can be severe when used with other CNS depressants
- Toxicity magnified with alcohol use
- Folate deficiency and hyperhomocysteinemia
- Can diminish systemic effects of exogenous or endogenous corticosteroids
- Bone and mineral loss with long-term use, increases vitamin D requirements
- May cause anesthesia at high doses: use with caution in patients with acute or chronic pain
- Increased tendency to fibrosis, including Dupuytren's contractures
- Reduces effectiveness of hormonal contraceptives

Do Not Use

- Patients with a proven allergy to primidone or phenobarbital, or patients with porphyria

Renal Impairment
- Usually a lower dose is required, but there are no clear guidelines on how much to decrease. For patients with creatinine clearance less than 10 mL/min, increase dosing interval by 50–100%. Consider supplemental dose post-dialysis

Hepatic Impairment
- Use with caution in patients with significant disease. Do not use in patients with hepatic encephalopathy

Cardiac Impairment
- No known effects

Elderly
- May need lower dose. More likely to experience CNS AEs and can increase fall risk

 Children and Adolescents
- Usual dose 2–6 mg/kg/day in 1–2 doses
- Commonly used for neonatal and febrile seizures
- In status epilepticus can give up to 30 mg/kg at rate no greater than 100 mg/min. Effective brain concentrations within 3 minutes
- May cause paradoxical excitement, aggression, tearfulness, or hyperkinetic states
- Can cause cognitive side effects in children when used to prevent febrile seizures

 Pregnancy
- Risk category D. High rate of fetal malformations, and infants can experience withdrawal after birth
- Risk of neonatal hemorrhage due to vitamin K deficiency. Supplement with folate and vitamin K 1 month prior and during delivery. Risks of stopping medication must outweigh risk to fetus
- Supplementation with 0.4 mg of folic acid before and during pregnancy is recommended

Breast Feeding
- Drug is found in mother's breast milk in substantial quantities
- Generally recommendations are to discontinue drug or bottle feed, but may assist in preventing infant withdrawal from drug
- Monitor infant for sedation, poor feeding, or irritability

Potential Advantages
- Effective for multiple types of epilepsy. Useful in refractory epilepsy
- Inexpensive. Long half-life
- Lower abuse potential than other barbiturates

Potential Disadvantages
- Sedation and multiple potential AEs
- Potent hepatic induction complicates therapy with other AEDs
- Unlike many other AEDs, not useful for mood disorders. May cause depression

Primary Target Symptoms
- Seizure frequency and severity
- Anxiety and alcohol withdrawal symptoms

 Pearls
- Commonly used in developing countries due to low cost and ability to treat multiple seizure types
- For patients with epilepsy, even with good seizure control, it may be worth changing to another agent due to potential AEs such as sedation, bone loss, and cognitive slowing
- In children, more effective than phenytoin in small studies for the prevention of febrile seizures, but cognitive AEs are common
- Less popular than benzodiazepines for alcohol withdrawal. Respiratory depression, especially when combined with alcohol, is a potential problem
- Use with extreme caution in patients with a history of substance abuse, depression, or suicidal tendencies

Suggested Reading

Abend NS, Dlugos DJ. Treatment of refractory status epilepticus: literature review and a proposed protocol. Pediatr Neurol 2008; 38(6):377–90.

Gaily E, Liukkonen E, Paetau R, Rekola R, Granström ML. Infantile spasms: diagnosis and assessment of treatment response by video-EEG. Dev Med Child Neurol 2001;43(10):658–67.

Hayner CE, Wuestefeld NL, Bolton PJ. Phenobarbital treatment in a patient with resistant alcohol withdrawal syndrome. Pharmacotherapy 2009;29(7):875–8.

PHENYTOIN

THERAPEUTICS

Brands

- Dilantin, Phenytek, Epanutin

Generic?
Yes

Class
- Antiepileptic drug (AED)

Commonly Prescribed for
(FDA approved in bold)
- **Generalized tonic-clonic and complex partial seizures (monotherapy or adjunctive in adults and children)**
- **Treatment of seizures during or following neurosurgery**
- **Status epilepticus**
- Trigeminal neuralgia
- Glossopharyngeal neuralgia
- Migraine prophylaxis
- Neuropathic pain
- Junctional epidermolysis bullosa
- Preeclampsia (alternative to magnesium sulfate)
- Cardiac arrhythmias (especially glycoside-induced)
- Myotonia

How the Drug Works

- Reduces hyperexcitability, likely by effect on sodium channels
- May modulate T-type calcium channels, but not in the thalamus (unlike AEDs used for absence seizures)

How Long Until It Works
- Seizures – may decrease by 2–3 weeks
- Trigeminal neuralgia – may start working in hours to weeks

If It Works
- Seizures – goal is the remission of seizures. Continue as long as effective and well-tolerated. Consider tapering and slowly stopping after 2 years without seizures, depending on the type of epilepsy
- Pain – goal is the reduction of pain severity and frequency. If trigeminal neuralgia remits on medication, periodically attempt to lower dose or discontinue

If It Doesn't Work
- Increase to highest tolerated dose
- Epilepsy: consider changing to another agent, adding a second agent or referral for epilepsy surgery evaluation. Check drug level
- Pain – try an alternative agent

Best Augmenting Combos for Partial Response or Treatment-Resistance

- Epilepsy: keep in mind drug interactions and their effect on levels

Tests
- During intravenous administration, continuous heart monitoring is required, with frequent blood pressure checks
- Obtain blood counts monthly for the first few months due to risk of blood dyscrasias

ADVERSE EFFECTS (AEs)

How Drug Causes AEs
- CNS side effects are probably caused by sodium channel effects

Notable AEs
- Nystagmus, ataxia, dysarthria, insomnia, nervousness, motor twitching, tremor, dizziness, impaired memory
- Gingival hyperplasia, rash (usually morbilliform), hirsutism, coarsening of facial features
- Pneumonia, sinusitis, rhinitis, asthma
- Tinnitus, diplopia, eye pain, taste loss
- Lymph node hyperplasia, chest pain, edema
- Soft tissue injury with intravenous use

Life-Threatening or Dangerous AEs

- Hypotension, cardiac conduction abnormalities with rapid intravenous administration. Can be fatal. Less likely with phosphenytoin
- May inhibit insulin release and cause hyperglycemia. Rare diabetes insipidus
- Blood dyscrasias (thrombocytopenia or agranulocytosis)
- Rare serious allergic rash (Stevens-Johnson syndrome, lupus erythematosus syndrome)
- Rare lymphoma or multiple myeloma
- Toxic hepatitis and liver damage

- May cause cerebellar atrophy with long-term use at high doses
- "Purple glove syndrome" is a rare complication associated with intravenous use. Extremities become swollen, discolored, and painful. May require amputation

Weight Gain
- Not Unusual

unusual not unusual common problematic

Sedation
- Commom

unusual not unusual common problematic

What to Do About AEs
- Side effects may decrease or remit after a longer time on a stable dose
- A small decrease in dose may improve side effects
- Stop drug for any hematologic abnormalities
- Recommend good oral hygiene to prevent gingival hyperplasia

Best Augmenting Agents for AEs
- Take with food to avoid GI AEs
- Most AEs only improve with stopping drug or lowering dose

DOSING AND USE

Usual Dosage Range
- Epilepsy: 300 – 600 mg/day for adults
- Trigeminal Neuralgia – 300–500 mg/day in divided doses

Dosage Forms
- Chewable tablets: 50 mg
- Capsules: 100 mg, extended release 30, 100, 200 and 300 mg
- Oral suspension: 125 mg/5 mL
- Injection: 50 mg/mL
- As prodrug fosphenytoin: 150 mg in 2 mL or 750 in 10 mL vials

How to Dose
- Start at 300 mg/day in 3 divided doses. Can use once daily with extended-release drug once a stable dose is established. Increase up to 600 mg/day

---

- Follow drug levels to determine effective dose and if compliance is in question
- For patients with hypoalbuminemia, kidney or liver disease, check free drug level
- Status epilepticus: 15–20 mg/kg load, followed by usual maintenance dose of 4–6 mg/kg/day
- Flush the medication with sterile saline after intravenous administration to avoid local skin irritation

 Dosing Tips
- Adverse events increase with dose
- Usual effective levels are 7–20 mg/L but vary from patient to patient
- Tube feeding can decrease absorption, give 2 hours before or after
- Drug takes 7–10 days to achieve steady state – wait to check levels

Overdose
- At concentrations > 20 mcg/mL: nystagmus
- At concentrations > 30 mcg/mL: ataxia
- At concentrations > 40 mcg/mL: diminished mental capacity, coma, hypotension, lack of pupillary reactivity
- Lethal dose is estimated to be 2–5 grams, with death from respiratory and circulatory depression

Long-Term Use
- Safe for long-term use

Habit Forming
- No

How to Stop
- Taper slowly. Abrupt withdrawal can lead to seizures in patients with epilepsy

Pharmacokinetics
- Oral peak plasma levels at 12 hours, intravenous within 1.5–3 hours. At higher doses, individual patients may not be able to metabolize drug, leading to high drug levels. This may produce toxic drug levels as half-life increases at higher concentrations. Plasma half-life ranges from 6–24 hours. About 90% protein bound. Metabolized in liver; metabolites are excreted in urine

Drug Interactions

- Potent inducer of P450 hepatic metabolism, particularly CYP2B6, CYP3A4
- Levels increase due to inhibition of metabolism (valproic acid, acute ethanol, allopurinol, amiodarone, omeprazole, cimetidine, fluconazole, benzodiazepines among others), displacement from protein binding sites (salicylates, tricyclic antidepressants, valproic acid) or unknown mechanisms (ibuprofen and phenothiazines)
- Levels decrease due to drugs that increase metabolism (carbamazepine, barbiturates, chronic ethanol, rifampin), decrease absorption (antacids) or unknown mechanisms (nitrofurantoin, pyridoxine, and many antineoplastics)
- Can increase metabolism of other drugs, including valproic acid, carbamazepine, amiodarone, mexiletine, theophylline, corticosteroids, cardiac glycosides, and estrogens and corticosteroids. Decreased levels of dopamine, levodopa, phenothiazines, among many others
- Can increase lithium toxicity (even with normal lithium serum levels)
- Decreased effectiveness of meperidine while increasing toxic metabolite
- May displace warfarin, leading to bleeding complications

⚠ **Other Warnings/ Precautions**

- CNS side effects increase when taken with other CNS depressants
- May decrease serum or free thyroxine concentrations
- Any unusual bleeding or bruising, fever, or mouth sores should raise concern for rare blood dyscrasias
- Use with caution in patients with acute intermittent porphyria

Do Not Use

- Patients with a proven allergy to phenytoin. Do not use in sinus bradycardia, sino-atrial block, 2nd or 3rd degree AV block, or in patients with Adams-Stokes syndrome

Renal Impairment

- Because phenytoin is highly protein bound, it is often easier to use than many other AEDs. No post-dialysis supplement is required

Hepatic Impairment

- Clearance may be decreased in patients with severe liver disease. Reduce dose

Cardiac Impairment

- Use with caution in hypotension or myocardial insufficiency, especially intravenously

Elderly

- May be more susceptible to CNS and cardiovascular side effects

 Children and Adolescents

- Usual dose is 4–8 mg/kg/day. Maximum 300 mg/day. Checking levels can help determine best dose
- Divide doses equally if possible. If not, give the larger dose at bedtime

 Pregnancy

- Risk category D. Fetal hydantoin syndrome includes craniofacial abnormalities, such as microcephaly and cleft lip and palate, and mild mental retardation. Clinically similar to fetal alcohol syndrome. Potential risk to fetus may be dose-related. Perhaps less likely to cause spinal malformations than valproate or carbamazepine
- Risk of neonatal hemorrhage due to vitamin K deficiency. Supplement with 10 mg per day 1 month before expected delivery
- Supplementation with 0.4 mg of folic acid before and during pregnancy is recommended
- Plasma levels may decrease, resulting in increased rate of seizures due to changes in metabolism. Check levels more frequently
- Risks of stopping medication must outweigh risk to fetus for patients with epilepsy. Seizures and potential status epilepticus place the woman and fetus at risk and can cause reduced oxygen and blood supply to the womb

• Patients taking phenytoin for conditions other than epilepsy should generally stop before considering pregnancy

Breast Feeding

• A small amount of drug is found in mother's breast milk
• Generally recommendations are to discontinue drug or bottle feed
• Monitor infant for sedation, poor feeding or irritability

THE ART OF NEUROPHARMACOLOGY

Potential Advantages

• Highly effective and relatively non-sedating. Low cost and available intravenously. Ease of monitoring drug levels

Potential Disadvantages

• Non-linear kinetics, drug interactions and CNS AEs
• Ineffective for many seizure types, including myoclonic, absence, and atonic seizures, Lennox-Gastaut and infantile spasms

Primary Target Symptoms

• Seizure frequency and severity

 Pearls

• Useful for many common epilepsy syndromes. Ability to monitor levels is useful in patients with frequent seizures requiring emergency visits
• Reduces risk of epileptic seizures associated with neurosurgery, especially if the doses are therapeutic, but does not reduce the incidence of post-traumatic epilepsy
• AE profile generally better than barbiturates, but worse than most newer AEDs
• In acute trigeminal neuralgia, often effective within days and may give as intravenous treatment in an emergency room setting (250 mg over 5 minutes). Effect of drug in chronic facial pain often decreases over time
• Fos-phenytoin is an alternative IV treatment for status epilepticus which is cleaved to phenytoin. It may be given 3 times faster or as IM injection without risk of "purple glove syndrome."
• Effective in some studies for treatment of neuropathic pain, such as diabetic neuropathy
• Effective treatment for myotonia (delayed relaxation of muscles after activity) in myotonia congenita or myotonic dystrophy patients who require pharmacologic treatment of their symptoms

 Suggested Reading

Cheshire WP. Fosphenytoin: an intravenous option for the management of acute trigeminal neuralgia crisis. J Pain Symptom Manage 2001;21(6):506–10.

Gilad R, Izkovitz N, Dabby R, Rapoport A, Sadeh M, Weller B, Lampl Y. Treatment of status epilepticus and acute repetitive seizures with i.v. valproic acid vs phenytoin. Acta Neurol Scand 2008;118(5):296–300.

Rozen TD. Trigeminal neuralgia and glossopharyngeal neuralgia. Neurol Clin 2004; 22(1):185–206. Review.

Trip J, Drost G, van Engelen BG, Faber CG. Drug treatment for myotonia. Cochrane Database Syst Rev 2006;(1):CD004762.

Tudur Smith C, Marson AG, Clough HE, Williamson PR. Carbamazepine versus phenytoin monotherapy for epilepsy. Cochrane Database Syst Rev 2002;(2):CD001911.

Walker M. Status epilepticus: an evidence based guide. BMJ 2005;331(7518):673–7.

PIZOTIFEN

THERAPEUTICS

Brands
• Sanomigran

Generic?
Yes

Class
• Antihistamine

Commonly Prescribed for
(FDA approved in bold)
• Migraine prophylaxis (children and adults)
• Cluster headache prophylaxis
• Treatment of serotonin syndrome
• Anxiety/social phobia

How the Drug Works
• An antihistamine and 5-HT2 receptor antagonist that is structurally related to tricyclic antidepressants. Has weak anticholinergic effects and may act as a calcium channel blocker at high doses. The relative importance of each action in headache prophylaxis is unclear. Prevention of cortical spreading depression may be the mechanism of action for all migraine preventatives

How Long Until It Works
• Migraines may decrease in as little as 2 weeks, but can take up to 2 months to see full effect

If It Works
• Migraine – goal is a 50% or greater decrease in migraine frequency or severity. Consider tapering or stopping if headaches remit for more than 6 months or if considering pregnancy

If It Doesn't Work
• Increase to highest tolerated dose
• Migraine: address other issues, such as medication-overuse, other coexisting medical disorders, such as anxiety, and consider changing to another agent or adding a second agent

Best Augmenting Combos for Partial Response or Treatment-Resistance
• Migraine: For some patients with migraine, low-dose polytherapy with 2 or more drugs

may be better tolerated and more effective than high-dose monotherapy. May use in combination with AEDs, antidepressants, natural products, and non-medication treatments, such as biofeedback, to improve headache control

Tests
• Monitor weight during treatment

ADVERSE EFFECTS (AEs)

How Drug Causes AEs
• Most are related to antihistamine and anticholinergic activity

Notable AEs
• Weight gain and sedation are most common
• Nausea, weakness, dry mouth, depression, sexual dysfunction, and urinary retention

Life-Threatening or Dangerous AEs
• Increased intraocular pressure
• Rare activation of mania or suicidal ideation
• Rare increase in seizures in patients with epilepsy
• Hypersensitivity reactions

Weight Gain
• Problematic

unusual   not unusual   common   problematic

Sedation
• Common

unusual   not unusual   common   problematic

What to Do About AEs
• Lower dose or switch to another agent. For serious AEs, do not use

Best Augmenting Agents for AEs
• Try magnesium for constipation. For migraine, consider using with agents that cause weight loss as an AE (e.g., topiramate)

DOSING AND USE

Usual Dosage Range
- 1.5–3 mg/day

Dosage Forms
- Tablets: 0.5 mg, 1.5 mg
- Elixir: 0.25 mg/ 5 mL

How to Dose
- Migraine/tension-type headache: Initial dose is either 0.5 mg 3 times daily or 1.5 mg at night. Increase if needed to 3 mg–4.5 mg daily. At doses above 3 mg/day, divide doses

 Dosing Tips
- Take largest dose at night to minimize drowsiness

Overdose
- CNS depression is most common, but hypotension, tachycardia, and respiratory depression may occur. Anticholinergic effects include fixed pupils, flushing, and hyperthermia

Long-Term Use
- Safe for long-term use

Habit Forming
- No

How to Stop
- No need to taper, but migraine often returns after stopping

Pharmacokinetics
- Rapid absorption with 78% bioavailability. Peak levels at 4–5 hours. Metabolized by glucuronidation. Most drug is excreted as metabolites in urine, but about 18% is excreted in feces. Elimination half-life of metabolite is 23 hours

 Drug Interactions
- Use with MAO inhibitors may increase toxicity and should be avoided
- May lower effectiveness of SSRIs due to serotonin antagonism
- Excess sedation with other CNS depressants (alcohol, barbiturates) can occur

 Other Warnings/ Precautions
- Tablets contain lactose and sucrose

Do Not Use
- Hypersensitivity to drug, angle-closure glaucoma, bladder neck obstruction, patients using MAO inhibitors, symptomatic prostatic hypertrophy

SPECIAL POPULATIONS

Renal Impairment
- No known effects

Hepatic Impairment
- May reduce metabolism. Titrate more slowly

Cardiac Impairment
- Rarely causes arrhythmias and ECG changes. Use with caution

Elderly
- More likely to experience AEs especially anticholinergic

 Children and Adolescents
- Drug has been used in children, usually age 7 and up, but may decrease alertness or produce paradoxical excitation

 Pregnancy
- Category B. Use only if potential benefit outweighs risk to the fetus

Breast Feeding
- Unknown if excreted in breast milk. Do not breast feed on drug

THE ART OF NEUROPHARMACOLOGY

Potential Advantages
- Commonly used migraine preventive, with efficacy in children and adults

Potential Disadvantages

- No large studies that demonstrate effectiveness. Sedation and weight gain

Primary Target Symptoms

- Headache frequency and severity

 Pearls

- Efficacy similar to flunarizine and nimodipine in some studies
- Small studies report effectiveness in preventing recurrent abdominal migraine in children
- Antiserotonin effects make pizotifen a potentially useful drug in the treatment of serotonin syndrome

 Suggested Reading

Barnes N, Millman G. Do pizotifen or propranolol reduce the frequency of migraine headache? Arch Dis Child 2004;89(7):684–5.

Christensen MF. Double blind placebo controlled trial of pizotifen syrup in the treatment of abdominal migraine. Arch Dis Child 1995; 73(2):183.

Silberstein SD. Preventive migraine treatment. Neurol Clin 2009;27(2):429–43.

Victor S, Ryan SW. Drugs for preventing migraine headaches in children. Cochrane Database Syst Rev 2003;(4):CD002761.

PRAMIPEXOLE

Brands
• Mirapex, Mirapexin

Generic?
No

 Class
• Dopamine agonist, non-ergot

Commonly Prescribed for
(FDA approved in bold)
• **Parkinson's disease (PD)**
• **Restless legs syndrome (RLS)**
• Fibromyalgia

 How the Drug Works
• Dopamine agonist, with high affinity for the D2 receptor. This action is likely the main reason for effectiveness in PD. Also binds with high affinity to D3 receptors, but the importance of this is unclear. The mechanism of action for RLS is probably related to D2 receptor agonism

How Long Until It Works
• PD – weeks
• RLS – days to weeks

If It Works
• PD – may require dose adjustments over time or augmentation with other agents. Most PD patients will eventually require carbidopa-levodopa to manage their symptoms
• RLS – safe for long-term use with dose adjustments

If It Doesn't Work
• PD – Bradykinesia, gait and tremor should improve. Non-motor symptoms including autonomic symptoms such as postural hypotension, depression, and bladder dysfunction do not improve. If the patient has significantly impaired functioning, add carbidopa-levodopa with or without pramipexole
• RLS – Rule out peripheral neuropathy, iron deficiency, thyroid disease. Change to another drug such as a benzodiazepine. Antiepileptic drugs (AEDs) such as

gabapentin or carbamazepine may also be beneficial. In severe cases consider opioids

 Best Augmenting Combos for Partial Response or Treatment-Resistance
• For suboptimal effectives add carbidopa-levodopa with or without a COMT inhibitor. MAO-B inhibitors may also be beneficial
• For younger patients with bothersome tremor: anticholinergics may help
• For severe motor fluctuations and/or dyskinesias with good "on" time, functional neurosurgery is an option. Adding pramipexole may allow reduction of total levodopa dose which can help dyskinesias
• Depression is common in PD and may respond to SSRIs
• Cognitive impairment/dementia is common in mid-late stage PD and may improve with acetylcholinesterase inhibitors
• For patients with late-stage PD experiencing hallucinations or delusions, withdraw pramipexole and consider oral atypical neuroleptics (quetiapine, olanzapine, clozapine). Acute psychosis is a medical emergency that may require hospitalization
• For RLS, can change to a different dopamine agonist or add another drug such as a benzodiazepine. AEDs such as gabapentin or carbamazepine may be beneficial. In severe cases consider opioids

Tests
• None required

How Drug Causes AEs
• Direct effect on dopamine receptors

Notable AEs
• Drowsiness, nausea, dizziness, hallucination, constipation, postural hypotension, weakness, edema, urinary frequency. Dyskinesia and hallucinations usually occur only with advanced PD patients

Life-Threatening or Dangerous AEs

- May cause somnolence or sudden-onset sleep, often without warning. Occurs more often than with ergot agonists or carbidopa-levodopa

Weight Gain

- Unusual

Sedation

- Common

What to Do About AEs

- Nausea can be problematic when initiating drug – titrate slowly
- Hallucinations or delusions may require stopping the medication
- Warn patients about the risks of sleeping while driving

Best Augmenting Agents for AEs

- Amantadine may help suppress dyskinesias
- Orthostatic hypotension: adjust dose or stop antihypertensives, add supplemental salt, and consider fludrocortisone or midodrine

---

DOSING AND USE

Usual Dosage Range

- PD – 1.5–4.5 mg daily, divided into 3 doses
- RLS – 0.25–0.5 mg daily, 2–3 hours before bedtime

Dosage Forms

- Tablets: 0.125, 0.25, 0.5, 1.0, 1.5 mg

How to Dose

- PD: Start at 0.125 mg 3 times daily with or without concomitant levodopa. Each week increase each dose by 0.125 mg until reaching 1.5 mg 3 times daily or desired clinical effect
- RLS: take 2–3 hours before bedtime. Start at 0.125 mg, and increase to 0.25 mg in 4–7 days. After another 4–7 days increase to

0.5 mg if needed. There is no evidence that increasing doses higher is more effective

 Dosing Tips

- Slow titration will minimize nausea and dizziness. Food delays the time to maximum plasma levels by 1 hour

Overdose

- Symptoms include somnolence, agitation, orthostatic hypotension, chest and abdominal pain, nausea, or dyskinesias. For cases of excessive CNS stimulation, neuroleptics can be effective

Long-Term Use

- Safe for long-term use. Effectiveness may decrease over time in PD (years) and RLS (months)

Habit Forming

- No

How to Stop

- Taper and discontinue over a period of 1 week for PD, but no taper is required in RLS patients. PD and RLS symptoms may worsen, but serious AEs from discontinuation are rare

Pharmacokinetics

- 15% protein binding. >90% bioavailability. Half-life is 8–12 hours. Peak action in 2 hours. Over 90% of drug is excreted unchanged in the urine

 Drug Interactions

- Increases the effect of levodopa
- Drugs that are eliminated by renal secretion (cimetidine, ranitidine, diltiazem, triamterene, verapamil, quinidine, quinine) decrease the clearance of pramipexole
- Dopamine antagonists such as phenothiazines, metoclopramide diminish effectiveness
- Use with caution in patients on antihypertensive medications due to risk of orthostatic hypotension

Other Warnings/ Precautions

- Dopamine agonists can precipitate impulse control disorders, such as pathological gambling

Do Not Use

- Hypersensitivity to the drug

SPECIAL POPULATIONS

Renal Impairment

- Decrease dose as follows:
- Creatinine clearance 30–59 mL/min: start at 0.125 mg twice a day to a maximum of 1.5 twice a day. Severe impairment with creatinine clearance 15–29 mL/min: start at 0.125 mg daily to a maximum of 1.5 mg daily. Use in hemodialyis patients is not recommended

Hepatic Impairment

- No known effects

Cardiac Impairment

- No known effects

Elderly

- There is reduced drug clearance, but no dose adjustment needed as the dose used is the lowest that provides clinical improvement

Children and Adolescents

- Not studied in children (PD is rare in pediatrics)

Pregnancy

- Category C. Use only if benefits of medication outweigh risks

Breast Feeding

- Inhibits prolactin secretion. Unknown if excreted in breast milk

THE ART OF NEUROPHARMACOLOGY

Potential Advantages

- PD: may delay need for carbidopa-levodopa and decreases risk of motor dyskinesias by 30%. This is especially important in younger PD patients. Unlike ergot-based agonists, no known risk of fibrotic complications. RLS: less risk of dependence compared to opioids or benzodiazepines and less augmentation than levodopa

Potential Disadvantages

- Less effective than carbidopa-levodopa for PD with more AEs such as hallucinations, somnolence and orthostatic hypotension. Patients with significant motor disability will require carbidopa-levodopa

Primary Target Symptoms

- PD – motor dysfunction including bradykinesia, hand function, gait and rest tremor
- RLS – pain, insomnia

Pearls

- Excellent drug for young patients with early PD. Favorable long-term AEs
- Using pramipexole (over levodopa) as initial treatment for PD has been associated with a lower risk of motor complications and dyskinesias
- First-line treatment for RLS with less augmentation or "rebound" than carbidopa-levodopa
- AE profile differs from ropinirole. More often associated with postural hypotension, dyskinesias and edema, but less likely to cause dizziness, syncope, nausea or respiratory problems
- For patients with mildly symptomatic disease, dopamine agonists are also appropriate for initial therapy, but for patients with significant disability, use carbidopa-levodopa early

Suggested Reading

Kvernmo T, Houben J, Sylte I. Receptor-binding and pharmacokinetic properties of dopaminergic agonists. Curr Top Med Chem 2008; 8(12):1049–67.

Lang AE. When and how should treatment be started in Parkinson disease? Neurology 2009;72 (7 Suppl):S39–43.

Varga LI, Ako-Agugua N, Colasante J, Hertweck L, Houser T, Smith J, Watty AA, Nagar S, Raffa RB. Critical review of ropinirole and pramipexole – putative dopamine D(3)-receptor selective agonists – for the treatment of RLS. J Clin Pharm Ther 2009;34(5):493–505.

Weiner WJ. Early diagnosis of Parkinson's disease and initiation of treatment. Rev Neurol Dis 2008;5(2):46–53; quiz 54–5.

PREDNISONE

THERAPEUTICS

Brands
- Sterapred, Cordrol, Orasone, Prednicot, Panasol, Meticorten, Deltasone

Generic?
Yes

Class
- Glucocorticoid, immunomodulator

Commonly Prescribed for
(FDA approved in bold)
- **Acute exacerbation of multiple sclerosis (MS)**
- **Optic neuritis**
- **Inflammatory myopathies: dermatomyositis (DM) and polymyositis (PM)**
- **Temporal arteritis (TA)**
- **Cerebral edema associated with brain tumor or head injury**
- **Asthma**
- **Chronic obstructive pulmonary disease**
- **Rheumatologic disorders: gouty arthritis, rheumatoid arthritis, bursitis (many others)**
- **Systemic lupus erythematosus**
- **Neoplastic disorders: Lymphoma and acute leukemia**
- **Hematologic disorders: hemolytic anemia, idiopathic thrombocytopenia purpura (many others)**
- **Allergic conditions, such as atopic dermatitis, drug hypersensitivity reactions**
- **Acute episodes in Crohn's disease and ulcerative colitis**
- **Nephrotic syndrome**
- **Tuberculous meningitis**
- Chronic inflammatory demyelinating polyneuropathy (CIDP)
- Myasthenia gravis (MG)
- Duchenne muscular dystrophy (DMD)
- Migraine headache
- Cluster headache
- Idiopathic intracranial hypertension
- Acute demyelinating encephalomyelitis (ADEM)
- Graves ophthalmopathy
- Ophthalmoplegic migraine

How the Drug Works
- Glucocorticoids have anti-inflammatory effects, modify immune responses to stimuli, and have numerous metabolic effects. Prednisone is a synthetic steroid with glucocorticoid and mineral corticoid activity

How Long Until It Works
- MS, migraine, cluster – days
- MG, DM, PM, CIDP – weeks to months
- TA – days

If It Works
- MS: Use for acute exacerbation that causes significant disability. In relapsing-remitting form, long-term disease-modifying treatments improve prognosis
- Migraine: Usually used for intractable headache or status migrainosus for short periods of time. After resolution, revert to safer preventive and abortive therapy
- Cluster: Start preventive therapy and prednisone at the beginning of a cycle
- MG: Weakness and fatigability improve. Decrease dose cautiously if clinical remission occurs
- DM/PM: Improves strength and mobility. Start a steroid-sparing agent if needed and taper dose cautiously with clinical remission
- CIDP: Improves strength and sensory symptoms and prevents disability. Decrease dose cautiously if clinical remission occurs
- TA: Monitor clinical response and sedimentation rate

If It Doesn't Work
- MS: If no improvement, question the diagnosis of relapsing-remitting MS
- Migraine: Start preventive therapy. Intravenous neuroleptics or dihydroergotamine may be needed to treat status migrainosus
- Cluster: Start preventive therapy
- MG: Start an adjunctive treatment or change to another modifying therapy. For acute exacerbations, consider plasma exchange or immune globulin
- DM/PM: Reconsider the diagnosis (inclusion body myositis, muscular dystrophy)
- CIDP: Immune globulin or plasma exchange are effective. Consider other less proven immune modulators
- TA: Reconsider diagnosis. Immunomodulatory drugs may be effective

Best Augmenting Combos for Partial Response or Treatment-Resistance

- MS: Use disease-modifying treatments to reduce relapses that require steroids
- Migraine/cluster: Antiemetics and migraine-specific agents may be used with prednisone for acute attacks
- MG: Use a steroid-sparing agent such as azathioprine, cyclosporine, mycophenolate mofetil, or cyclophosphamide. Treat acute exacerbations, usually with plasma exchange or immune globulin, and continue symptomatic treatment, such as pyridostigmine
- DM/PM: Combine with corticosteroid-sparing agents such as methotrexate or azathioprine
- CIDP: Combine with corticosteroid-sparing agent, immune globulin or plasma exchange
- TA: Combine with corticosteroid-sparing agent

Tests

- Monitor blood pressure, blood glucose and electrolytes with long-term therapy

ADVERSE EFFECTS (AEs)

How Drug Causes AEs

- Most AEs are due to immunosuppression, metabolic or endocrine effects

Notable AEs

- Convulsion, vertigo, paresthesias, aggravation of psychiatric conditions, insomnia
- Amenorrhea, cushingoid state, increased sweating, increased insulin requirement in diabetics, hyperglycemia
- Pancreatitis, abdominal distension, esophagitis, bowel perforation, weight gain
- Cataracts, glaucoma
- Impaired wound healing, petechiae, erythema, hirsutism
- Sodium and fluid retention, hypokalemia, metabolic acidosis
- Muscle weakness, myopathy, muscle mass loss, tendon rupture
- Thrombophlebitis, hypertension

 Life-Threatening or Dangerous AEs

- Fractures, aseptic necrosis of femoral or humoral heads
- Hypokalemia may cause cardiac arrhythmias
- Diabetic ketoacidosis, hyperosmolar coma
- May mask symptoms of infection and prevent ability of patient to prevent dissemination. May activate latent amebiasis or tuberculosis. May prolong coma in cerebral malaria
- Adrenal suppression with long-term use
- Psychosis with clouded sensorium, severe depression, personality changes, or insomnia, usually within 15–30 days after starting treatment. Female sex and higher doses are risk factors

Weight Gain

- Problematic

unusual   not unusual   common   problematic

Sedation

- Unusual

unusual   not unusual   common   problematic

What to Do About AEs

- For diseases such as migraine or MS, avoid using for prolonged periods of time and stop for most significant AEs
- In diseases requiring long-term treatment, consider using corticosteroid-sparing agents – often starting these treatments with prednisone to reduce the dose requirement and possibly allow discontinuation as clinical symptoms improve
- Weight-bearing exercises are recommended to promote bone protection and minimize muscle wasting
- Weight gain – avoid other medications that may exacerbate, dietary modification
- Hypertension – convert to a glucocorticoid with less sodium-retaining potency, such as methylprednisolone or dexamethasone

Best Augmenting Agents for AEs

- With prolonged treatment, use daily calcium and vitamin D supplements and bisphosphonates to prevent osteoporosis and fractures, and H2 blocker or proton pump inhibitors to prevent peptic ulcers

DOSING AND USE

Usual Dosage Range
- 5–200 mg daily (The range of doses varies dramatically depending on the disease being treated.)

Dosage Forms
- Tablets: 1 mg, 2.5 mg, 5 mg, 10 mg, 20 mg, 50 mg
- Oral solution: 5 mg/5 mL, 5 mg/mL

How to Dose
- MS: Give 200 mg for 1 week for acute exacerbations, followed by 80 mg every other day for 1 month. Other regimens using lower doses may also be effective
- Migraine: No standard regimen. Usually used for less than 1 week for status migrainosus at doses of 10–60 mg daily with rapid taper
- Cluster: Often used for 2–3 weeks at a time. Doses of 10–80 mg/day appear effective. Start with a higher dose and taper over 1–3 weeks
- MG: In outpatients, start at 20 mg daily and increase by 5 mg every 3–5 days until reaching target dose of 1.0 mg/kg/day (usually 50–100 mg) over 4–8 weeks. Then after 1 month at goal dose, slowly taper every month as clinical symptoms improve, either by lowering the daily dose or decreasing doses only on alternate days until patients are taking only every other day
- DM/PM – Start at 1 mg/kg (up to 80 mg) daily for 4–6 weeks, usually in combination with a steroid-sparing agent. Decrease by 10 mg a week until taking 40 mg, then by 5 mg a week until taking 20 mg. Then decrease by only 2.5 mg a week until at 10 mg and by 1 mg every 2 weeks until at 5 mg per day. Taper very slowly at lower doses and monitor strength during treatment
- CIDP – Start at 1–1.5 mg/kg per day (usually 50–80 mg and not greater than 100 mg). Taper by 5–10 mg per month in clinically stable patients. For some patients, tapering to an alternate day regimen is an alternative. For example, patients may taper by 20 mg every other day (60–40 then 60–20 then 60–0) every month. Taper more slowly at doses of 15 mg/day and below. For recurrence of clinical symptoms, a temporary increase to previous dose is often effective
- DMD – Give 0.75 mg/kg per day or alternatively 5 mg/kg every other day
- TA – Start at 40–60 mg daily. Start tapering every 2–4 weeks as symptoms permit, but taper more slowly at doses of 20 mg or less. Most patients will require 9–12 months of treatment and symptoms often reappear with a too rapid taper

Dosing Tips
- Give with food to avoid GI upset
- In patients improving on long-term treatment, consider converting to every-other-day dosing to reduce AEs

Overdose
- Large doses often produce cushingoid changes, including moonface, central obesity, hirsutism, acne, hypertension, osteoporosis, sexual dysfunction, diabetes, hyperlipidemia, peptic ulcer, and electrolyte and fluid imbalance

Long-Term Use
- Often used for long periods of time but long-term AEs may be significant and steroid-sparing agents are often used in MG or DM

Habit Forming
- No

How to Stop
- Taper rapidly for exacerbation of acute disorder, such as MS
- Taper very slowly over months and monitor for recurrence of symptoms in chronic disorders, such as MG or DM
- Acute adrenal insufficiency can occur with too rapid withdrawal. Symptoms include nausea, anorexia, hypoglycemia, dizziness, orthostatic hypotension, fever, and myalgias. Return of normal adrenal and pituitary function may take up to 9 months

Pharmacokinetics
- Half-life 60 minutes. Hepatic metabolism to prednisolone, which has a half-life of 115–212 min. Protein binding 70–90%
- Prednisone 5 mg is equal to prednisolone 5 mg, cortisone 25 mg, dexamethasone 0.75 mg, and methylprednisolone 4 mg

Drug Interactions
- Do not give live vaccines during therapy with high doses

- Estrogens, oral contraceptives, and ketoconazole may decrease clearance and increase levels
- Barbiturates may reduce effects
- Rifampin, ephedrine, and phenytoin may increase clearance and reduce effects
- Prednisone may increase digitalis or cyclosporine toxicity
- May cause severe hypokalemia with potassium-depleting diuretics
- Reduces salicylate levels and effectiveness
- May inhibit growth-promoting effect of somatrem
- May decrease levels of isoniazid
- May alter activity of oral anticoagulants or theophylline

 Other Warnings/ Precautions

- May suppress reactions to skin tests
- Although occasionally used for chronic active hepatitis, may actually be harmful for hepatitis B

Do Not Use

- Hypersensitivity to drug, systemic fungal infection

SPECIAL POPULATIONS

Renal Impairment

- Patients are more likely to develop edema with steroids. Use with caution

Hepatic Impairment

- No known effects

Cardiac Impairment

- Associated with left ventricular free wall rupture after recent myocardial infarction. Use with caution

Elderly

- Consider lower doses due to lower plasma volumes and decreased muscle mass. Monitor blood pressure, glucose, and electrolytes at least every 6 months

 Children and Adolescents

- Appears safe. Frequently used in asthma, DMD, but may cause growth problems with long-term use

 Pregnancy

- Category C. Relatively lower placental transport compared to other steroids. May cause hypoadrenalism in infants

Breast Feeding

- Appears in breast milk and may suppress growth. Avoid breast feeding with high-dose, long-term treatment

THE ART OF NEUROPHARMACOLOGY

Potential Advantages

- Highly effective treatment for acute MS, TA, and migraine and cluster headache. Relatively fast-acting disease-modifying treatment for many neuromuscular conditions

Potential Disadvantages

- Effectiveness varies depending on the disorder. Numerous AEs, especially with long-term use

Primary Target Symptoms

- Depending on disorder: Treating and preventing neurological complications in MS, TA, reducing pain in headache disorders, improving weakness in neuromuscular conditions

 Pearls

- Although generally effective for improving symptoms and functioning after acute MS exacerbations, does not improve long-term outcome or disease course. Use for serious symptoms such as weakness, inability to ambulate and not for pure sensory symptoms
- MS patients hospitalized with acute symptoms typically will receive intravenous treatment with methylprednisolone (usually 1 g up to 5 days) or dexamethasone
- Cardiac arrhythmias are most common with rapid intravenous administration of methylprednisolone (1 g in 10 minutes) rather than with oral prednisone therapy
- In MG, prednisone may produce remission in about 30% of patients and improve symptoms in another 50%. Benefit begins in

2–3 weeks and peaks at 4–6 months. Often combined with other immunotherapies

- About half of MG patients experience worsening after initiating steroid treatment, with a minority requiring intubation. This usually begins within 5–6 days after starting treatment and may persist for another week
- Because of the risk of initial deterioration, initiate treatment with high-dose steroid mainly in inpatients receiving concurrent treatment with immune globulin or plasma exchange. In other patients, start at a lower dose
- Short courses of intravenous corticosteroids are typically used in cases of ADEM or transverse myelitis
- In TA, initiating treatment with intravenous corticosteroids for 2–5 days may improve long-term outcome
- TA typically responds dramatically to prednisone and it is important to begin treatment early to avoid visual complications. Still, given the need for long-term treatment, it is important to confirm diagnosis with temporal artery biopsy
- The treatment of CNS vasculitis is similar to that of MG or DM. Usual starting dose is 1 mg/kg/day. Cyclophosphamide is an alternative treatment
- In DMD, daily prednisone or prednisolone therapy appears to have an anabolic effect, improves muscle strength and forced vital capacity, and prevents loss of ambulation for up to 3 years. Non-ambulatory patients are more likely to experience weight gain. Deflazcort, a prednisone derivative, also appears effective and is less likely to cause weight gain. The optimal age for starting prednisone in DMD is unknown
- An alternative treatment for intractable migraine during pregnancy, due to lack of safe preventive or abortive treatment. Use short-term for bouts of status migrainosus
- When effective in migraine, patients usually improve within 24 hours
- May reduce the duration of attacks of ophthalmoplegic migraine, which may be a recurrent demyelinating neuropathy rather than migraine
- Corticosteroids (often dexamethasone) are commonly used in emergency room settings for severe migraine, and may reduce recurrence. However, they may be associated with greater AEs than standard migraine treatment and do not usually resolve medication-overuse headache
- Steroids are effective in the majority of patients with cluster headache. Effective regimens include dexamethasone 4–8 mg/day, and prednisolone. The majority of patients achieve at least some improvement, but due to long AEs, steroids are generally tapered over 2–3 weeks. The majority of patients experience recurrence after completing the taper, so preventive therapy should be started when initiating treatment
- Shorter corticosteroid courses, to reduce AEs, may be appropriate in cluster headache depending on disease severity and frequency of cycles: for patients with frequent cycles (more than 1/year) consider a taper of 10 days or less
- Prednisone and other corticosteroids may be helpful for symptoms of idiopathic intracranial hypertension, but withdrawal can actually precipitate worsening. Avoid using, especially since weight gain from frequent use may exacerbate the disease
- Dexamethasone is usually used for the treatment of cerebral edema related to primary or metastatic brain tumors or head trauma

Suggested Reading

Burton JM, O'Connor PW, Hohol M, Beyene J. Oral versus intravenous steroids for treatment of relapses in multiple sclerosis. Cochrane Database Syst Rev 2009;(3):CD006921.

Campbell C, Jacob P. Deflazacort for the treatment of Duchenne Dystrophy: a systematic review. BMC Neurol 2003;3:7.

Diener HC. How to treat medication-overuse headache: prednisolone or no prednisolone? Neurology 2007;69(1):14–15.

Dodick DW, Capobianco DJ. Treatment and management of cluster headache. Curr Pain Headache Rep 2001;5(1):83–91.

Manzur AY, Kuntzer T, Pike M, Swan A. Glucocorticoid corticosteroids for Duchenne muscular dystrophy. Cochrane Database Syst Rev 2008;(1):CD003725.

Mazlumzadeh M, Hunder GG, Easley KA, Calamia KT, Matteson EL, Griffing WL, Younge BR, Weyand CM, Goronzy JJ. Treatment of giant cell arteritis using induction therapy with high-dose glucocorticoids: a double-blind, placebo-controlled, randomized prospective clinical trial. Arthritis Rheum 2006;54(10):3310–18.

Merlini L, Cicognani A, Malaspina E, Gennari M, Gnudi S, Talim B, Franzoni E. Early prednisone treatment in Duchenne muscular dystrophy. Muscle Nerve 2003;27(2):222–7.

Pageler L, Katsarava Z, Diener HC, Limmroth V. Prednisone vs. placebo in withdrawal therapy following medication overuse headache. Cephalalgia 2008;28(2):152–6.

Vincent A, Leite MI. Neuromuscular junction autoimmune disease: muscle specific kinase antibodies and treatments for myasthenia gravis. Curr Opin Neurol 2005;18(5):519–25.

PREGABALIN

THERAPEUTICS

Brands
• Lyrica, Zeegap

Generic?
No

Class
• Anti-epileptic drug (AED)

Commonly Prescribed for
(FDA approved in bold)
• **Partial-onset seizures (adjunctive for adults)**
• **Neuropathic pain associated with post-herpetic neuralgia**
• **Neuropathic pain associated with diabetic peripheral neuropathy**
• **Fibromyalgia**
• Migraine prophylaxis
• Facial pain
• Panic disorder
• Mania or bipolar disorder
• Generalized anxiety disorder
• Alcohol/benzodiazepine withdrawal

How the Drug Works
• Structural analog of GABA that binds at the $\alpha_2\delta$ subunit and reduces calcium influx. Changes calcium channel function but not a channel blocker
• Reduces release of excitatory neurotransmitters, such as glutamate, noradrenaline and substance P
• Inactive at GABA receptors and does not affect GABA uptake or degradation

How Long Until It Works
• Seizures – 2 weeks
• Pain/anxiety – days-weeks
• Fibromyalgia – often in the first week

If It Works
• Seizures – goal is the remission of seizures. Continue as long as effective and well-tolerated. Consider tapering and slowly stopping after 2 years without seizures, depending on the type of epilepsy
• Pain – goal is reduction of pain. Usually reduces but does not cure pain and there is recurrence off the medication. Consider tapering for conditions that may improve

over time, i.e., post-herpetic neuralgia or fibromyalgia

If It Doesn't Work
• Epilepsy: consider changing to another agent, adding a second agent or referral for epilepsy surgery evaluation
• Pain: If not effective in 2 months, consider stopping or using another agent

Best Augmenting Combos for Partial Response or Treatment-Resistance
• Epilepsy: No major drug interactions with other AEDs. Using in combination may worsen CNS side effects or weight gain
• Neuropathic pain: Can use with tricyclic antidepressants, SNRIs, other AEDs or opioids to augment treatment response. Proven to decrease opioid requirements in patients with post-herpetic neuralgia
• Anxiety: Usually used as an adjunctive agent with SSRIs, SNRIs, MAO inhibitors, or benzodiazepines

Tests
• No regular blood tests are recommended

ADVERSE EFFECTS (AEs)

How Drug Causes AEs
• CNS AEs are probably caused by interaction with calcium channel function

Notable AEs
• Sedation, dizziness, fatigue, blurred vision
• Myoclonus, usually mild and does not cause discontinuation
• Weight gain, nausea, constipation, peripheral edema, pruritus
• Decreased libido, erectile dysfunction. May impair fertility in men
• Euphoria and confusion

Life-Threatening or Dangerous AEs
• Associated with decreased platelet counts, increased creatinine kinase, and mild PR interval prolongation in clinical trials, although rarely of clinical significance

Weight Gain
• Common

Sedation
• Common

• May wear off with time

What to Do About AEs
• Decrease dose or take a higher dose at night to avoid sedation
• Switch to another agent

Best Augmenting Agents for AEs
• Adding a second agent unlikely to decrease side effects

DOSING AND USE

Usual Dosage Range
• Epilepsy: 150–600 mg/day
• Neuropathic pain: 100–600 mg/day, usually 300 mg or less
• Fibromyalgia: 300–450 mg/day

Dosage Forms
• Capsules: 25 mg, 50 mg, 75 mg, 100 mg, 150 mg, 200 mg, 300 mg

How to Dose
• Start at 150 mg in 2–3 divided doses, can double dose every 3–7 days to 300 mg and 600 mg or goal dose

 Dosing Tips
• Slow increase will improve tolerability. Increase evening dose first
• Use a slower titration for patients on other medications that can increase CNS AEs
• Most patients take twice daily, but may be better tolerated initially using 3 times a day dosing, especially during titration phase
• Rate of absorption decreased with food

Overdose
• No reported deaths. Patients taking higher than recommended dose experience no more side effects than patients taking recommended doses

Long-Term Use
• Safe for long-term use

Habit Forming
• Unlikely in most but occasionally in patients with a history of substance abuse

How to Stop
• Taper slowly
• Abrupt withdrawal can lead to seizures in patients with epilepsy

Pharmacokinetics
• Renal excretion without being metabolized. Linear kinetics. Half-life 5–7 hours. Does not bind to plasma proteins

 Drug Interactions
• No significant interactions, may increase CNS side effects of other medications

 Other Warnings/ Precautions
• Sedation and dizziness can increase risk of falls in elderly patients

Do Not Use
• Patients with a proven allergy to pregabalin or gabapentin
• May cause problems in patients with galactose intolerance or Lapp lactase deficiency (due to the capsule containing galactose)

SPECIAL POPULATIONS

Renal Impairment
• Renal excretion means that lower dose is needed and that hemodialysis will remove Adjust dose based on creatinine clearance: below 15 mL/min, 25–75 mg/day, 15–30 mL/min 50–150 mg/day, 30–60 mL/min 75–300 mg/day

Hepatic Impairment
• No known effects

Cardiac Impairment
• No known effects

Elderly

- May need lower dose. More likely to experience AEs

 Children and Adolescents

- Safety and efficacy unknown

 Pregnancy

- Risk category C. Some teratogenicity in animal studies. Patients taking for pain or anxiety should generally stop before considering pregnancy
- Supplementation with 0.4 mg of folic acid before and during pregnancy is recommended

Breast Feeding

- Some drug is found in mother's breast milk
- Generally recommendations are to discontinue drug or bottle feed
- Monitor infant for sedation, poor feeding or irritability

THE ART OF NEUROPHARMACOLOGY

Potential Advantages

- Linear kinetics compared to gabapentin and easy to titrate. Proven efficacy for multiple types of pain and anxiety as well as epilepsy. May help sleep. Relatively low AEs

Potential Disadvantages

- Dosing twice daily. Weight gain. Ineffective against most primary generalized epilepsies

Primary Target Symptoms

- Seizure frequency and severity
- Pain
- Anxiety

 Pearls

- Advantages compared to gabapentin include twice-daily dosing, and more clinical trials demonstrating efficacy for pain
- Easier to titrate quickly compared to tricyclic antidepressants, gabapentin
- Good evidence for multiple types of neuropathic pain. May avoid opioid use
- No evidence of benefit beyond 300 mg dose and more AEs for post-herpetic neuralgia or diabetic peripheral neuropathy
- 50 mg of pregabalin is equivalent to 300 mg of gabapentin, but at higher gabapentin doses, this ratio does not apply
- First drug with FDA approval to treat fibromyalgia. Improved sleep, vitality and fatigue as well as pain
- Schedule V controlled substance. Recreational drug users report euphoria with high doses similar to diazepam

 Suggested Reading

Jensen TS, Madsen CS, Finnerup NB. Pharmacology and treatment of neuropathic pains. Curr Opin Neurol 2009;22(5):467–74.

Lyseng-Williamson KA, Siddiqui MA. Pregabalin: a review of its use in fibromyalgia. Drugs 2008; 68(15):2205–23.

Moore RA, Straube S, Wiffen PJ, Derry S, McQuay HJ. Pregabalin for acute and chronic pain in adults. Cochrane Database Syst Rev 2009;(3):CD007076.

Shneker BF, McAuley JW. Pregabalin: a new neuromodulator with broad therapeutic indications. Ann Pharmacother 2005; 39(12):2029–37.

Warner G, Figgitt DP. Pregabalin: as adjunctive treatment of partial seizures. CNS Drugs 2005;19(3):265–72; discussion 273–4.

PRIMIDONE

THERAPEUTICS

Brands
• Mysoline

Generic?
Yes

 Class
• Antiepileptic drug (AED)

Commonly Prescribed for
(FDA approved in bold)
• **Generalized tonic-clonic, psychomotor, and partial seizures (monotherapy and adjunctive, children and adults)**
• Essential tremor
• Long QT syndrome
• Psychosis

 How the Drug Works
• Primidone and its 2 metabolites (phenobarbital and phenylethylmalonamide) raise seizure thresholds or alter seizure patterns
• The exact mechanism of action is unknown but likely enhances GABA-A receptor activity
• Depresses glutamate excitability, alters sodium, calcium and potassium channel conductance

How Long Until It Works
• Seizures – should decrease by 2 weeks
• Essential tremor – should improve tremors in 1–2 weeks

If It Works
• Seizures – goal is the remission of seizures. Continue as long as effective and well-tolerated. Consider tapering and slowly stopping after 2 years without seizures, depending on the type of epilepsy
• Essential tremors – tremors improve but usually do not remit. Use lowest effective dose

If It Doesn't Work
• Increase to highest tolerated dose
• Epilepsy: consider changing to another agent, adding a second agent or referral for epilepsy surgery evaluation. When adding a second agent, keep in mind drug interactions

 Best Augmenting Combos for Partial Response or Treatment-Resistance
• Epilepsy: drug interactions complicate multi-drug therapy. Primidone itself is a second-line agent in developed countries due to AE profile

Tests
• CBC, hepatic and kidney function panels at baseline and every 6 months

ADVERSE EFFECTS (AEs)

How Drug Causes AEs
• CNS AEs are probably caused by effects of increased GABA activity and alteration of ion channel function
• Vitamin D deficiency is caused by induction of metabolism

Notable AEs
• Ataxia, vertigo, sedation, nystagmus, diplopia
• Nausea, vomiting, anorexia
• Irritability, emotional disturbances, confusion, rash
• 20–25% of patients experience an idiosyncratic reaction with nausea and drowsiness and even obtundation – often on the first dose

 Life-Threatening or Dangerous AEs
• Megaloblastic anemia, rarely agranulocytosis
• Respiratory depression: use with caution in patients with asthma or pulmonary disease

Weight Gain
• Common

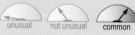

Sedation
• Problematic

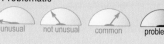

What to Do About AEs

- A small dose decrease may improve CNS AEs
- Do not take the first dose of medication alone, due to risk of idiosyncratic reaction
- Megaloblastic anemia: treat with folate

Best Augmenting Agents for AEs

- No treatment for most AEs other than lowering dose or stopping drug

DOSING AND USE

Usual Dosage Range

- Epilepsy: 500–1000 mg/day (as monotherapy)
- Essential tremor: 250–750 mg/day, in 2–3 divided doses

Dosage Forms

- Tablets: 50 mg and 250 mg

How to Dose

- Epilepsy as monotherapy: start at 100–125 mg at bedtime for 3 days, then increase to 100–125 mg twice daily. On day 7 increase to 100–125 mg three times daily. on day 10, 250 mg 3 times daily to maintenance dose
- Essential tremor: titrate slower and with lower doses
- When adding to other AEDs start at 100–125 mg at bedtime and titrate more slowly
- When changing from another AED to primidone, the transition should take at least 2 weeks

 Dosing Tips

- Primidone may induce its own metabolism
- Check a serum level (goal 5–12 mcg/mL) for optimal dosage

Overdose

- Similar to barbiturates. Respiratory depression, ataxia, nystagmus, tachycardia, hypotension, hypothermia can all occur

Long-Term Use

- Safe for long-term use with periodic laboratory monitoring

Habit Forming

- Tolerance, psychological and physical dependence can occur, especially with long-term use at high doses. Use with caution in patients with depression or history of substance abuse

How to Stop

- Taper slowly
- Abrupt withdrawal can lead to seizures in patients with epilepsy

Pharmacokinetics

- Hepatic metabolism: 15–25% is metabolized to phenobarbital, a potent hepatic P450 CYP3A4 inducer. Half-life of primidone is 10–12 hours but its metabolites have a half-life of several days. Renal excretion. Bioavailability is about 100%
- May reduce folate by inhibiting dihydrofolate reductase
- Primidone itself has minimal protein binding, but the phenobarbital metabolite is about 50% protein bound

 Drug Interactions

- Phenobarbital metabolite is a potent inducer of hepatic P450 metabolism. Lowers levels of many medications including warfarin, lamotrigine, tricyclic antidepressants, corticosteroids, methadone, cyclosporine, ACTH, vitamin D, verapamil, and nifedipine among many others
- Variable effect on phenytoin metabolism
- Many AEDs inhibit CYP2C9 or CYP2C19 and can increase serum levels of primidone/phenobarbital, including phenytoin, valproic acid, carbamazepine, and felbamate
- Acetazolamide, ethosuximide, and antacids can lower levels

 Other Warnings/ Precautions

- CNS AEs can be severe when used with other CNS depressants
- Toxicity magnified with alcohol use
- Folate deficiency and hyperhomocysteinemia
- Bone and mineral loss with long-term use, increases vitamin D requirements
- May cause anesthesia at high doses: use with caution in patients with chronic pain
- Reduces effectiveness of hormonal contraceptives

Do Not Use
• Patients with a proven allergy to primidone or phenobarbital, or in patients with porphyria

Renal Impairment
• Decrease dosing intervals as follows. Creatinine clearance 10–50 mL/min give 2–3 times daily, < 10 mL/min 1–2 times daily, and for patients on hemodialysis give a supplemental dose after each session

Hepatic Impairment
• Use with caution in patients with moderate-severe disease

Cardiac Impairment
• No known effects

Elderly
• May need lower dose. More likely to experience CNS AEs which can limit effectiveness in essential tremor

 Children and Adolescents
• In children under age 8, start with 50 mg at night for 3 days. Then increase to 50 mg twice daily for 3 days, then 100 mg twice daily for 3 days and increase to maintenance dose
• Usual dose 125–250 mg three times daily or 10–25 mg/kg/day
• May cause paradoxical excitement, aggression, tearfulness, or hyperkinetic states. Cognitive side effects can limit use

 Pregnancy
• Risk category D. High rate of fetal malformations and infants can experience withdrawal after birth. Risk of neonatal hemorrhage due to vitamin K deficiency. Supplement with folate and vitamin K prior to and during delivery. Risks of stopping medication must outweigh risk to fetus for patients with epilepsy

• Patients taking for tremor should generally stop before considering pregnancy
• Supplementation with 0.4 mg of folic acid before and during pregnancy is recommended

Breast Feeding
• Drug is found in mother's breast milk in substantial quantities
• Generally recommendations are to discontinue drug or bottle feed
• Monitor infant for sedation, poor feeding or irritability

Potential Advantages
• Effective for multiple types of epilepsy. Useful in refractory epilepsy
• Less toxic than phenobarbital
• Proven effectiveness for essential tremor

Potential Disadvantages
• Sedation and multiple potential side effects
• Potent hepatic induction complicates therapy with other AEDs
• Unlike many other AEDs, not useful for mood disorders. May cause depression

Primary Target Symptoms
• Seizure frequency and severity
• Tremor

 Pearls
• Commonly used in developing countries due to low cost and ability to treat multiple seizure types
• Effective in essential tremor, but AEs limit use in the elderly patients most likely to have the disorder
• May be useful for some patients with primary orthostatic tremor or dystonic tremor
• QTc prolongation by AEDs is one suggested mechanism of sudden death in epilepsy but this is not proven. Primidone may shorten QTc interval in some patients with long QT syndrome

Suggested Reading

Beghi E. Efficacy and tolerability of the new antiepileptic drugs: comparison of two recent guidelines. Lancet Neurol 2004;3(10):618–21.

Ondo WG. Essential tremor: treatment options. Curr Treat Options Neurol 2006;8(3):256–67.

Rincon F, Louis ED. Benefits and risks of pharmacological and surgical treatments for essential tremor: disease mechanisms and current management. Expert Opin Drug Saf 2005;4(5):899–913.

Serrano-Dueñas M. Use of primidone in low doses (250 mg/day) versus high doses (750 mg/day) in the management of essential tremor. Double-blind comparative study with one-year follow-up. Parkinsonism Relat Disord 2003;10 (1):29–33.

Sun MZ, Deckers CL, Liu YX, Wang W. Comparison of add-on valproate and primidone in carbamazepine-unresponsive patients with partial epilepsy. Seizure 2009;18(2):90–3.

PROCHLORPERAZINE

THERAPEUTICS

Brands
- Compazine, Stemetil, Buccastem

Generic?
Yes

Class
- Antipsychotic, antiemetic

Commonly Prescribed for
(FDA approved in bold)
- **Schizophrenia**
- **Nonpsychotic anxiety in adults**
- **Severe nausea and vomiting**
- Migraine
- Vertigo and labyrinthine disorders
- Mania in bipolar disorder

How the Drug Works
- Dopamine receptor antagonist with greater action at D2 receptors. Also blocks serotonin 2A receptors, alpha-adrenergic receptors and is an antihistamine

How Long Until It Works
- Injection effective within 10 minutes, oral 1–2 hours

If It Works
- Use at lowest effective dose
- Monitor QT corrected (QTc) interval
- Continue to assess effect of the medication and if it is still needed

If It Doesn't Work
- Increase dose, or discontinue and change to another agent

Best Augmenting Combos for Partial Response or Treatment-Resistance
- Migraine: often combined with NSAIDs and triptans or ergots
- Nausea and vomiting: corticosteroids

Tests
- Monitor weight, blood pressure, lipids, and fasting glucose with frequent chronic use.

Obtain blood pressure and pulse before initial IV use and monitor QTc with ECG

ADVERSE EFFECTS (AEs)

How Drug Causes AEs
- Motor AEs and prolactinemia – blocking of D2 receptors
- Hypotension – blocking of alpha-1 adrenergic receptors

Common AEs
- Most common: Dizziness, sedation, dry mouth, constipation, skin changes
- Tachycardia, hypo- or hypertension
- Akathisia, parkinsonism

Life-Threatening or Dangerous AEs
- Tardive dyskinesias
- ECG changes including prolongation of QTc. Rarely cardiac arrest

Weight Gain
- Common

unusual not unusual common problematic

- With frequent use

Sedation
- Common

unusual not unusual common problematic

What to Do About AEs
- Rarely causes ECG changes. Use with caution if QTc is above 450 (women) or 440 (men) and do not administer with QTc greater than 500
- If excessive sedation occurs, use only as a rescue agent for inpatients or when patients can lie down or sleep

Best Augmenting Agents for AEs
- Give fluids to avoid hypotension, tachycardia, and dizziness
- Give anticholinergics (diphenhydramine or benztropine) or benzodiazepines for extrapyramidal reactions

DOSING AND USE

Usual Dosage Range
- Migraine/vertigo: 5–80 mg/daily (oral, IM, IV) or 25–100 mg/daily (rectal)

Dosage Forms
- Tablets: 5 mg, 10 mg
- Sustained-release capsules: 10 mg
- Syrup: 5 mg/5 mL
- Injection: 5 mg/mL
- Buccal tablets: 3 mg
- Suppositories: 2.5 mg, 5 mg, 25 mg

How to Dose
- Migraine/vertigo: Give IV, IM, oral, or suppository. Non-oral routes are useful for severe vomiting. Give 5–10 mg 3–4 times daily as needed for nausea, vertigo, or headache. Alternatively give 25 mg rectally up to 2 times daily

Dosing Tips
- Migraine/vertigo: Effective in hospitalized patients while monitoring blood pressure, pulse, and daily ECG

Overdose
- CNS depression, hypotension, and extrapyramidal reactions are most common. Respiratory suppression or death is rare

Long-Term Use
- Safe for long-term use but may cause irreversible AEs (tardive dyskinesias) with frequent use

Habit Forming
- No

How to Stop
- No need to taper

Pharmacokinetics
- Hepatic metabolism via CYP2D6 and 3A4. Half-life 4–8 hours depending on route. 91–99% protein bound

Drug Interactions
- Use with CNS depressants (barbiturates, opiates, general anesthetics) potentiates CNS AEs
- Anticholinergics may decrease effects

- CYP450 3A4 (ketoconazole, fluoxetine, nefazodone, duloxetine), and 2D6 (duloxetine, paroxetine) inhibitors may increase levels
- May enhance effects of antihypertensives
- Use with alcohol or diuretics may increase hypotension
- May decrease effectiveness of dopaminergic agents
- May reduce effectiveness of anticoagulants

Other Warnings/ Precautions
- Use cautiously in patients with Parkinson's disease or Lewy body dementia
- Neuroleptic malignant syndrome is characterized by fever, rigidity, confusion and autonomic instability, and is more common with IV antipsychotic treatment

Do Not Use
- Hypersensitivity to drug, CNS depression/coma, or QTc greater than 500

SPECIAL POPULATIONS

Renal Impairment
- No dose adjustment needed

Hepatic Impairment
- Use with caution

Cardiac Impairment
- May worsen orthostatic hypotension

Elderly
- More likely to experience movement AEs or hypotension

Children and Adolescents
- Efficacy and safety unknown for children under age 2. Base dose on weight. 9–13 kg: 2.5 mg up to 3 times daily. 14–17 kg: 2.5 mg 3–4 times daily. 18–38 kg: 2.5–5 mg up to 3 times daily

Pregnancy
- Category C. Extrapyramidal signs have been reported with phenothiazine use during

pregnancy. Use only for intractable headache or vomiting

Breast Feeding

• Probably found in breast milk

THE ART OF NEUROPHARMACOLOGY

Potential Advantages

• Effective medication for intractable migraine, vomiting, or vertigo. Less sedation and orthostasis than other neuroleptics

Potential Disadvantages

• Not as effective orally. Potential for movement disorders, especially with frequent use

Primary Target Symptoms

• Headache, vertigo, and nausea

Pearls

• In acute migraine, prochlorperazine suppositories are an effective treatment for severe headache with nausea.
• Pretreat or combine with diphenydramine, 25–50 mg, to reduce rate of akathisia and dystonic reactions. Benztropine is also useful and may be given orally or IM
• In outpatients with severe or daily headache, may be used daily for short periods of time (3–10 days) as a bridge treatment before preventive medication becomes effective
• May be effective and considered safe in the treatment of migraine in pregnancy

Suggested Reading

Friedman BW, Esses D, Solorzano C, Dua N, Greenwald P, Radulescu R, Chang E, Hochberg M, Campbell C, Aghera A, Valentin T, Paternoster J, Bijur P, Lipton RB, Gallagher EJ. A randomized controlled trial of prochlorperazine versus metoclopramide for treatment of acute migraine. Ann Emerg Med 2008;52(4):399–406.

Khatri R, Hershey AD, Wong B. Prochlorperazine – treatment for acute confusional migraine. Headache 2009; 49(3):477–80.

Siow HC, Young WB, Silberstein SD. Neuroleptics in headache. Headache 2005; 45(4):358–71.

Tanen DA, Miller S, French T, Riffenburgh RH. Intravenous sodium valproate versus prochlorperazine for the emergency department treatment of acute migraine headaches: a prospective, randomized, double-blind trial. Ann Emerg Med 2003;41(6):847–53.

PROPRANOLOL

THERAPEUTICS

Brands
- Inderal, Inderal-LA, InnoPran XL

Generic?
Yes

Class
- Antihypertensive, beta-blocker (non-selective)

Commonly Prescribed for
(FDA approved in bold)
- **Migraine prophylaxis**
- **Essential tremor**
- **Hypertension**
- **Angina pectoris due to coronary atherosclerosis**
- **Cardiac arrhythmias (including supraventricular arrhythmias, ventricular tachycardia, digitalis intoxication)**
- **Myocardial infarction**
- **Hypertrophic subaortic stenosis**
- **Pheochromocytoma**
- Akathisia (antipsychotic induced)
- Parkinsonian tremor
- Congestive heart failure
- Tetralogy of Fallot
- Hyperthyroidism (adjunctive)
- Generalized anxiety disorder
- Post-traumatic stress disorder
- Prevention of variceal bleeding

How the Drug Works
- Migraine: Proposed mechanisms include inhibition of adrenergic pathway, interaction with serotonin system and receptors, inhibition of nitric oxide production, and normalization of contingent negative variation. Prevention of cortical spreading depression may be the mechanism of action for all migraine preventives
- Tremor: effectiveness is likely due to peripheral beta-2 receptor antagonism

How Long Until It Works
- Migraines – within 2 weeks, but can take up to 3 months on a stable dose to see full effect
- Tremor – within days

If It Works
- Migraine – goal is a 50% or greater decrease in migraine frequency or severity. Consider tapering or stopping if headaches remit for more than 6 months or if considering pregnancy
- Tremor – reduction in the severity of tremor, allowing greater functioning with daily activities and clearer speech

If It Doesn't Work
- Increase to highest tolerated dose
- Migraine: Address other issues, such as medication overuse, other coexisting medical disorders, such as anxiety, and consider changing to another drug or adding a second drug
- Tremor: Coadministration with primidone up to 250 mg/day can augment response. Second-line medications include benzodiazepines, such as clonazepam, gabapentin, topiramate, methazolamide, nadolol, and botulinum toxin (useful for voice and hand tremor.) For truly refractory patients, thalamotomy or deep brain stimulation of the ventral intermediate nucleus of the thalamus are options
- Alternatives for tremor include hand weights and eliminating caffeine. Low doses of alcohol reduce tremor, but is not generally recommended

Best Augmenting Combos for Partial Response or Treatment-Resistance

- Migraine: For some patients, low-dose polytherapy with 2 or more drugs may be better tolerated and more effective than high-dose monotherapy. May use in combination with AEDs, antidepressants, natural products, and non-pharmacologic treatments, such as biofeedback, to improve headache control
- Tremor: Can use in combination with primidone or second-line medications

Tests
- None required

ADVERSE EFFECTS (AEs)

How Drug Causes AEs
- Antagonism of beta receptors

Notable AEs

- Bradycardia, hypotension, hyper- or hypoglycemia, weight gain
- Bronchospasm, cold/flu symptoms, sinusitis, pneumonias
- Dizziness, vertigo, fatigue/tiredness, depression, sleep disturbances
- Sexual dysfunction, decreased libido, dysuria, urinary retention, joint pain
- Exacerbation of symptoms in peripheral vascular disease and Raynaud's syndrome

 ## Life-Threatening or Dangerous AEs

- In acute CHF, may further depress myocardial contractility
- Can blunt premonitory symptoms of hypoglycemia in diabetes and mask clinical signs of hyperthyroidism
- Non-selective beta-blockers such as propranolol can inhibit bronchodilation, making them contraindicated in asthma, severe COPD
- Do not use in pheochromocytoma unless alpha-blockers are already being used
- Risk of excessive myocardial depression in general anesthesia

Weight Gain

- Common

Sedation

- Common

What to Do About AEs

- Lower dose, change to extended-release formulation, or switch to another agent

Best Augmenting Agents for AEs

- When patients have significant benefit from beta-blocker therapy but hypotension limits treatment, consider alpha-agonists (midodrine) or volume expanders (fludrocortisones) for symptomatic relief

---

DOSING AND USE

Usual Dosage Range

- 40–400 mg/day

Dosage Forms

- Tablets: 10, 20, 40, 60, 80, 90 mg
- ER capsules: 60, 80, 120, 160 mg
- Oral solution: 4 or 8 mg/mL
- Injection: 1 mg/mL

How to Dose

- Migraine: Initial dose 40 mg/day in divided doses or once daily in extended-release preparations for most patients. Gradually increase over days to weeks to usual effective dose: 40–400 mg/day
- Tremor: Start 40 mg twice a day. The dosage may be gradually increased as needed to 120–320 mg/day in 2 to 3 divided doses

 ## Dosing Tips

- For extended-release capsules, give once daily at bedtime consistently, with or without food. Doses above 120 mg had no additional antihypertensive effect in clinical trials
- Food can enhance bioavailability

Overdose

- Bradycardia, hypotension, low-output heart failure, shock, seizures, coma, hypoglycemia, apnea, cyanosis, respiratory depression, and bronchospasm. Epinephrine and dopamine are used to treat toxicity

Long-Term Use

- Safe for long-term use

Habit Forming

- No

How to Stop

- Do not abruptly discontinue. Gradually reduce dosage over 1–2 weeks. May exacerbate angina, and there are reports of tachyarrhythmias or myocardial infarction with rapid discontinuation in patients with cardiac disease

Pharmacokinetics

- Half-life 3–5 hours, 8–11 in extended-release form. Bioavailability is 30%, 9–18% for long-acting. Hepatic metabolism to hydroxypropranolol (also pharmacologically active). 90% protein binding. Good CNS penetration due to high lipid solubility

Drug Interactions

- Cimetidine, oral contraceptives, ciprofloxacin, hydralazine, hydroxychloroquine, loop diuretics, certain SSRIs (with CYP2D6 metabolism), and phenothiazines can increase levels and/or effects of propranolol
- Use with calcium channel blockers can be synergistic or additive, use with caution
- Barbiturates, penicillins, rifampin, calcium and aluminum salts, thyroid hormones, and cholestyramine can decrease effects of beta-blockers
- NSAIDs, sulfinpyrazone, and salicylates inhibit prostaglandin synthesis and may inhibit the antihypertensive activity of beta-blockers
- Propranolol can increase AEs of gabapentin and benzodiazapines
- Propranolol can increase levels of lidocaine, resulting in toxicity and increase the anticoagulant effect of warfarin
- Increased postural hypotension with prazosin and peripheral ischemia with ergot alkaloids
- Sudden discontinuation of clonidine while on beta-blockers or when stopping together can cause life-threatening increases in blood pressure

Other Warnings/ Precautions

- May elevate blood urea, serum transaminases, alkaline phosphatase, and LDH
- Rare development of antinuclear antibodies (ANA)
- May worsen symptoms of myasthenia gravis
- Can lower intraocular pressure, interfering with glaucoma screening test

Do Not Use

- Sinus bradycardia, greater than first-degree heart block, cardiogenic shock
- Bronchial asthma, severe COPD
- Proven hypersensitivity to beta-blockers

atenolol are eliminated by the kidney and require dose adjustment. Use with caution

Hepatic Impairment

- Hepatic metabolism causes increased drug levels and half-life with significant hepatic disease. Use with caution

Cardiac Impairment

- Do not use in acute shock, MI, hypotension, and greater than first-degree heart block, but indicated in clinically stable patients post-MI to reduce risk of reinfarction starting 1–4 weeks after event. Metoprolol, another beta-blocker, is commonly used to reduce mortality and hospitalization for patients with stable CHF in patients already receiving ACE inhibitors and diuretics

Elderly

- Use with caution. May increase risk of stroke

Children and Adolescents

- Usual dose in children is 2–4 mg/kg in 2 divided doses. Maximum 16 mg/kg/day. Clinical trials for migraine prophylaxis did not include children. When stopping, taper slowly over 1–2 weeks

Pregnancy

- Category C. Embryotoxic in animal studies only at doses much higher than maximum recommended human doses. May reduce perfusion of the placenta. Use if potential benefit outweighs risk to the fetus. Most beta-blockers are class C, except atenolol, which is D, and acebutolol, pindolol, and sotalol, which are B

Breast Feeding

- Not recommended. Propranolol is found in breast milk, due to high lipid solubility, more than many other beta-blockers

SPECIAL POPULATIONS

Renal Impairment

- No significant changes in half-life or concentration, even with severe failure. Among beta-blockers, nadolol, sotalol, and

THE ART OF NEUROPHARMACOLOGY

Potential Advantages

- Proven effectiveness in migraine and ability to treat coexisting conditions, such as hypertension or anxiety. For tremor, less sedation than primidone and benzodiazepines

Potential Disadvantages
- Multiple potential undesirable AEs, including bradycardia, hypotension and fatigue

Primary Target Symptoms
- Migraine frequency and severity
- Tremor

Pearls
- Alternative beta-blockers for migraine: Metoprolol 100–200 mg/day, timolol 20–60 mg/day (FDA approved), atenolol 50–200 mg/day, nadolol 20–160 mg/day
- Beta-blockers that are partial agonists, with intrinsic sympathomimetic activity, are not effective in migraine prophylaxis. These include acebutolol, alprenolol, and pindolol

- Often used in combination with other drugs in migraine. Using to treat migraine may allow patients to better tolerate medications that cause tremor, such as valproate
- Not effective for cluster headache
- May worsen depression, but helpful for anxiety
- 50–70% of patients with essential tremor receive some relief, usually with about 50% improvement or greater
- Beta-1 selective antagonists are less effective in essential tremor but metoprolol may be an option in patients with asthma or severe COPD
- Recent studies have downgraded beta-blockers as a first-line treatment for hypertension compared with other classes due to lack of effectiveness, increased rate of stroke in elderly, and risk of provoking type II diabetes

Suggested Reading

Law MR, Morris JK, Wald NJ. Use of blood pressure lowering drugs in the prevention of cardiovascular disease: meta-analysis of 147 randomised trials in the context of expectations from prospective epidemiological studies. BMJ 2009;338:b1665.

Lyons KE, Pahwa R. Pharmacotherapy of essential tremor: an overview of existing and upcoming agents. CNS Drugs 2008;22 (12):1037–45.

Ramadan NM. Current trends in migraine prophylaxis. Headache 2007;47 (Suppl 1): S52–7.

Silberstein SD. Preventive migraine treatment. Neurol Clin 2009;27(2):429–43.

Taylor FR. Weight change associated with the use of migraine-preventive medications. Clin Ther 2008;30(6):1069–80.

PYRIDOSTIGMINE

THERAPEUTICS

Brands
- Mestinon, Mestinon Timespan, Regonal

Generic?
Yes

Class
- Cholinesterase inhibitor, peripheral

Commonly Prescribed for
(FDA approved in bold)
- **Myasthenia gravis (MG)**
- **Reversal of non-depolarizing muscle relaxants**

How the Drug Works
- Improves symptoms of MG by preventing the metabolism of acetylcholine by cholinesterase. This improves neuromuscular transmission in MG

How Long Until It Works
- Orally about 30 minutes, intramuscular form within 15 minutes, intravenously within 5 minutes

If It Works
- Continue to use to reduce symptoms of MG. Often combined with disease-modifying therapy such as immunosuppression or thymectomy

If It Doesn't Work
- Increase to the maximal dose: if no effect, question the diagnosis of MG. Remove potential offending medications. Consider immunosuppression or thymectomy

Best Augmenting Combos for Partial Response or Treatment-Resistance
- Generally not combined with other symptomatic treatments. For refractory MG, add immunotherapy

Tests
- None

ADVERSE EFFECTS (AEs)

How Drug Causes AEs
- Cholinergic properties of the drug

Notable AEs
- Muscarinic AEs include diarrhea, abdominal cramps, nausea, increased salivation, miosis, increased bronchial secretions, rash, worsening of bronchial asthma and diaphoresis. Nicotinic AEs, including fasciculations and muscle cramping, are less bothersome

Life-Threatening or Dangerous AEs
- Bradycardia – possibly leading to hypotension – is most common with IV use
- Cholinergic crisis – worsening weakness, usually with overdose of drug and severe cholinergic AEs – is very rare

Weight Gain
- Unusual

Sedation
- Unusual

What to Do About AEs
- Lower to tolerable dose, take with food

Best Augmenting Agents for AEs
- Treat GI AEs with anticholinergic that do not affect nicotinic receptors (so no weakness): *Glycopyrrolate* 1 mg, Probanthine 15 mg or *Hyoscyamine* sulfate 0.125 mg. Use 3 times a day or take with each pyridostigmine dose. For diarrhea try *loperamide* or *diphenoxylate* hydrochloride-atropine. To prevent bradycardia and excessive secretions with IV form, use atropine 0.6–1.2 mg IV immediately prior

DOSING AND USE

Usual Dosage Range
- MG – 180–1500 mg/day in divided doses. The average dose is 600 mg/day

- Reversal of non-depolarizing muscle relaxants: 10 – 20 mg

Dosage Forms
- Tablets: 60 mg
- Extended-release tablets: 180 mg
- Syrup: 60 mg/5 mL
- Injection: 5 mg/mL in 2 mL amps

How to Dose
- Start at 60 mg 3 times a day. Increase as tolerated each day with 3–6 times-daily dosing(120 mg every 2–3 hours) until having significant relief of MG symptoms or until AEs become bothersome. Usual most effective dose is 600 mg but varies from patient to patient
- Extended-release form is very useful for patients with difficulties on awakening. Use once or twice daily (total 180–1080 mg). Wait at least 6 hours between doses

Dosing Tips
- Take with food to reduce GI AEs

Overdose
- Symptoms may include abdominal pain, diarrhea and vomiting, excessive salivation, cold sweating, pallor, urinary urgency, blurry vision, muscle fasciculations, anxiety or panic, and paralysis. Treat with atropine IV 0.5 to 1 mg initially and use up to 10 mg

Long-Term Use
- Safe for long-term use

Habit Forming
- No

How to Stop
- No need to taper but MG symptoms will likely worsen

Pharmacokinetics
- Poorly absorbed from GI tract. Onset of action 20–45 minutes orally with duration of action 3–6 hours and half-life about 4 hours. IM/IV forms: duration 2–4 hours, onset of action in < 15 minutes IM and < 5 minutes IV. Drug excreted in urine up to 72 hours after administration

Drug Interactions
- Do not combine with other cholinesterase inhibitors
- May increase neuromuscular blocking effects of succinylcholine
- Magnesium may depress skeletal muscle effect and reduce drug effectiveness
- Corticosteroids may decrease drug effect, and increase drug effect with discontinuation
- Antiarrhythmics and local/general anesthetics decrease drug effectiveness and can cause generalized MG complications

Do Not Use
- Known hypersensitivity to the cholinesterase inhibitors. Mechanical intestinal or urinary obstruction

SPECIAL POPULATIONS

Renal Impairment
- No known effects

Hepatic Impairment
- No known effects

Cardiac Impairment
- Use with caution in MG patients with bradycardia, arrhythmias, hypotension or AV block

Elderly
- May have slower clearance of drug

Children and Adolescents
- Safe for use. Congenital MG usually presents in the first 2 years of life. These patients do not have antibodies (anti-Ache or Musk) or respond to immunosuppressants. Neonatal MG occurs in 12% of the pregnancies with a mother with MG. Symptoms start in the first 2 days and resolve within a few weeks. Juvenile MG starts in childhood but after the peripartum period

Pregnancy
- Category C. Use only if benefits of medication outweigh risks

Breast Feeding

• Excreted in breast milk. Do not use

THE ART OF NEUROPHARMACOLOGY

Potential Advantages

• Fewer AEs than other cholinesterase inhibitors for the symptomatic treatment of MG. Serious AEs are rare

Potential Disadvantages

• Does not cure MG. Need for frequent dosing. Eventually loses efficacy

Primary Target Symptoms

• To improve weakness, visual problems, respiratory symptoms associated with MG

Pearls

• Patients can occasionally develop drug resistance. Monitor symptoms and increase dose as needed
• Most cases of MG crisis are caused by worsening of the disease itself or some additional factor, such as infection. Cholinergic crisis is rare, especially if patients are taking the usual prescribed doses of pyridostigmine (less than 1500 mg/day)
• In crisis (i.e., when patients are intubated) there is no need to give drug. May prolong intubation due to increased secretions. Usually restarted after extubation
• To supplement oral dose before or during surgery, during labor or post-partum or during MG crisis, give 1/30 the usual oral dose either IM or as a slow IV infusion
• Avoid using telithromycin, aminoglycosides, interferon alpha, penicillamine, intravenous magnesium and intravenous lidocaine in MG patients. Use beta-blockers, fluroquinolones, and CNS depressants such as opioids or muscle relaxants with caution. Neuromuscular blocking agents can be used for anesthesia but in MG could delay extubation or recovery of muscle strength
• Occasionally used postoperatively for distention or urinary retention
• Can be used for orthostatic hypotension, by increasing ganglionic sympathetic traffic
• Extended-release form is used at bedtime, due to cholinergic AEs with frequent use

Suggested Reading

Argov Z. Management of myasthenic conditions: nonimmune issues. Curr Opin Neurol 2009; 22(5):493–7.

Gales BJ, Gales MA. Pyridostigmine in the treatment of orthostatic intolerance. Ann Pharmacother 2007;41(2):314–8.

Hetherington KA, Losek JD. Myasthenia gravis: myasthenia vs. cholinergic crisis. Pediatr Emerg Care 2005;21(8):546–8.

Kirmani JF, Yahia AM, Qureshi AI. Myasthenic crisis. Curr Treat Options Neurol 2004;6(1):3–15.

QUETIAPINE

THERAPEUTICS

Brands
- Seroquel, Ketipinor, Seroquel XR

Generic?
In some countries

 Class
- Atypical antipsychotic

Commonly Prescribed for
(FDA approved in bold)
- **Schizophrenia**
- **Bipolar disorder (depression and acute mania)**
- **Major depressive disorder (adjunctive)**
- Psychosis in patients with Parkinson's disease (PD) or dementia with Lewy bodies (DLB)
- Obsessive-compulsive disorder
- Autism
- Alcoholism
- Tourette syndrome
- Insomnia
- Anxiety

 How the Drug Works
- Blocks D2 receptor similar to other neuroleptics, but also blocks serotonin 2A receptors, which improves motor side effects and perhaps depression and cognitive problems
- May also affect serotonin 1A and other receptors, contributing to efficacy for cognitive and affective symptoms in some patients

How Long Until It Works
- Psychosis – may be effective in days, more commonly takes weeks or months to determine best dose and achieve best clinical effect. Usually 4–6 weeks
- Insomnia – may be effective immediately

If It Works
- Continue to use at lowest required dose. Most patients with schizophrenia see a reduction in psychosis with quetiapine (and other neuroleptics), but some patients, including many with PD and DLB, may improve more than 50%

If It Doesn't Work
- Increase dose

- In psychosis related to PD or DLB, reduce dose or eliminate offending medications, such as dopamine agonists or amantadine
- If not effective consider changing to clozapine. In PD and DLB, avoid long-term use of conventional antipsychotics
- Insomnia: if no sedation occurs despite adequate dosing, change to another agent

 Best Augmenting Combos for Partial Response or Treatment-Resistance
- Patients with affective disorders, such as bipolar disorder, may respond to mood stabilizing anticonvulsants, lithium, or benzodiazepines. In PD and DLB, cholinesterase inhibitors may improve symptoms (particularly in DLB).

Tests
- Prior to starting treatment and periodically during treatment, monitor weight, blood pressure, lipids, and fasting glucose due to risk of metabolic syndrome

ADVERSE EFFECTS (AEs)

How Drug Causes AEs
- Motor AEs – blocking of D2 receptors
- Sedation, weight gain – blocking of histamine 1 receptors
- Hypotension – blocking of alpha-1 adrenergic receptors
- Dry mouth, constipation – blocking of muscarinic receptors

Notable AEs
- Most common: sedation, weight gain, constipation, dry mouth,
- Less common: dizziness, tachycardia, nausea, akathisia, elevation of hepatic transaminases. May increase risk of cataracts

 Life-Threatening or Dangerous AEs
- Tardive dyskinesias (lower than other neuroleptics)
- Severe weight gain and metabolic syndrome/ diabetes
- Neuroleptic malignant syndrome (rare compared with conventional antipsychotics)

Weight Gain
- Common

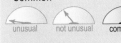

Sedation
- Problematic

What to Do About AEs
- Take at night: for many disorders there is no need for daytime dosing. Medical management for obesity, including weight loss and exercise, may help combat weight gain

Best Augmenting Agents for AEs
- Most AEs cannot be improved with an augmenting agent

DOSING AND USE

Usual Dosage Range
- Bipolar disorder/schizophrenia: 150–800 mg/day
- Psychosis in PD/DLB: 25–200 mg/day

Dosage Forms
- Capsules: 25 mg, 50 mg, 100 mg, 200 mg, 300 mg
- Extended release: 50 mg, 150 mg, 200 mg, 300 mg, 400 mg

How to Dose
- Start at 25 mg twice a day for acute psychosis or mania. If not tolerated, give larger dose in the evening. Increase by 25–50 mg (twice a day) every 1–2 days until effective dose is reached
- For depression or psychosis with PD or DLB, consider dosing all the medication at night. Start PD and DLB patients with psychosis on 12.5 mg at night and increase by 12.5 mg every 1–2 days until symptoms improve. Most patients respond to a lower dose (average 50–75 mg/day)
- Titrate more rapidly when treating acute mania or schizophrenia – up to 800 mg/day in some cases

Dosing Tips
- Patients with bipolar disorder (mania or depression) often need a high dose (over 400 mg/day) to achieve best results. Elderly and children often need lower doses

Overdose
- Sedation, hypotension, bradycardia, and dysarthria have been reported. Death is rare

Long-Term Use
- Safe for long-term use with appropriate monitoring

Habit Forming
- No, although may be used by addicts to manage drug withdrawal

How to Stop
- No need to taper, but psychosis or insomnia often recurs

Pharmacokinetics
- Hepatic metabolism to inactive metabolites via CYP450 3A and 2D6. Half-life 6–7 hours, and steady state reached in 2 days

Drug Interactions
- CYP3A and 2D6 inhibitors (ketoconazole, erythromycin, ciprofloxacin, duloxetine) and valproate may increase levels
- Enzyme inducers, such as phenobarbital, carbamazepine, phenytoin, increase clearance and may lower levels
- Quetiapine may slightly lower levels of valproate and lorazepam

Other Warnings/ Precautions
- May increase risk of cataracts, aspiration pneumonia, and priapism

Do Not Use
- Proven hypersensitivity to quetiapine

Renal Impairment
• No dose adjustment needed

Hepatic Impairment
• Use with caution. May need to lower dose

Cardiac Impairment
• May worsen orthostatic hypotension. Use with caution

Elderly
• Start with lower doses. Clearance reduced by about 40%

Children and Adolescents
• Efficacy and safety unknown, but occasionally used for affective disorders. Monitor for weight gain and other AEs

Pregnancy
• Category C. Probably safer than anticonvulsants during pregnancy for bipolar disorder. PD and DLB are uncommon in women of childbearing age. Use only if benefit outweighs risks

Breast Feeding
• Unknown if found in breast milk. Use while breast feeding is generally not recommended

THE ART OF NEUROPHARMACOLOGY

Potential Advantages
• Useful in controlling psychosis associated with PD at relatively low doses without risk of drug-induced parkinsonism or tardive dyskinesias. No risk of blood dyscrasias

Potential Disadvantages
• Probably less effective than clozapine. Does not usually improve motor symptoms of PD. Risk of weight gain and metabolic syndrome

Primary Target Symptoms
• Psychosis, depression, mania, and insomnia

Pearls
• Clozapine, formerly the first-line agent for psychosis with PD, is now often a second-line agent due to risk of agranulocytosis. Use low doses and titrate much more slowly when treating PD or DLB with neuroleptics compared to patients with mania or schizophrenia
• Previous studies suggested usefulness in treating psychosis in patients with Alzheimer's dementia, but subsequently shown to worsen cognitive function with significant AEs
• Often effective at low doses for insomnia, but not recommended as a first-line option. Atypical antipsychotics increase mortality when used to treat dementia-related psychosis

Suggested Reading

Keating GM, Robinson DM. Spotlight on quetiapine in bipolar depression. CNS Drugs 2007;21(8):695–7.

Kurlan R, Cummings J, Raman R, Thal L; Alzheimer's Disease Cooperative Study Group. Quetiapine for agitation or psychosis in patients with dementia and parkinsonism. Neurology 2007;68(17):1356–63.

Miyasaki JM, Shannon K, Voon V, Ravina B, Kleiner-Fisman G, Anderson K, Shulman LM, Gronseth G, Weiner WJ; Quality Standards Subcommittee of the American Academy of Neurology. Practice parameter: evaluation and treatment of depression, psychosis, and dementia in Parkinson disease (an evidence-based review): report of the Quality Standards Subcommittee of the American Academy of Neurology. Neurology 2006;66(7):996–1002.

Ondo WG, Tintner R, Voung KD, Lai D, Ringholz G. Double-blind, placebo-controlled, unforced titration parallel trial of quetiapine for dopaminergic-induced hallucinations in Parkinson's disease. Mov Disord 2005; 20(8):958–63.

Poewe W. When a Parkinson's disease patient starts to hallucinate. Pract Neurol 2008; 8(4):238–41.

Rabey JM, Prokhorov T, Miniovitz A, Dobronevsky E, Klein C. Effect of quetiapine in psychotic Parkinson's disease patients: a double-blind labeled study of 3 months' duration. Mov Disord 2007;22(3):313–8.

Srisurapanont M, Disayavanish C, Taimkaew K. Quetiapine for schizophrenia. Cochrane Database Syst Rev 2000;(3):CD000967.

QUININE SULFATE

THERAPEUTICS

Brands
- Formula Q, Legatrim, Qualaquin

Generic?
Yes

Class
- Antimalarial, neuromuscular drug

Commonly Prescribed for
(FDA approved in bold)
- **Malaria**
- Symptomatic myotonia (myotonia congenita, myotonic dystrophy)
- Leg cramps

How the Drug Works
- Quinine has several actions on skeletal muscle. Increases the refractory period by acting on the muscle membrane and sodium channel, decreases motor end-plate excitability, and affects the distribution of calcium within the muscle fiber

How Long Until It Works
- 1–2 hours

If It Works
- Continue to use

If It Doesn't Work
- Change to an alternative agent

Best Augmenting Combos for Partial Response or Treatment-Resistance
- Myotonia: Anticonvulsants, such as phenytoin and carbamazepine, are effective. The antiarrhythmic drug mexiletine (also a sodium channel blocker) is an alternative

Tests
- Obtain baseline ECG due to risk of cardiac arrhythmia (common in myotonic dystrophy)

ADVERSE EFFECTS (AEs)

How Drug Causes AEs
- Drug effect of blocking sodium channels

Notable AEs
- "Cinchonism" is a common set of AEs seen in most patients; includes headache, flushing, vertigo, hearing difficulties, tinnitus, blurry vision, and nausea. More severe symptoms include vomiting, abdominal pain, deafness, and blindness
- Hypersensitivity reactions include flushing, pruritus, rash, fever, tinnitus, and dyspnea
- Chest pain, orthostatic hypotension, hypoglycemia, anorexia, jaundice, and abnormal liver function tests

Life-Threatening or Dangerous AEs
- Cardiac arrhythmias, including atrioventricular block, atrial fibrillation, QTc prolongation, ventricular fibrillation, ventricular tachycardia, torsades de pointes, and cardiac arrest
- Hemolysis associated with glucose-6-phosphate dehydrogenase deficiency
- Severe hypersensitivity (angioedema)
- Rarely asthma or pulmonary edema

Weight Gain
- Unusual

unusual   not unusual   common   problematic

Sedation
- Unusual

unusual   not unusual   common   problematic

What to Do About AEs
- Lower dose for most AEs, but discontinue for serious AEs

Best Augmenting Agents for AEs
- Most AEs cannot be improved by an augmenting agent

DOSING AND USE

Usual Dosage Range
- 260–2000 mg/day

Dosage Forms
- Tablets: 260 mg
- Capsules: 200 mg, 260 mg, 324 mg, 325 mg

How to Dose
- Take 1–2 tablets or capsules at night and as needed during the day, up to 3 times daily

 Dosing Tips
- Take with food to reduce GI irritation

Overdose
- Tinnitus, dizziness, rash, intestinal cramping, and headache are common. At higher doses fever, vomiting, convulsions and apprehension occur. Blindness, hearing loss, arrhythmia and death may occur. Gastric lavage or emesis are indicated and acidification of urine will enhance elimination

Long-Term Use
- Safe for long-term use. Continue to assess need for use

Habit Forming
- No

How to Stop
- No need to taper

Pharmacokinetics
- Peak action 1–3 hours, half-life 4–5 hours. Most drug does not cross blood-brain barrier. 70–90% protein bound. Mostly hepatic metabolism

 Drug Interactions
- Antacids delay or decrease absorption
- Cimetidine reduces clearance and increases half-life
- Mefloquine coadministration may cause convulsions
- Rifampin increases hepatic clearance and lowers level
- Urinary alkalinizers, such as acetazolamide, sodium bicarbonate, increase levels

- Quinine enhances the action and levels of oral anticoagulants, digoxin, and succinylcholine
- May potentiate the effects of neuromuscular blocking agents

 Other Warnings/ Precautions
- May produce an elevated value for urinary 17-ketogenic steroids

Do Not Use
- Known hypersensitivity, pregnancy, glucose-6-phosphate dehydrogenase deficiency, myasthenia gravis

SPECIAL POPULATIONS

Renal Impairment
- Drug concentrations are increased with severe renal failure. Reduce dose and take twice a day or less. The effect of mild-moderate disease on drug levels is unknown

Hepatic Impairment
- Use with caution. Patients with severe disease may need a lower dose

Cardiac Impairment
- Risk of cardiac arrhythmias. Use with caution and consider alternative treatments

Elderly
- No known effects

 Children and Adolescents
- Appears safe in the treatment of malaria, but not studied for myotonia

 Pregnancy
- Category X with multiple congenital malformations, including deafness. Do not use

Breast Feeding
- Small amounts are excreted in breast milk. Use with caution

THE ART OF NEUROPHARMACOLOGY

Potential Advantages
• Effective treatment for disabling muscle cramps

Potential Disadvantages
• Risk of cardiac arrhythmias

Primary Target Symptoms
• Symptoms of myotonia (muscle pain, stiffness, weakness, dysphagia), pain

 Pearls

• Many patients with myotonia (delayed relaxation of muscles after activity) do not require pharmacologic treatment of their symptoms
• Weakness in myotonia is usually in the arms or hands
• Sodium channel blockers, such as phenytoin, mexiletine or tricyclic antidepressants, are now first-line treatment due to the risk of quinine precipitating cardiac arrhythmias. Benzodiazepines, calcium channel blockers, taurine, and prednisone and physical therapy may be beneficial for some patients

 Suggested Reading

Cleland JC, Griggs RC. Treatment of neuromuscular channelopathies: current concepts and future prospects. Neurotherapeutics 2008;5(4):607–12.

Duff HJ, Mitchell LB, Wyse DG, Gillis AM, Sheldon RS. Mexiletine/quinidine combination therapy: electrophysiologic correlates of anti-arrhythmic efficacy. Clin Invest Med 1991; 14(5):476–83.

Meola G, Sansone V. Treatment in myotonia and periodic paralysis. Rev Neurol (Paris) 2004; 160(5 Pt 2):S55–69.

RASAGILINE

THERAPEUTICS

Brands
- Azilect

Generic?
No

Class
- Monoamine oxidase type B (MAO-B) inhibitor

Commonly Prescribed for
(FDA approved in bold)
- Parkinson's disease (PD)
- Alzheimer's (AD) and other dementias

How the Drug Works
- Selectively blocks monoamine oxidase type B (MAO-B) and inhibits metabolism of dopamine, increasing its effectiveness. At higher doses, may affect MAO-A as well as -B and inhibit metabolism of norepinephrine, serotonin, and tyramine, as well as dopamine

How Long Until It Works
- PD – weeks

If It Works
- PD – may require dose adjustments over time or augmentation with other agents. Most PD patients will eventually require carbidopa-levodopa to manage their symptoms

If It Doesn't Work
- Bradykinesia, gait, and tremor should improve. If the patient has significantly impaired functioning, consider adding a dopamine agonist and/or carbidopa-levodopa

Best Augmenting Combos for Partial Response or Treatment-Resistance
- For suboptimal effectiveness consider adding a dopamine agonist and/or carbidopa-levodopa with or without a catechol-o-methyl transferase (COMT) inhibitor
- For younger patients with bothersome tremor: anticholinergics may help

- For severe motor fluctuations and/or dyskinesias with good "on" time, functional neurosurgery is an option
- Cognitive impairment/dementia is common in mid-late stage PD and may improve with acetylcholinesterase inhibitors
- For patients with late-stage PD experiencing hallucinations or delusions, consider oral atypical neuroleptics (quetiapine, clozapine). Acute psychosis is a medical emergency that may require hospitalization and short-term use of neuroleptics

Tests
- Monitor for any changes in blood pressure

ADVERSE EFFECTS (AEs)

How Drug Causes AEs
- Increases concentration of peripheral and CNS dopamine. At higher doses affects serotonin and norepinephrine levels

Notable AEs
- In studies, as monotherapy, rasagiline had fewer side effects than placebo. Nausea, hallucinations, confusion, lightheadedness, loss of balance, abdominal pain, orthostatic hypotension, weight loss are uncommon but may occur. Can exacerbate existing dyskinesias

Life-Threatening or Dangerous AEs
- Rasagiline currently has a warning regarding possible hypertensive crisis when used in combination with foods containing tyramine. Tyramine-containing foods include aged cheeses, liver, sauerkraut, cured and processed meats, soy, chianti wine, and vermouth. Recent studies however demonstrate that rasagiline has a lower tyramine sensitivity factor than selegiline, which has no tyramine warning. Therefore, it is likely safe to consume tyramine-containing foods while taking rasagiline at therapeutic doses. It is expected that the FDA will withdraw the tyramine warning in light of the tyramine sensitivity studies

Weight Gain
• Unusual

Sedation
• Unusual

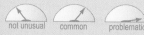

What to Do About AEs
• Lower the dose or change to alternative PD medications

Best Augmenting Agents for AEs
• Orthostatic hypotension: adjust dose or stop antihypertensives, add supplemental salt, and consider fludrocortisone or midodrine

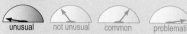

DOSING AND USE

Usual Dosage Range
• PD – 0.5–1 mg daily

Dosage Forms
• Tablets: 0.5 mg, 1 mg

How to Dose
• Regular tablets: Start at 0.5 mg daily and increase to 1 mg daily in a few days if tolerated for desired clinical effect. After 3–4 days, may attempt to lower dose of carbidopa-levodopa

 Dosing Tips
• Food has no effect on metabolism

Overdose
• At doses above 1 mg, rasagiline may become less selective and may inhibit MAO-A as well as MAO-B. This increases the risk of hypertensive crisis. Symptoms include dizziness, insomnia, hypotension or hypertension, headache, sedation, respiratory depression, and death. Symptoms of overdose can be delayed up to 12 hours, and maximal worsening may not occur until the next day

Long-Term Use
• Safe for long-term use. Effectiveness may decrease over time in PD

Habit Forming
• No

How to Stop
• No need to taper

Pharmacokinetics
• Hepatic metabolism via CYP1A2, with metabolites excreted in urine. Linear pharmacokinetics. Bioavailability 36% and protein binding 90%. Peak plasma levels at about 30 minutes

 Drug Interactions
• Increases the effect of levodopa, potentially requiring dose adjustments
• CYP1A2 inhibitors, such as tacrine, mexiletine, and atazanavir, increase plasma concentration
• Do not use meperidine within 2 weeks of drug
• Opioid analgesics, including methadone, tramadol, propoxyphene, and dextromethorphan, may also cause reactions
• Rasagiline has a warning with respect to possible serotonin syndrome when used in combination with TCAs, SSRIs, and SNRIs. Amitriptyline, citalopram, sertraline, trazodone, paroxetine and escitalopram were allowed in studies with rasagiline and there were no reports of serotonin syndrome. Physicians should use their clinical judgment when using rasagiline with antidepressants. Do not use within 5 weeks of fluoxetine due to fluoxetine's long half-life
• Dopamine antagonists, such as phenothiazines, metoclopramide, may diminish effectiveness
• Use with caution in patients on antihypertensive medications due to risk of orthostatic hypotension
• At higher doses can potentially interact with sympathomimetics. These include intravenous dopamine, norepinephrine and epinephrine, methylphenidate, nasal decongestants, sinus medications, asthma inhalers, and some weight loss treatments

 Other Warnings/ Precautions
• Cutaneous melanoma is more common in PD, but it is unclear if this is a medication effect or not

• Discontinue 14 days prior to elective surgery in the event that sympathomimetic agents are needed during anesthesia

Do Not Use

• Known hypersensitivity to the drug. Patients using meperidine, fluoxetine or patients with pheochromocytoma

SPECIAL POPULATIONS

Renal Impairment

• No known effects

Hepatic Impairment

• In patients with mild impairment, give 0.5 mg daily dose. Do not use in patients with moderate-severe impairment

Cardiac Impairment

• No known effects

Elderly

• Rasagiline is safe in the elderly, with no reports of increased adverse effects

Children and Adolescents

• Not studied in children (PD is rare in pediatrics)

Pregnancy

• Category C. Use only if benefits of medication outweigh risks

Breast Feeding

• Unknown if excreted in breast milk. Do not use

THE ART OF NEUROPHARMACOLOGY

Potential Advantages

• May delay need for carbidopa-levodopa or allow reduction of dose. Good initial treatment. Better tolerated (less nausea, fewer neuropsychiatric adverse events, less somnolence) than dopamine agonists. Potential, but unproven, neuroprotective effect

Potential Disadvantages

• Potentially less effective for motor symptoms than other PD treatments. Patients with significant motor disability or patients older than 75 may require carbidopa-levodopa. Multiple potential drug interactions

Primary Target Symptoms

• PD – motor dysfunction, including bradykinesia, hand function, gait and rest tremor

 Pearls

• Well-tolerated monotherapy and adjunctive medication for PD. Favorable long-term AEs
• MAO-B inhibitors have drawn interest as possible neuroprotective or disease-modifying agents in PD and AD. Two large studies of rasagiline have demonstrated possible disease-modifying benefits in PD
• Putative neuroprotective mechanisms of rasagiline include stabilization of mitochondrial membrane potential, reduction of oxidative stress, which leads to apoptosis, increasing activity of antioxidative enzymes superoxide dismutase and catalase, and increasing glial cell-derived neurotrophic factor, nerve growth factor, and brain-derived neurotrophic factor
• Rasagiline appears to facilitate the conversion of amyloid precursor protein into intracellular soluble APP-alpha, which may be neuroprotective in AD. Still, rasagiline is not proven to have neuroprotective properties
• MAO inhibitors may inhibit cholinesterase and be useful for the treatment of AD. There have not been clinical trials to support use to date
• Unlike selegiline, rasagiline does not have methamphetamine metabolites
• In clinical trials, patients taking 1 mg/day did not follow dietary restrictions and no AEs related to tyramine occurred. At a dose of 1 mg or less, the drug is selective for MAO-B and dietary restrictions are likely unnecessary

Suggested Reading

Elmer LW, Bertoni JM. The increasing role of monoamine oxidase type B inhibitors in Parkinson's disease therapy. Expert Opin Pharmacother 2008;9(16):2759–72.

Naoi M, Maruyama W. Functional mechanism of neuroprotection by inhibitors of type B monoamine oxidase in Parkinson's disease. Expert Rev Neurother 2009;9(8):1233–50.

Olanow CW, Hauser RA, Jankovic J, Langston W, Lang A, Poewe W, Tolosa E, Stocchi F, Melamed E, Eyal E, Rascol O. A randomized, double-blind, placebo-controlled, delayed start study to assess rasagiline as a disease modifying therapy in Parkinson's disease (the ADAGIO study): rationale, design, and baseline characteristics. Mov Disord 2008;23(15):2194–201.

Oldfield V, Keating GM, Perry CM. Rasagiline: a review of its use in the management of Parkinson's disease. Drugs 2007; 67(12):1725–47.

RESERPINE

THERAPEUTICS

Brands
• Harmonyl

Generic?
Yes

Class
• Antiadrenergic, synaptic vesicle blocker, antidopaminergic, antimonoaminergic

Commonly Prescribed for
(FDA approved in bold)
• **Hypertension**
• **Psychotic states**
• Gilles de la Tourette syndrome (GTS) or tics
• Chorea and dyskinesias in Huntington's disease
• Hemiballism
• Dystonia (especially tardive)
• Myoclonus

How the Drug Works
• Depleting agent that depletes stores of catecholamines (dopamine, norepinephrine) and serotonin in the brain and adrenal medulla. Depression of sympathetic nerve function lowers heart rate and blood pressure

How Long Until It Works
• Hypertension – less than a week
• Psychosis, movement disorders – effects can be seen within a few days

If It Works
• In neurologic conditions, continue to assess effect of the medication and determine if still needed

If It Doesn't Work
• Chorea: Consider benzodiazepines and anticonvulsants (valproate). Neuroleptics are usually effective. Tetrabenazine (another antiadrenergic) is often better tolerated
• Generalized dystonia: Anticholinergics, baclofen, or benzodiazepines may be effective. Surgical treatments (including pallidotomy, thalamotomy, deep brain stimulation, myotomy, rhizotomy, or peripheral denervation) are reserved for refractory cases

• GTS/tics – neuroleptics and alpha-2 adrenergic agonists are often effective

Best Augmenting Combos for Partial Response or Treatment-Resistance
• AEs, such as CNS depression, often increase when used with other agents, but if tolerated consider combinations with anticonvulsants or benzodiazepines

Tests
• Monitor blood pressure and pulse

ADVERSE EFFECTS (AEs)

How Drug Causes AEs
• Related to depletion of catecholamines and serotonin

Notable AEs
• Bradycardia, edema, angina-like symptoms
• Drowsiness, dizziness, depression, nightmares
• Nausea, dry mouth, anorexia, impotence, dyspnea, nasal congestion
• Rash, purpura

Life-Threatening or Dangerous AEs
• Hypersensitivity reactions
• Deafness, optic atrophy
• Parkinsonism and extrapyramidal tract dysfunction (less common than neuroleptics)

Weight Gain
• Common

unusual / not unusual / **common** / problematic

Sedation
• Problematic

unusual / not unusual / common / **problematic**

What to Do About AEs
• Stop drug for serious AEs, and use the lowest needed dose

Best Augmenting Agents for AEs
• Most AEs cannot be improved by an augmenting agent

DOSING AND USE

Usual Dosage Range
- 0.1–1 mg/day once daily

Dosage Forms
- Tablets: 0.1 mg, 0.25 mg

How to Dose
- Hypertension: start 0.5–1 mg once daily for 1–2 weeks, but many patients are able to lower dose to 0.1–0.25 mg daily
- Psychosis and movement disorders: start 0.5 mg per day and adjust upward or downward based on patient response to 0.1–1.0 mg per day

 Dosing Tips
- Patients should be aware that drug has slow onset of action and prolonged effects

Overdose
- Severe sedation ranging from drowsiness to coma. Flushing, conjunctival injection, papillary constriction, and hypotension are common. Bradycardia and respiratory depression in severe cases. Treat symptomatically and observe for 72 hours due to long-acting effects

Long-Term Use
- Safe, but patients often discontinue due to AEs

Habit Forming
- No

How to Stop
- No need to taper

Pharmacokinetics
- Half-life is 33 hours with IV administration. Bioavailability is about 50% and protein binding is about 96%. Metabolism of drug is unknown

 Drug Interactions
- Do not use with MAO inhibitors
- Tricyclic antidepressants may decrease antihypertensive effect
- Use with digitalis or quinidine may precipitate cardiac arrhythmias
- Use with caution with direct- or indirect-acting sympathomimetics. Reserpine

prolongs the action of direct-acting amines (epinephrine, isoproterenol) and inhibits the action of indirect-acting amines (ephedrine, tyramine, amphetamines)

 Other Warnings/ Precautions
- Increases GI motility and secretions. May precipitate biliary colic
- May cause depression that persists for months after use and may be severe enough to result in suicide

Do Not Use
- Proven hypersensitivity, depression or history of suicidal tendencies, active peptic ulcer, ulcerative colitis, patients receiving electroconvulsive therapy

SPECIAL POPULATIONS

Renal Impairment
- Patients with renal insufficiency may adjust poorly to lowered blood pressure

Hepatic Impairment
- No known effects

Cardiac Impairment
- Avoid using in patients with cardiac arrhythmias, especially those taking digitalis or quinidine

Elderly
- No known effects

 Children and Adolescents
- Not recommended for hypertension but occasionally used for the treatment of generalized dystonias. Monitor for parkinsonism and hypotension

 Pregnancy
- Category C. Crosses placental barrier. Use only if there is a clear need

Breast Feeding
- Excreted in breast milk and may cause respiratory difficulties and anorexia. Use only if clearly needed

THE ART OF NEUROPHARMACOLOGY

Potential Advantages
- A useful drug for hypertensive patients with psychosis and many movement disorders without risk of tardive dyskinesia

Potential Disadvantages
- More AEs than tetrabenazine and most other treatments

Primary Target Symptoms
- Reduction in severity of psychosis, chorea, dystonia, myoclonus, or tics

 Pearls
- Effective treatment for hyperkinetic movement disorders such as tics, chorea, dyskinesias, and tardive dystonias
- Compared to tetrabenazine, has a longer half-life and greater peripheral effects (GI AEs and hypotension). In refractory dystonia, reserpine with trihexyphenidyl and pimozide may be effective

 Suggested Reading

Fernandez HH, Friedman JH. Classification and treatment of tardive syndromes. Neurologist 2003;9(1):16–27.

Paleacu D, Giladi N, Moore O, Stern A, Honigman S, Badarny S. Tetrabenazine treatment in movement disorders. Clin Neuropharmacol 2004;27(5):230–3.

Shamon SD, Perez MI. Blood pressure lowering efficacy of reserpine for primary hypertension. Cochrane Database Syst Rev 2009;(4): CD007655.

Simpson GM. The treatment of tardive dyskinesia and tardive dystonia. J Clin Psychiatry 2000;61 (Suppl 4): 39–44.

RILUZOLE

THERAPEUTICS

Brands
- Rilutek

Generic?
No

Class
- Neuromuscular drug, centrally acting

Commonly Prescribed for
(FDA approved in bold)
- **Amyotrophic lateral sclerosis (ALS)**

How the Drug Works
- The mode of action is unknown, but the effect in ALS is felt to be from glutamate antagonism. Putative mechanisms include inhibition of glutamate release, interference with transmitter binding at excitatory amino acid receptors, and inactivation of voltage-gated sodium channels. In animal models, appears to be neuroprotective in mice with human superoxide dismutase mutations and has sedative and myorelaxant properties at large doses

How Long Until It Works
- Steady state is reached in 5 days, but it can take months to assess any clinical effect from the drug

If It Works
- ALS is a degenerative disease and deterioration is the general rule. Riluzole can increase survival or time to tracheostomy but is not a cure

If It Doesn't Work
- It is difficult to determine if the treatment is effective, especially because ALS progression varies greatly from patient to patient. Supportive care is the mainstay of current ALS treatment. This may include monitoring and treatment of gait, swallowing and respiratory difficulties

Best Augmenting Combos for Partial Response or Treatment-Resistance
- No other medication is indicated for the treatment of ALS progression

Tests
- Measure serum transaminases, including ALT levels, at baseline and monthly for 3 months. Then evaluate every 3 months for the first year and periodically after that. Once ALT exceeds 5 times normal, begin checking weekly, and discontinue if ALT exceeds 10 times normal or clinical symptoms, such as jaundice, occur

ADVERSE EFFECTS (AEs)

How Drug Causes AEs
- Unknown

Notable AEs
- Nausea, weakness, dizziness, diarrhea, abdominal pain, pneumonia, tremor, anorexia, somnolence, and paresthesias. Elevation of hepatic transaminases

Life-Threatening or Dangerous AEs
- Neutropenia and hepatic effects. Neutropenia is uncommon (less than 1/1000 in clinical trials). Hepatic transaminase elevation is common (about 50% of patients will experience one elevated level) but usually clinically insignificant

Weight Gain
- Unusual

Sedation
- Unusual

What to Do About AEs
- Check blood counts on all patients with febrile illness and treat aggressively

Best Augmenting Agents for AEs
- AEs cannot be improved with use of augmenting agents

DOSING AND USE

Usual Dosage Range
- ALS – 50 mg every 12 hours

Dosage Forms
- Tablets: 50 mg

How to Dose
- Start at 50 mg dose twice daily

 Dosing Tips
- Taking with a high-fat meal will reduce absorption

Overdose
- Unknown

Long-Term Use
- Safe for long-term use

Habit Forming
- No

How to Stop
- No need to taper

Pharmacokinetics
- Metabolized by CYP450 1A2 isozyme. 60% bioavailability and 96% protein bound. Elimination half-life is about 12 hours. Drug excreted in urine and feces. Female patients generally metabolize more slowly and Japanese patients appear to have about 50% slower clearance of drug, even when adjusting for body weight

 Drug Interactions
- CYP1A2 inhibitors (caffeine, amitriptyline, quinolones, theophyline) increase levels of riluzole and 1A2 inducers (rifampin, omeprazole, cigarette smoke, and charcoal-broiled food) lower levels. The effect of riluzole itself on CYP1A2 activity is unknown

Do Not Use
- Known hypersensitivity to the drug

SPECIAL POPULATIONS

Renal Impairment
- Severe renal disease may slow drug clearance. Use with caution

Hepatic Impairment
- Use with caution due to known hepatic risks of riluzole. Significant hepatic impairment may increase drug levels

Cardiac Impairment
- No known effects

Elderly
- No known effects. AEs similar to younger patients in those with normal renal and hepatic function

 Children and Adolescents
- Not studied in children (ALS is rare in pediatrics)

 Pregnancy
- Category C. Use only if benefits of medication outweigh risks

Breast Feeding
- Unknown if excreted in breast milk. Do not use

THE ART OF NEUROPHARMACOLOGY

Potential Advantages
- Only medication approved for the treatment of ALS. Relatively well-tolerated

Potential Disadvantages
- Lack of effectiveness and cost. Patients or caregivers expecting dramatic improvement from the drug are likely to be disappointed

Primary Target Symptoms
- Survival and delay of need for tracheostomy

 Pearls
- Well-tolerated with few major AEs, but does not reverse ALS symptoms or the disease itself
- Do not expect noticeable clinical improvement
- In clinical trials, extended life 3 to 6 months on average and delayed need for tracheostomy

Suggested Reading

Bensimon G, Doble A. The tolerability of riluzole in the treatment of patients with amyotrophic lateral sclerosis. Expert Opin Drug Saf 2004; 3(6):525–34.

Cheung YK, Gordon PH, Levin B. Selecting promising ALS therapies in clinical trials. Neurology 2006;67(10):1748–51.

Corcia P, Meininger V. Management of amyotrophic lateral sclerosis. Drugs 2008; 68(8):1037–48.

Miller RG, Mitchell JD, Lyon M, Moore DH. Riluzole for amyotrophic lateral sclerosis (ALS)/ motor neuron disease (MND). Cochrane Database Syst Rev 2007;(1):CD001447.

RITUXIMAB

THERAPEUTICS

Brands
- Rituxan, MabThera

Generic?
No

Class
- Immunosuppressant, immunomodulator, monoclonal antibody

Commonly Prescribed for
(FDA approved in bold)
- **B-cell non-Hodgkin lymphoma (NHL)**
- **Rheumatoid arthritis**
- Myasthenia gravis (MG)
- Multiple sclerosis (MS) (relapsing-remitting)
- Multifocal motor neuropathy
- Anti-myelin-associated glycoprotein (MAG) neuropathy
- Chronic inflammatory demyelinating polyneuropathy (CIDP)
- Neuromyelitis optica
- Dermatomyositis
- Opsoclonus myoclonus
- Sarcoidosis
- Chronic lymphocytic leukemia
- Waldenstrom macroglobulinemia
- Thrombocytopenic purpura

How the Drug Works
- Binds to the CD 20 antigen on pre-B and mature B lymphocytes, inducing apoptosis. The antigen is expressed in greater than 90% of B-cell NHL but not on stem cells, pro-B-cells, plasma cells or normal tissues. B-cells are felt to be important in the pathogenesis of rheumatoid arthritis, MS, MG, and many other autoimmune diseases
- Rituximab may also decrease other biologic markers of inflammation, such as c-reactive protein, serum amyloid protein, and rheumatoid factor

How Long Until It Works
- By 2 weeks, but effect on disease may take months

If It Works
- May allow reduction in dose or discontinuation of steroids or other agents in the treatment of MG, MS, or other neurological conditions

If It Doesn't Work
- Usually used as an adjunctive agent in conjunction with steroids or other agents in MG, but other agents such as azathioprine, mycophenolate mofetil, and cyclosporine are often used instead. In MS, used as an alternative to other agents for refractory relapsing-remitting patients

Best Augmenting Combos for Partial Response or Treatment-Resistance
- Often combined with prednisone or other steroids for treatment of MG, allowing eventual decrease in dose. Occasionally combined with other immunosuppressive agents for many autoimmune diseases, but AEs may increase

Tests
- Obtain complete blood counts before beginning and during therapy, more frequently if patient develops cytopenia

ADVERSE EFFECTS (AEs)

How Drug Causes AEs
- Serious AEs are related to infusion reactions, immunosuppression, and lymphopenia

Notable AEs
- Infusion reactions in 32% usually take place with the first infusion and may include fever, chills, angioedema, bronchospasm, or blood pressure changes. Infection (mostly respiratory tract infections) fever, chills, weakness, itching, headache, and dyspepsia

Life-Threatening or Dangerous AEs
- Not uncommon: Severe lymphopenia lasting a few weeks, occurs in about 40% of patients. Neutropenia, leukopenia, and anemia are less common. Reactivation of hepatitis B. Severe mucocutaneous reactions, including Stevens-Johnson syndrome. Severe infection or sepsis. Tumor lysis syndrome
- Rare: JC virus infection leading to progressive multifocal leukoencephalopathy. Bowel obstruction and perforation

Weight Gain
• Unusual

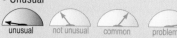

Sedation
• Unusual

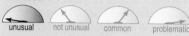

What to Do About AEs
• Give slowly or stop infusion for serious AEs. Treat infections appropriately

Best Augmenting Agents for AEs
• For infusion reactions, pretreat with acetaminophen and antihistamines. Pretreatment with IV glucocorticoids may also help

DOSING AND USE

Usual Dosage Range
• 375 mg/m^2 once weekly for 4–8 doses

Dosage Forms
• Injection: 10 mg/mL

How to Dose
• In most cases, given once weekly for 4–8 weeks. Start infusion at a lower rate 50 mg/h and increase by rate of 50 mg/h every 30 minutes to a maximum of 400 mg/h. If tolerated, start at 100 mg/h during subsequent treatments

 Dosing Tips
• Do not mix with other drugs. Infusion should be given by staff familiar with potential AEs

Overdose
• Unknown

Long-Term Use
• Usually used on a short-term basis for refractory disorders

Habit Forming
• No

How to Stop
• No need to taper, but monitor for recurrence of neurological disorder

Pharmacokinetics
• B-cells rapidly decrease after administration and peripheral B-lymphocytes are nearly depleted by 2 weeks. Most patients continue to have B-cell depletion for 6 months, but most have normal B-cell levels 1 year after treatment

 Drug Interactions
• Combining with cisplatin causes renal toxicity
• Use with immunosuppressant agents requires close monitoring for infection or other AEs

Do Not Use
• Known hypersensitivity to the drug or its components

SPECIAL POPULATIONS

Renal Impairment
• No contraindications, but rituximab can cause renal toxicity. Use with caution in patients with preexisting renal disease

Hepatic Impairment
• No known effects

Cardiac Impairment
• No known effects

Elderly
• Older patients with B-cell lymphomas were more likely to experience supraventricular arrhythmias and pulmonary reactions on rituximab

 Children and Adolescents
• Effectiveness and safety are unknown

 Pregnancy
• Category C. Do not use in individuals considering pregnancy. Use contraception during and 12 months after treatment

Breast Feeding

- Discontinue until drug levels are not detectable

THE ART OF NEUROPHARMACOLOGY

Potential Advantages

- Mechanism of action different than most immunosuppressive agents for neurological disorders

Potential Disadvantages

- Not a first-line agent in any neurological disorder due to lack of proven efficacy and serious AEs

Primary Target Symptoms

- Preventive treatment of complications from diseases such as MG or MS

Pearls

- There are several case reports describing the use of rituximab in refractory MG, including those with MuSK antibodies. Its actions on B cells distinguish rituximab from other agents that act on the cell cycle inhibiting production of B and T lymphocytes (azathioprine, cyclophosphamide, methotrexate, and mycophenolate mofetil)

or immunosuppression of T-cells (cyclosporine and tacrolimus). The relative efficacy of rituximab compared to other agents is unknown

- Less proven in MS as compared to natalizumab, another monoclonal antibody. It is unknown if other monoclonal antibodies, such as alemtuzumab and daclizumab, are effective. There is an active clinical trial underway looking into the efficacy of rituximab in MS
- In a small study of 16 children with opsoclonus myoclonus and an increased percentage of CD20 B-cells in CSF, 4 infusions of rituximab 375 mg/m^2 were given in combination with ACTH or immunoglobulins. Treatment allowed reduction in ACTH dose with few relapses
- Open-label studies demonstrate effectiveness in the treatment of immune-mediated neuropathies, such as multifocal motor and vasculitic neuropathies. In anti-MAG neuropathy, treatment improved clinical symptoms, electrophysiological findings, and anti-MAG antibody titers
- Studies of rituximab for the treatment of chronic inflammatory demyelinating polyneuropathy show mixed results
- Case reports indicate usefulness in the treatment of anti- *N*-methyl-D-aspartate (NMDA) encephalitis, a rare autoimmune, usually paraneoplastic, disease

Suggested Reading

Finsterer J. Treatment of immune-mediated, dysimmune neuropathies. Acta Neurol Scand 2005;112(2):115–25.

Ishiura H, Matsuda S, Higashihara M, Hasegawa M, Hida A, Hanajima R, Yamamoto T, Shimizu J, Dalmau J, Tsuji S. Response of anti-NMDA receptor encephalitis without tumor to immunotherapy including rituximab. Neurology 2008;71(23):1921–3.

Muraro PA, Bielekova B. Emerging therapies for multiple sclerosis. Neurotherapeutics 2007;4(4):676–92.

Rizvi SA, Bashir K. Other therapy options and future strategies for treating patients with multiple sclerosis. Neurology 2004;63 (12 Suppl 6):S47–54.

Zebardast N, Patwa HS, Novella SP, Goldstein JM. Rituximab in the management of refractory myasthenia gravis. Muscle Nerve 2010; 41(3):375–8.

RIVASTIGMINE

THERAPEUTICS

Brands
- Exelon, Prometax

Generic?
No

Class
- Cholinesterase inhibitor

Commonly Prescribed for
(FDA approved in bold)
- **Alzheimer dementia (AD) (mild or moderate)**
- **Dementia associated with Parkinson's Disease (PD)**
- Dementia with Lewy Bodies (DLB)
- Vascular dementia

How the Drug Works
- Increases the concentration of acetylcholine through reversible inhibition of acetylcholinesterase, which increases availability of acetylcholine. Also inhibits butyrylcholinesterase. A deficiency of cholinergic function is felt to be important in producing the signs and symptoms of AD. May interfere with amyloid deposition
- Although symptoms of AD can improve, rivastigmine does not prevent disease progression

How Long Until It Works
- Typically 2–6 weeks at a given dose, but effect is best observed over a period of months

If It Works
- Continue to use but symptoms of dementia usually continue to worsen

If It Doesn't Work
- Non-pharmacologic measures are the basis of dementia treatment. Maintain regular schedules and routines. Avoid prolonged travel, unnecessary medical procedures or emergency room visits, crowds, and large social gatherings
- Limit drugs with sedative properties such as opioids, hypnotics, antiepileptic drugs and tricyclic antidepressants

- Treat other disorders which can worsen symptoms such as hyperglycemia or urinary difficulties

 ### Best Augmenting Combos for Partial Response or Treatment-Resistance
- Addition of the NMDA receptor antagonist memantine may be beneficial
- Treat depression or apathy, if present, with SSRIs. Avoid tricyclic antidepressants in demented patients due to risk of confusion
- For significant confusion and agitation avoid typical neuroleptics (especially in DLB) because of the risk of neuroleptic malignant syndrome. Atypical antipsychotics (risperidone, quetiapine, olanzapine, clozapine) can be used instead

Tests
- None required

ADVERSE EFFECTS (AEs)

How Drug Causes AEs
- Acetylcholinesterase and butyrylcholinesterase inhibition in the CNS and PNS

Notable AEs
- GI AEs (nausea/vomiting, diarrhea, anorexia, increased gastric acid secretion and weight loss) are most common
- Fatigue, depression, dizziness, increased sweating and headache

 ### Life-Threatening or Dangerous AEs
- Rarely bradycardia or heart block causing syncope. Generalized convulsions. Increases gastric acid secretions which can predispose to GI bleeding

Weight Gain
- Unusual

unusual · not unusual · common · problematic
- Weight loss is more common

Sedation
- Unusual

unusual · not unusual · common · problematic

What to Do About AEs

- In patients with dementia, determining if AEs are related to medication or another medical condition can be difficult. For CNS side effects, discontinuation of non-essential centrally acting medications may help. If a bothersome AE is clearly drug-related then lower the dose (especially for GI AEs), titrate more slowly or discontinue

Best Augmenting Agents for AEs

- Most AEs do not respond to adding other medications

DOSING AND USE

Usual Dosage Range

- 6–12 mg/day in 2 divided doses for oral formulations, or 4.6 or 9.5 mg 1 transdermal patch per day

Dosage Forms

- Capsules: 1.5, 3, 4.5 and 6 mg
- Oral solution: 2 mg/mL in a 120 mL bottle
- Patches: 4.6 mg/24 hour and 9.5 mg/24 hour

How to Dose

- Start at 1.5 mg twice a day. Increase at a minimum of 2 weeks by 3 mg/day to a maximum of 12 mg/day in 2 divided doses
- Transdermal patch: start 4.6-mg/24-hour patch applied once daily. After 4 weeks increase to one 9.5-mg/24-hour patch daily if well-tolerated

 Dosing Tips

- Slow titration can reduce AEs. Nausea is most common in the titration phase. Food slows absorption

Overdose

- Symptoms of cholinergic crisis can occur: nausea/vomiting, salivation, hypotension, diaphoresis, convulsions, bradycardia/collapse. May cause muscle weakness and respiratory failure. Atropine with an initial dose of 1–2 mg IV is a potential antidote

Long-Term Use

- Safe for long-term use. Effectiveness may decrease over time as the dementing illness progresses

Habit Forming

- No

How to Stop

- Abrupt discontinuation can produce worsening of dementia symptoms, memory and behavioral disturbances. Taper slowly

Pharmacokinetics

- Elimination half-life 1–2 hours. No hepatic interactions or CYP-450 interactions. Metabolites are excreted in urine

 Drug Interactions

- Increases the effect of anesthetics such as succinylcholine. Stop before surgery
- Anticholinergics interfere with effect of drug
- Other cholinesterase inhibitors and cholinergic agonists (bethanechol) may cause a synergistic effect
- Bradycardia may occur when used with beta-blockers
- Nicotine increases drug clearance

Do Not Use

- Known hypersensitivity to the drug or carbamate derivatives

SPECIAL POPULATIONS

Renal Impairment

- Variable changes in clearance with moderate and severe disease. No dose adjustment needed

Hepatic Impairment

- Patients with severe disease have 60% reduced clearance but not clinically significant. No dose adjustment needed

Cardiac Impairment

- Syncope has been reported

Elderly

- No known effects

 Children and Adolescents

- Not studied. AD does not occur in children

Pregnancy

- Category B. Use only if benefits of medication outweigh risks

Breast Feeding

- Unknown if excreted in breast milk. Do not use

THE ART OF NEUROPHARMACOLOGY

Potential Advantages

- Proven effectiveness for AD and PD dementia. Low risk of the hepatotoxicity seen with other acetylcholinesterases (tacrine) and fewer drug interactions than donepezil. Available as a transdermal patch. Additional inhibition of butyrylcholinesterase may increase effectiveness

Potential Disadvantages

- Cost and minimal effectiveness. Does not prevent progression of AD or other dementia. GI AEs

Primary Target Symptoms

- Confusion, agitation, memory, performing activities of daily living

 Pearls

- May be used in combination with memantine with good effect, but combining with other cholinesterase inhibitors is not recommended
- In most clinical trials, medication treatments for AD patients had a similar rate of benefit
- May be useful for both behavioral problems in AD (delusion, anxiety and apathy for example) as well as memory disturbance
- PD patients may benefit from lower doses than in AD (less than 6 mg/day)
- Usually the effect of rivastigmine is not dramatic, but patients with DLB might show more benefit. Effective for the cognitive and behavioral symptoms (agitation, apathy, hallucinations) of DLB
- When changing from one cholinesterase inhibitor to another, avoid a washout period which could precipitate clinical deterioration
- Butyrylcholinesterase inhibition may be more beneficial in later stages of AD when gliosis occurs
- May be more selective for the form of acetylcholinesterase in the hippocampus (G1)

 Suggested Reading

Bentué-Ferrer D, Tribut O, Polard E, Allain H. Clinically significant drug interactions with cholinesterase inhibitors: a guide for neurologists. CNS Drugs 2003;17(13):947–63.

Chitnis S, Rao J. Rivastigmine in Parkinson's disease dementia. Expert Opin Drug Metab Toxicol 2009;5(8):941–55. Review.

Cummings J, Lefèvre G, Small G, Appel-Dingemanse S. Pharmacokinetic rationale for the rivastigmine patch. Neurology 2007;69 (4 Suppl 1):S10–3.

Downey D. Pharmacologic management of Alzheimer disease. J Neurosci Nurs 2008;40(1):55–9.

Stahl SM. The new cholinesterase inhibitors for Alzheimer's disease, Part 1: their similarities are different. J Clin Psychiatry 2000;61(10):710–11.

RIZATRIPTAN

THERAPEUTICS

Brands
• Maxalt

Generic?
No

 Class
• Triptan

Commonly Prescribed for
(FDA approved in bold)
• Migraine

 How the Drug Works
• Selective 5-HT1 receptor agonist, working predominantly at the B and D receptor subtypes. Effectiveness may be due to blocking the transmission of pain signals from the trigeminal nerve to the trigeminal nucleus caudalis and preventing release of inflammatory neuropeptides rather than just causing vasoconstriction

How Long Until It Works
• 1 hour or less

If It Works
• Continue to take as needed. Patients taking acute treatment more than 2 days/week are at risk for medication-overuse headache, especially if they have migraine

If It Doesn't Work
• Treat early in the attack – triptans are less likely to work after the development of cutaneous allodynia, a marker of central sensitization
• For patients with partial response or reoccurrence, add an NSAID
• Change to another agent

 Best Augmenting Combos for Partial Response or Treatment-Resistance
• NSAIDs or neuroleptics are often used to augment response

Tests
• None required

ADVERSE EFFECTS (AEs)

How Drug Causes AEs
• Direct effect on serotonin receptors

Notable AEs
• Tingling, flushing, sensation of burning, dizziness, sensation of pressure, palpitations, heaviness, nausea

 Life-Threatening or Dangerous AEs
• Rare cardiac events including acute MI, cardiac arrhythmias, and coronary artery vasospasm have been reported with rizatriptan

Weight Gain
• Unusual

unusual | not unusual | common | problematic

Sedation
• Unusual

unusual | not unusual | common | problematic

What to Do About AEs
• In most cases, only reassurance is needed. Lower dose, change to another triptan or use an alternative headache treatment

Best Augmenting Agents for AEs
• Treatment of nausea with antiemetics is acceptable. Other AEs improve with time

DOSING AND USE

Usual Dosage Range
• 5–10 mg, maximum 20 mg/day

Dosage Forms
• Tablets: 5 and 10 mg
• Orally disintegrating tablets: 5 and 10 mg

How to Dose
• Tablets: Most patients respond best at 10 mg oral dose. Give 1 pill at the onset of an attack and repeat in 2 hours for a partial response or the headache returns. Maximum 30 mg/day. Limit 10 days per month

Dosing Tips
- Treat early in attack

Overdose
- May cause hypertension, cardiovascular symptoms. Other possible symptoms include seizure, tremor, extremity erythema, cyanosis or ataxia. For patients with angina, perform ECG and monitor for ischemia for at least 12 hours

Long-Term Use
- Monitor for cardiac risk factors with continued use

Habit Forming
- No

How to Stop
- No need to taper. Patients who overuse triptans often experience withdrawal headaches lasting up to several days

Pharmacokinetics
- Half-life 2 hours. Tmax 1–2.5 hours, longer with orally disintregrating tablets. Bioavailability is 40%. Metabolism mostly by MAO A isoenzyme. 14% protein binding

Drug Interactions
- MAO inhibitors may make it difficult for drug to be metabolized. Theoretical interactions with SSRI/SNRI. It is unclear that triptans pose any risk for the development of serotonin syndrome in clinical practice
- Concurrent propranolol use increases peak concentrations – use the 5 mg dose
- Use with sibutramine, a weight loss drug, can cause a serotonin syndrome including weakness, irritability, myoclonus and confusion

⚠ Other Warnings/ Precautions
- For phenylketonurics: Tablets contain phenylalanine

Do Not Use
- Within 2 weeks of MAO inhibitors, or 24 hours of ergot-containing medications such as dihydroergotamine
- Patients with proven hypersensitivity to sumatriptan, known cardiovascular disease, uncontrolled hypertension, or Prinzmetal's angina
- Rizatriptan was not studied in patients with hemiplegic and basilar migraine
- May worsen symptoms in ischemic bowel disease

SPECIAL POPULATIONS

Renal Impairment
- Concentration increases in those with severe renal impairment (creatinine clearance less than 2 mL/min). May be at increased cardiovascular risk

Hepatic Impairment
- Drug metabolism decreased with hepatic disease. Do not use with severe hepatic impairment

Cardiac Impairment
- Do not use in patients with known cardiovascular or peripheral vascular disease

Elderly
- May be at increased cardiovascular risk

Children and Adolescents
- Safety and efficacy have not been established
- Triptan trials in children were negative, due to higher placebo response

Pregnancy
- Category C. Use only if potential benefit outweighs risk to the fetus. Pregnancy registry studies ongoing. Migraine often improves in pregnancy, and other acute agents (opioids, neuroleptics, prednisone) have more proven safety

Breast Feeding
- Rizatriptan is found in breast milk. Use with caution

THE ART OF NEUROPHARMACOLOGY

Potential Advantages

- Effective and fast acting, even compared to other oral triptans. May be drug of choice for patients with relatively short-lasting migraines. AE similar to other triptans. Less risk of abuse than opioids or barbiturate-containing treatments. Available as melt formulation

Potential Disadvantages

- Cost, potential for medication-overuse headache. Relatively short half-life, even compared to other triptans

Primary Target Symptoms

- Headache pain, nausea, photo- and phonophobia

 Pearls

- Early treatment of migraine is most effective
- Compared to other triptans, it has the highest 2-hour pain-free response
- May not be effective when taken during aura, before headache begins
- In patients with "status migrainosus" (migraine lasting more than 72 hours) neuroleptics and DHE are more effective
- Triptans were not originally studied for use in the treatment of basilar or hemiplegic migraine
- Patients taking triptans more than 10 days/month are at increased risk of medication-overuse headache which is less responsive to treatment
- Chest and throat tightness are usually benign and may be related to esophageal spasm rather than cardiac ischemia. These symptoms occur more commonly in patients without cardiac risk factors

 ### Suggested Reading

Dodick D, Lipton RB, Martin V, Papademetriou V, Rosamond W, MaassenVanDenBrink A, Loutfi H, Welch KM, Goadsby PJ, Hahn S, Hutchinson S, Matchar D, Silberstein S, Smith TR, Purdy RA, Saiers J; Triptan Cardiovascular Safety Expert Panel. Consensus statement: cardiovascular safety profile of triptans (5-HT agonists) in the acute treatment of migraine. Headache 2004;44(5):414–25.

Ferrari MD, Roon KI, Lipton RB, Goadsby PJ. Oral triptans (serotonin 5-HT (1B/1D) agonists) in acute migraine treatment: a meta-analysis of 53 trials. Lancet 2001;358(9294):1668–75.

Freitag F, Diamond M, Diamond S, Janssen I, Rodgers A, Skobieranda F. Efficacy and tolerability of coadministration of rizatriptan and acetaminophen vs rizatriptan or acetaminophen alone for acute migraine treatment. Headache 2008;48(6):921–30.

Gladstone JP, Gawel M. Newer formulations of the triptans: advances in migraine management. Drugs 2003;63(21):2285–305.

O'Quinn S, Mansbach H, Salonen R. Comparison of rizatriptan and sumatriptan. Headache 1999;39(1):59–60.

ROPINIROLE

THERAPEUTICS

Brands
• Requip, Adartrel

Generic?
Yes

Class
• Dopamine agonist, non-ergot

Commonly Prescribed for
(FDA approved in bold)
• **Parkinson's disease (PD)**
• **Restless legs syndrome (RLS)**

How the Drug Works
• Dopamine agonist, with high affinity for the D2 receptor. This action is likely the main reason for effectiveness in PD. Also binds with high affinity to D3 receptors, but the importance of this is unclear. The mechanism of action for RLS is probably related to D2 receptor agonism

How Long Until It Works
• PD – weeks
• RLS – days to weeks

If It Works
• PD – may require dose adjustments over time or augmentation with other agents. Most PD patients will eventually require carbidopa-levodopa to manage their symptoms
• RLS – safe for long-term use with dose adjustments

If It Doesn't Work
• PD – Bradykinesia, gait and tremor should improve. Non-motor symptoms including autonomic symptoms such as postural hypotension, depression, and bladder dysfunction do not improve. If the patient has significantly impaired functioning, add carbidopa-levodopa with or without ropinirole
• RLS – Rule out peripheral neuropathy, iron deficiency, thyroid disease. Change to another drug such as a benzodiazepine. Antiepileptic drugs (AEDs) such as gabapentin or carbamazepine may also be beneficial. In severe cases consider opioids

Best Augmenting Combos for Partial Response or Treatment-Resistance
• For suboptimal effectiveness add carbidopa-levodopa with or without a COMT inhibitor. MAO-B inhibitors may also be beneficial
• For younger patients with bothersome tremor: anticholinergics may help
• For severe motor fluctuations and/or dyskinesias with good "on" time, functional neurosurgery is an option
• Depression is common in PD and may respond to SSRIs
• Cognitive impairment/dementia is common in mid-late stage PD and may improve with acetylcholinesterase inhibitors
• For patients with late-stage PD experiencing hallucinations or delusions, withdraw ropinirole and consider oral atypical neuroleptics (quetiapine, olanzapine, clozapine). Acute psychosis is a medical emergency that may require hospitalization
• For RLS, can change to a different dopamine agonist or add another drug such as a benzodiazepine. AEDs such as gabapentin or carbamazepine may be beneficial. In severe cases consider opioids

Tests
• None required

ADVERSE EFFECTS (AEs)

How Drug Causes AEs
• Direct effect on dopamine receptors

Notable AEs
• Nausea/vomiting, dizziness, hallucination, constipation, somnolence, abdominal pain/discomfort, diaphoresis, anxiety, viral infection, pharyngitis, dyskinesias, and orthostatic hypotension

Life-Threatening or Dangerous AEs
• May cause somnolence or sudden-onset sleep, often without warning. Occurs more often than with ergot agonists or carbidopa-levodopa. Rare syncope or cardiac arrhythmias, most commonly bradycardia

Weight Gain
• Unusual

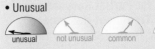

Sedation
• Common

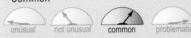

What to Do About AEs
• Nausea can be problematic when initiating drug – titrate slowly
• Hallucinations or delusions may require stopping the medication
• Warn patients about the risks of sleeping while driving

Best Augmenting Agents for AEs
• Amantadine may help suppress dyskinesias
• Orthostatic hypotension: adjust dose or stop antihypertensives, add supplemental salt, and consider fludrocortisone or midodrine
• Urinary incontinence: reducing PM fluids, voiding schedules, oxybutynin, desmopressin nasal spray, hyoscyamine sulfate, urological evaluation

---

DOSING AND USE

Usual Dosage Range
• PD – 3–24 mg daily, divided into 3 daily doses or once daily with XL formulation
• RLS – 4 mg or less 1–3 hours before bedtime

Dosage Forms
• Tablets: 0.25 mg, 0.5 mg, 1 mg, 2 mg, 3 mg, 4 mg, 5 mg
• Extended-release tablets: 2 mg, 4 mg, 8 mg

How to Dose
• PD (Immediate release): Start at 0.25 mg 3 times daily. Each week increase each dose by 0.25 mg until reaching 1 mg 3 times daily at week 4. After week 4 increase each dose by 0.5 mg per week if needed until taking 9 mg/day, then by 1 mg each dose until taking a maximum of 24 mg/day in 3 divided doses to reach desired clinical effect
• PD (Extended release): Start at 2 mg/day for 1–2 weeks, then increase by 2 mg every week until symptomatic relief or maximum of 24 mg/day

---

• RLS: take 1–3 hours before bedtime. Start at 0.25 mg, and increase to 0.5 mg in 2–3 days. After 1 week increase to 1.0 mg and after that increase by 0.5 mg every week until at 4 mg at bedtime

 Dosing Tips
• Slow titration will minimize nausea and dizziness

Overdose
• Symptoms include somnolence, agitation, orthostatic hypotension, abdominal pain, nausea, or dyskinesias. For cases of excessive CNS stimulation, neuroleptics can be effective

Long-Term Use
• Safe for long-term use. Effectiveness may decrease over time in PD (years) and RLS (months)

Habit Forming
• No

How to Stop
• Taper and discontinue over a period of 1 week. PD and RLS symptoms may worsen, but serious AEs from discontinuation are rare

Pharmacokinetics
• Extensive metabolism in liver by CVP 1A2 enzyme. 55% bioavailability. Half-life is 6 hours

 Drug Interactions
• Increases the effect of levodopa
• Estrogen, especially ethinyl estradiol, can reduce clearance of drug
• CYP1A2 inhibitors (ciprofloxacin, cimetidine, diltiazem, erythromycin, mexiletine, fluvoxamine, tacrine) increase ropinirole concentration
• Dopamine antagonists such as phenothiazines, metoclopramide diminish effectiveness
• Use with caution in patients on antihypertensive medications due to risk of orthostatic hypotension
• Smoking induces CYP1A2 and increases drug clearance

Other Warnings/ Precautions

- Dopamine agonists can precipitate impulse control disorders, such as pathological gambling

Do Not Use

- Hypersensitivity to the drug

SPECIAL POPULATIONS

Renal Impairment

- Dose does not seem to be affected but not studied in patients with severe disease

Hepatic Impairment

- Drug has hepatic metabolism but impairment does not appear to affect drug clearance. Use with caution

Cardiac Impairment

- Infrequently causes cardiac arrhythmias, rarely ventricular tachycardia. Use with caution

Elderly

- There is reduced drug clearance, but no dose adjustment needed as the dose used is the lowest that provides clinical improvement

 Children and Adolescents

- Not studied in children (PD is rare in pediatrics)

 Pregnancy

- Category C. Teratogenic in some animal studies. Use only if benefits of medication outweigh risks

Breast Feeding

- Inhibits prolactin secretion. Unknown if excreted in breast milk

THE ART OF NEUROPHARMACOLOGY

Potential Advantages

- PD: may delay need for carbidopa-levodopa and decreases risk of motor dyskinesias by 30%. This is especially important in younger PD patients. Available in 1/day dosing. Unlike ergot-based agonists, no known risk of fibrotic complications
- RLS: less risk of dependence compared to opioids or benzodiazepines and less augmentation than levodopa

Potential Disadvantages

- Less effective than carbidopa-levodopa for PD with more AEs such as hallucinations, somnolence and orthostatic hypotension. Patients with significant motor disability will require carbidopa-levodopa

Primary Target Symptoms

- PD – motor dysfunction including bradykinesia, hand function, gait and rest tremor
- RLS – pain, insomnia

 Pearls

- Excellent drug for young patients with early PD. Favorable long-term AEs
- First-line treatment for RLS with less augmentation or "rebound" than carbidopa-levodopa
- AE profile differs from pramipexole. Less often associated with postural hypotension, dyskinesias and edema, but more likely to cause dizziness, syncope, nausea or respiratory problems
- For patients with mildly symptomatic disease, dopamine agonists are also appropriate for initial therapy, but for patients with significant disability, use carbidopa-levodopa early

Suggested Reading

Chitnis S. Ropinirole treatment for restless legs syndrome. Expert Opin Drug Metab Toxicol 2008;4(5):655–64.

Kvernmo T, Houben J, Sylte I. Receptor-binding and pharmacokinetic properties of dopaminergic agonists. Curr Top Med Chem 2008;8(12):1049–67.

Lang AE. When and how should treatment be started in Parkinson disease? Neurology 2009;72 (7 Suppl):S39–43.

Varga LI, Ako-Agugua N, Colasante J, Hertweck L, Houser T, Smith J, Watty AA, Nagar S, Raffa RB. Critical review of ropinirole and pramipexole – putative dopamine D(3)-receptor selective agonists – for the treatment of RLS. J Clin Pharm Ther 2009;34(5):493–505.

Weiner WJ. Early diagnosis of Parkinson's disease and initiation of treatment. Rev Neurol Dis 2008;5(2):46–53; quiz 54–5.

RUFINAMIDE

THERAPEUTICS

Brands
- Banzel, Inovelon

Generic?
No

 ### Class
- Antiepileptic drug (AED)

Commonly Prescribed for
(FDA approved in bold)
- **Lennox-Gastaut syndrome (LGS) (adjunctive for age 4 and older)**
- Partial-onset seizures with and without generalization in adults and adolescents

 ### How the Drug Works
- The exact mechanism is unknown but likely related to modulation of sodium channel activity and membrane stabilization. Rufinamide prolongs the inactive state of the sodium channel

How Long Until It Works
- Seizures – should decrease by 2 weeks

If It Works
- Seizures – goal is the remission of seizures. Continue as long as effective and well-tolerated

If It Doesn't Work
- Increase to highest tolerated dose
- Epilepsy: consider changing to another agent, adding a second agent or referral for epilepsy surgery evaluation

 ### Best Augmenting Combos for Partial Response or Treatment-Resistance
- Generally used adjunctively in combination with other AEDs for refractory epilepsy

Tests
- No regular blood tests are recommended

ADVERSE EFFECTS (AEs)

How Drug Causes AEs
- CNS AEs are probably caused by effects on sodium channels

Notable AEs
- Sedation, anorexia, nausea/vomiting, headache, dizziness, tremor, nasopharyngitis, influenza

 ### Life-Threatening or Dangerous AEs
- Suicidal ideation
- Blood dyscrasias including leukopenia
- Bundle branch and first-degree AV block infrequently occurred in clinical trials but the relationship of this to rufinamide is unclear

Weight Gain
- Unusual

unusual | not unusual | common | problematic

Sedation
- Not unusual

unusual | not unusual | common | problematic

What to Do About AEs
- Decrease dose
- Taking drug in fasting state will lower absorption and may reduce both AEs and effectiveness

Best Augmenting Agents for AEs
- Most AEs cannot be improved by use of augmenting agent

DOSING AND USE

Usual Dosage Range
- Epilepsy: 1600–3200 mg/day in adults

Dosage Forms
- Tablets: 200 or 400 mg

How to Dose
- Start at a daily dose of 400–800 mg/day in 2 divided doses. Increase dose by 400–800 mg/day every 2 days until a maximum of 3200 mg/day in 2 divided doses. Typical dose is 3200 mg

Dosing Tips
- Drug absorption is significantly enhanced by taking with food
- Tablet is easily crushed and given with food

Overdose
- Unknown effect. Use induction of emesis or gastric lavage to remove drug. Hemodialysis will help remove some drug

Long-Term Use
- Safe for long-term use

Habit Forming
- No

How to Stop
- Taper slowly (25% of dose every 2 days)
- Abrupt withdrawal can lead to seizures in patients with epilepsy

Pharmacokinetics
- Extensive hepatic metabolism but not via CYP450 system. Half-life is 6–10 hours and peak levels at 4–6 hours. Food increases absorption. Protein binding is 34%. Renally excreted

Drug Interactions
- Rufinamide has no significant effect on CYP450 enzymes. It is a weak inhibitor of CYP2E1 and a weak inducer of CYP3A4 enzymes but does not typically change concentrations of other medications
- Half-life of drug is lower when using with phenytoin or carbamazepine compared to valproate. Valproate can increase rufinamide concentration up to 70%
- Lowers levels of oral contraceptives by about 20%

Do Not Use
- Patients with a proven allergy to rufinamide or familial short QT syndrome

Renal Impairment
- No dose adjustments needed, but hemodialysis will remove some of the drug

Hepatic Impairment
- No known effects but use with severe disease is not recommended

Cardiac Impairment
- No known effects

Elderly
- No known effects

Children and Adolescents
- Approved for use in children 4 and older with LGS
- Start at 10 mg/kg/day in 2 divided doses. Increase by about 10 mg/kg every other day as tolerated to effective dose. Maximum 3200 mg/day or 45 mg/kg/day (whichever is less.)

Pregnancy
- Risk category C. Use only if risks of stopping drug outweigh potential risk to fetus
- Supplementation with 0.4 mg of folic acid before and during pregnancy is recommended

Breast Feeding
- Some drug found in mother's breast milk
- Consider discontinuing drug or bottle feeding
- Monitor infant for sedation, poor feeding or irritability

Potential Advantages
- Effective in refractory epilepsy, safe to use with other AEDs and wide therapeutic window

Potential Disadvantages
- Few indications and lack of evidence for the treatment of many types of epilepsy, including generalized epilepsies. Unknown effectiveness as monotherapy

Primary Target Symptoms
- Seizure frequency and severity

Pearls

- Second- or third-line agent in refractory epilepsy. Lack of drug interactions and wide therapeutic index with unique structure (tiazole derivative). Often LGS is not amenable to surgery so multiple AED regimens are common

- In trials of rufinamide in subjects with LGS seizures decreased by over 30% and atonic seizures ("drop attacks") decreased by over 40%. Drop attacks are a major source of injury in LGS
- In patient with treatment-resistant partial-onset seizures, rufinamide reduced seizure frequency by over 20% from baseline as adjunctive therapy

Suggested Reading

Cheng-Hakimian A, Anderson GD, Miller JW. Rufinamide: pharmacology, clinical trials, and role in clinical practice. Int J Clin Pract 2006;60(11):1497–501.

Ferrie CD, Patel A. Treatment of Lennox-Gastaut Syndrome (LGS). Eur J Paediatr Neurol 2009;13(6):493–504.

Perucca E, Cloyd J, Critchley D, Fuseau E. Rufinamide: clinical pharmacokinetics and concentration-response relationships in patients with epilepsy. Epilepsia 2008;49(7):1123–41.

SELEGILINE

THERAPEUTICS

Brands
• Zelapar, Eldepryl, Emsam

Generic?
Yes (as oral)

Class
• Monoamine oxidase type B (MAO-B) inhibitor

Commonly Prescribed for
(FDA approved in bold)
• **Parkinson's disease (PD)**
• **Major depressive disorder, treatment-refractory (patch only)**
• Anxiety disorders
• Alzheimer's and other dementias
• Migraine

How the Drug Works
• Selectively blocks monoamine oxidase type B (MAO-B) and inhibits metabolism of dopamine, increasing its effectiveness. At higher doses, starts to affect MAO-A as well as -B and inhibits metabolism of norepinephrine, serotonin, and tyramine, as well as dopamine

How Long Until It Works
• PD – weeks
• Depression, anxiety: usually months

If It Works
• PD – may require dose adjustments over time or augmentation with other agents. Most PD patients will eventually require carbidopa-levodopa to manage their symptoms

If It Doesn't Work
• Bradykinesia, gait, and tremor should improve. If the patient has significantly impaired functioning, add carbidopa-levodopa with or without a dopamine agonist

Best Augmenting Combos for Partial Response or Treatment-Resistance
• For suboptimal effectiveness, add carbidopa-levodopa with or without a COMT inhibitor or a dopamine agonist

• For younger patients with bothersome tremor: anticholinergics may help
• For severe motor fluctuations and/or dyskinesias with good "on" time, functional neurosurgery is an option
• Cognitive impairment/dementia is common in mid-late stage PD and may improve with acetylcholinesterase inhibitors
• For patients with late-stage PD experiencing hallucinations or delusions, consider oral atypical neuroleptics (quetiapine, olanzapine, clozapine). Acute psychosis is a medical emergency that may require hospitalization and short-term use of neuroleptics

Tests
• Monitor for any changes in blood pressure

ADVERSE EFFECTS (AEs)

How Drug Causes AEs
• Increases concentration of peripheral and CNS dopamine. At higher doses affects serotonin and norepinephrine levels

Notable AEs
• Nausea, hallucinations, confusion, lightheadedness, loss of balance, insomnia, orthostatic hypotension, hypertension, weight gain

Life-Threatening or Dangerous AEs
• Hypertensive crisis, especially at higher doses that prevent breakdown of tyramine. Tyramine-containing foods include aged cheeses, liver, sauerkraut, cured and processed meats, soy, alcohol (especially chianti wine and vermouth), and avocado

Weight Gain
• Common

Sedation
• Unusual

What to Do About AEs
- Lower the dose or change to alternative PD medications

Best Augmenting Agents for AEs
- Orthostatic hypotension: adjust dose or stop antihypertensives, add supplemental salt, and consider fludrocortisone or midodrine

DOSING AND USE

Usual Dosage Range
- PD – 10 mg daily, divided into 2 daily doses taken at breakfast and lunch
- Depression – only the transdermal patch is indicated for the treatment of depression

Dosage Forms
- Tablets: 5 mg
- Capsules: 5 mg
- Orally disintegrating tablets: 1.25 mg
- Transdermal patch: 6, 9 or 12 mg per 24 hours

How to Dose
- Regular tablets: Start at 2.5 mg (regular tablets) twice daily (usually at breakfast and lunch) and increase to 5 mg twice a day in a few days if tolerated. After 3–4 days, may attempt to lower dose of carbidopa-levodopa
- Orally disintegrating tablets: Start at 1.25 mg in the morning before breakfast, and increase to 2.5 mg daily if tolerated and desired benefit not achieved
- Transdermal patch: Start at 6 mg per 24 hours. Increase every 2 weeks until desired effect achieved in 3 mg increments to a maximum of 12 mg/day

 Dosing Tips
- Take orally disintegrating tablets before breakfast
- At doses above 10 mg, selegiline starts to become less selective and starts to have more MAO-A inhibition. This increases the risk of hypertensive crisis

Overdose
- Symptoms include dizziness, insomnia, hypotension or hypertension, headache, sedation, respiratory depression, and death. Symptoms of overdose can be delayed up to 12 hours, and maximal worsening may not occur until the next day

Long-Term Use
- Safe for long-term use. Effectiveness may decrease over time in PD

Habit Forming
- No

How to Stop
- No need to taper. Drug wears off in 2–3 weeks

Pharmacokinetics
- Orally disintregrating tablets (Tmax 10–15 minutes) have a more rapid absorption and greater bioavailability than the swallowed tablets (Tmax 40–90 minutes). The 2.5 mg disintregrating tablets have an effect similar to 10 mg of the regular tablets. Hepatic metabolism with metabolites, including L-methamphetamine and L-amphetamine. Metabolites are then excreted in the urine

 Drug Interactions
- Increases the effect of levodopa, potentially requiring dose adjustments
- Multiple adverse CNS reactions reported when used with meperidine, including convulsions, coma, and death. Do not use meperidine within 2 weeks of drug
- Other analgesics, including methadone, tramadol, propoxyphene, and dextromethorphan, may also cause reactions
- Do not use within 2 weeks of tricyclic antidepressants, SSRIs, or SNRIs due to risk of serotonin syndrome (hyperthermia, myoclonus, rigidity, autonomic instability, mental status changes, or death.) Do not use within 5 weeks of fluoxetine
- Tramadol can increase risk of seizures
- Dopamine antagonists such as phenothiazines, metoclopramide may diminish effectiveness
- Use with caution in patients on antihypertensive medications due to risk of orthostatic hypotension
- At higher, non-selective doses can potentially interact with CNS stimulants due

to amphetamine metabolites. These include intravenous dopamine, norepinephrine and epinephrine, methylphenidate, nasal decongestants, sinus medications, asthma inhalers, diet pills or weight loss treatments, and even levodopa

Other Warnings/ Precautions

- Orally disintegrating tablets contain phenylalanine

Do Not Use

- Known hypersensitivity to the drug. Patients using meperidine, tricyclic antidepressants, SSRIs, or SNRIs

SPECIAL POPULATIONS

Renal Impairment

- No known effects

Hepatic Impairment

- May require lowering of dose

Cardiac Impairment

- No known effects

Elderly

- Start at a lower dose with careful titration. More likely to experience AEs

Children and Adolescents

- Not studied in children (PD is rare in pediatrics) and not recommended under age 16

Pregnancy

- Category C. Use only if benefits of medication outweigh risks

Breast Feeding

- Unknown if excreted in breast milk. Do not use

THE ART OF NEUROPHARMACOLOGY

Potential Advantages

- May delay need for carbidopa-levodopa or allow reduction of dose. Good initial treatment for patients with no cognitive dysfunction and significant disability. Better tolerated (less nausea) than dopamine agonists. May be useful for PD patients with comorbid depression

Potential Disadvantages

- Less effective than most PD treatments, including dopamine agonists, for motor dysfunction. Patients with significant motor disability, cognitive impairment, or patients older than 75 will require carbidopa-levodopa. Multiple drug interactions at doses greater than 10 mg limit titration and effectiveness

Primary Target Symptoms

- PD – motor dysfunction, including bradykinesia, hand function, gait and rest tremor

Pearls

- Well-tolerated adjunctive medication for PD. Favorable long-term AEs
- MAO-Is have drawn interest as possible neuroprotective agents in PD. Selegiline delays the need for levodopa compared to placebo, but this could be due to the symptomatic benefit of the drug. Newer studies of neuroprotection are evaluating rasagiline, another MAO-B inhibitor, which does not have methamphetamine as a metabolite
- May be useful in combination with other agents, such as donepezil, for the treatment of Alzheimer's dementia
- For depression, use the transdermal patch. For PD, use oral selegiline
- At a dose of 10 mg or less, the drug is selective for MAO-B and dietary restrictions do not come into play
- MAO-I may be useful for the treatment of refractory migraine, but does not appear effective in some patients

Suggested Reading

Chen JJ, Swope DM. Pharmacotherapy for Parkinson's disease. Pharmacotherapy 2007;27(12 Pt 2):161S–173S.

Fernandez HH, Chen JJ. Monoamine oxidase-B inhibition in the treatment of Parkinson's disease. Pharmacotherapy 2007;27(12 Pt 2): 174S–185S.

Frampton JE, Plosker GL. Selegiline transdermal system in major depressive disorder: profile report. CNS Drugs 2007;21(6):521–4.

Kuritzky A, Zoldan Y, Melamed E. Selegeline, a MAO B inhibitor, is not effective in the prophylaxis of migraine without aura – an open study. Headache 1992;32(8):416.

Löhle M, Storch A. Orally disintegrating selegiline for the treatment of Parkinson's disease. Expert Opin Pharmacother 2008;9(16):2881–91.

Yamada M, Yasuhara H. Clinical pharmacology of MAO inhibitors: safety and future. Neurotoxicology 2004;25(1–2):215–21.

SUMATRIPTAN, SUMATRIPTAN/NAPROXEN

Brands
• Imitrex, Treximet, Imigran, Sumarel

Generic?
Yes, with the exception of sumatriptan/naproxen

 Class
• Triptan

Commonly Prescribed for
(FDA approved in bold)
• **Migraine**
• **Cluster headache (injection only)**

 How the Drug Works
• Selective 5-HT1 receptor agonist, working predominantly at the B and D receptor subtypes. Effectiveness may be due to blocking the transmission of pain signals from the trigeminal nerve to the trigeminal nucleus caudalis and preventing release of inflammatory neuropeptides rather than just causing vasoconstriction
• Naproxen is an NSAID (cyclo-oxygenase inhibitor) which inhibits synthesis of prostaglandins, a mediator of inflammation

How Long Until It Works
• Oral or NS– 1 hour or less. SC – within 10–30 minutes

If It Works
• Continue to take as needed. Patients taking acute treatment more than 2 days/week are at risk for medication-overuse headache, especially if they have migraine

If It Doesn't Work
• Treat early in the attack – triptans are less likely to work after the development of cutaneous allodynia, a marker of central sensitization
• Use SC injection instead
• For patients with partial response or reoccurrence, use sumatriptan/naproxen combination
• Change to another agent

 Best Augmenting Combos for Partial Response or Treatment-Resistance
• NSAIDs or neuroleptics are often used to augment response
• Use sumatriptan/naproxen combination

Tests
• None required

How Drug Causes AEs
• Direct effect on serotonin receptors

Notable AEs
• Injection-site reaction/pain (SC), bad taste (NS), tingling, flushing, sensation of burning, dizziness, sensation of pressure, heaviness, nausea
• Sumatriptan/naproxen: Includes NSAID AEs such as dyspepsia, fluid retention, GI distress

 Life-Threatening or Dangerous AEs
• Rare cardiac events including acute MI, cardiac arrhythmias, and coronary artery vasospasm have been reported with sumatriptan
• Sumatriptan/naproxen: GI bleed, renal insufficiency, inhibition of platelet aggregation

Weight Gain
• Unusual

unusual / not unusual / common / problematic

Sedation
• Unusual

unusual / not unusual / common / problematic

What to Do About AEs
• In most cases, only reassurance is needed. Lower dose, change to the oral form if AE with SC injection, change to another triptan or use an alternative headache treatment

Best Augmenting Agents for AEs
• Treatment of nausea with antiemetics is acceptable. Other AEs improve with time

DOSING AND USE

Usual Dosage Range
- 25–100 mg, maximum 200 mg/day (oral)

Dosage Forms
- Tablets: 25, 50 and 100 mg
- Sumatriptan/Naproxen: 85 /550 mg
- Nasal Spray: 5 and 20 mg
- SC: 4 and 6 mg (Sumarel 6 mg only)

How to Dose
- Tablets: Most patients respond best at 100 mg oral dose. Give 1 pill at the onset of an attack and repeat in 2 hours for a partial response or if headache returns. Maximum 200 mg/day. Limit 10 days per month
- Injections: May repeat injections in 1 hour. Maximum 12 mg/day

 Dosing Tips
- Treat early in attack. For patients with cluster use SC. For patients with significant nausea/vomiting consider SC or NS

Overdose
- May cause hypertension, cardiovascular symptoms. Other possible symptoms include seizure, tremor, extremity erythema, cyanosis or ataxia. For patients with angina, perform ECG and monitor for ischemia for at least 10 hours

Long-Term Use
- Monitor for cardiac risk factors with continued use

Habit Forming
- No

How to Stop
- No need to taper. Patients who overuse triptans often experience withdrawal headaches lasting up to several days

Pharmacokinetics
- Half-life 2 hours. Tmax 1.5 hours except for SC (10–15 minutes) and 1 hour for sumatriptan/naproxen. Bioavailability is 96% for SC, 14–20% for the other forms. Metabolism mostly by MAO-A isoenzyme. 14–21% protein binding

 Drug Interactions
- MAO inhibitors may make it difficult for drug to be metabolized
- Theoretical interactions with SSRI/SNRI. It is unclear that triptans pose any risk for the development of serotonin syndrome in clinical practice

Do Not Use
- Within 2 weeks of MAO inhibitors, or 24 hours of ergot-containing medications such as dihydroergotamine
- Patients with proven hypersensitivity to sumatriptan, known cardiovascular disease, uncontrolled hypertension, or Prinzmetal's angina
- Sumatriptan was not studied in patients with hemiplegic and basilar migraine
- May worsen symptoms in ischemic bowel disease

SPECIAL POPULATIONS

Renal Impairment
- Do not use with severe renal impairment (creatinine clearance less than 15 mL/min). May be at increased cardiovascular risk

Hepatic Impairment
- Drug metabolism decreased with hepatic disease. Do not use with severe hepatic impairment

Cardiac Impairment
- Do not use in patients with known cardiovascular or peripheral vascular disease

Elderly
- May be at increased cardiovascular risk. Half-life is longer

 Children and Adolescents
- Safety and efficacy have not been established
- Triptan trials in children were negative, due to higher placebo response

Pregnancy

- Category C. Use only if potential benefit outweighs risk to the fetus. Pregnancy registry studies ongoing. Migraine often improves in pregnancy, and other acute agents (opioids, neuroleptics, prednisone) have more proven safety

Breast Feeding

- Sumatriptan is found in breast milk at low doses. Use with caution

THE ART OF NEUROPHARMACOLOGY

Potential Advantages

- Available as SC, proven for cluster headache. Most well-studied triptan. Less risk of abuse than opioids or barbiturate-containing treatments. Added efficacy with naproxen-containing formulation

Potential Disadvantages

- Potential for medication-overuse headache, relatively short half-life

Primary Target Symptoms

- Headache pain, nausea, photo- and phonophobia

 Pearls

- Early treatment of migraine is most effective. Subcutaneous sumatriptan is more effective than other triptans, but has the most AEs
- May not be effective when taking during aura, before headache begins
- In patients with "status migrainosus" (migraine lasting more than 72 hours) neuroleptics and DHE are more effective
- Triptans were not originally studied for use in the treatment of basilar or hemiplegic migraine
- Patients taking triptans more than 10 days/month are at increased risk of medication-overuse headache which is less responsive to treatment. Patients with cluster headache who have migraine may also be at risk
- Chest and throat tightness are usually benign and may be related to esophageal spasm rather than cardiac ischemia. These symptoms occur more commonly in patients without cardiac risk factors
- Sumavel uses a needle-free SC delivery system with efficacy similar to usual SC injection and may be prefered for patients unable to administer needles for acute attacks

 Suggested Reading

Brandes JL, Kudrow D, Stark SR, O'Carroll CP, Adelman JU, O'Donnell FJ, Alexander WJ, Spruill SE, Barrett PS, Lener SE. Sumatriptan-naproxen for acute treatment of migraine: a randomized trial. JAMA 2007;297(13):1443–54.

Ferrari MD, Roon KI, Lipton RB, Goadsby PJ. Oral triptans (serotonin 5-HT(1B/1D) agonists) in acute migraine treatment: a meta-analysis of 53 trials. Lancet 2001;358(9294):1668–75.

Göbel H, Heinze A, Stolze H, Heinze-Kuhn K, Lindner V. Open-labeled long-term study of the efficacy, safety, and tolerability of subcutaneous sumatriptan in acute migraine treatment. Cephalalgia 1999;19(7):676–83; discussion 626.

Scholpp J, Schellenberg R, Moeckesch B, Banik N. Early treatment of a migraine attack while pain is still mild increases the efficacy of sumatriptan. Cephalalgia 2004;24(11):925–33.

Wenzel RG, Tepper S, Korab WE, Freitag F. Serotonin syndrome risks when combining SSRI/SNRI drugs and triptans: is the FDA's alert warranted? Ann Pharmacother 2008;42(11):1692–6.

TETRABENAZINE

THERAPEUTICS

Brands
• Nitoman, Xenazine

Generic?
Yes

Class
• Antiadrenergic, antidopaminergic, synaptic vesicle blocker, antimonoaminergic

Commonly Prescribed for
(FDA approved in bold)
• **Chorea in Huntington's disease (HD)**
• **Dyskinesias in HD**
• Psychosis
• Hemiballism
• Dystonia (especially tardive)
• Myoclonus
• Gilles de la Tourette syndrome (GTS) or tics
• Hypertension

How the Drug Works
• Depleting agent that reversibly depletes stores of monoamines (dopamine, norepinephrine, serotonin, and histamine) from nerve terminals and blocks post-synaptic dopamine receptors. Effectiveness is likely related to dopamine depletion

How Long Until It Works
• Usually less than 1 week

If It Works
• In neurologic conditions, continue to assess effect of the medication, determine if still needed and adjust to optimal dose

If It Doesn't Work
• Chorea: Consider benzodiazepines and anticonvulsants (valproate). Neuroleptics are usually effective. Reserpine is an alternative depleting agent
• Generalized dystonia: Anticholinergics, baclofen, or benzodiazepines may be effective. Surgical treatments (including pallidotomy, thalamotomy, deep brain stimulation, myotomy, rhizotomy, or peripheral denervation) are reserved for refractory cases
• GTS/tics – Neuroleptics and alpha-2 adrenergic agonists are often effective

Best Augmenting Combos for Partial Response or Treatment-Resistance

• Chorea – combine with anticonvulsants, neuroleptics, or benzodiazepines
• Dystonia – combine with anticholinergics or benzodiazepines
• GTS/tics – Combine with neuroleptics for refractory cases

Tests
• At doses of 50 mg or greater, test patients for the CYP-450 2D6 gene to determine if they are poor, intermediate, or extensive metabolizers

ADVERSE EFFECTS (AEs)

How Drug Causes AEs
• Related to monoamine depletion

Notable AEs
• Drowsiness, fatigue, dizziness, depression, anxiety, insomnia
• Parkinsonism, akathisia, orthostatic hypotension, nausea
• Upper respiratory tract infection, dyspnea, dysuria

Life-Threatening or Dangerous AEs
• Falls and resulting trauma
• Neuroleptic malignant syndrome
• Parkinsonism and extrapyramidal tract dysfunction (less common than neuroleptics)
• QTc prolongation (usually mild)
• Dysphagia

Weight Gain
• Common

unusual   not unusual   common   problematic

Sedation
• Common

unusual   not unusual   common   problematic

What to Do About AEs
• Reducing doses improves most AEs

Best Augmenting Agents for AEs
• Most AEs cannot be improved by an augmenting agent

DOSING AND USE

Usual Dosage Range
- 50–200 mg/day

Dosage Forms
- Tablets: 12.5 mg, 25 mg

How to Dose
- Start at 12.5 mg daily in the AM and increase to 12.5 mg twice a day in 1 week. Increase as needed by 12.5 mg/week and dose 3–4 times daily. Avoid single doses over 50 mg. Most patients require doses of 100 mg or less

Dosing Tips
- Food has no effect on absorption

Overdose
- Reported symptoms include acute dystonia, oculogyric crisis, nausea and vomiting, sweating, sedation, hypotension, confusion, diarrhea, hallucinations, and tremor

Long-Term Use
- Safe, but monitor for long-term AEs

Habit Forming
- No

How to Stop
- No need to taper but symptoms usually reappear

Pharmacokinetics
- Rapidly metabolized to metabolites, predominantly by CYP-450 2D6 isoenzymes and mostly excreted in urine. Half-life about 10 hours

Drug Interactions
- Do not use with monoamine oxidase (MAO) inhibitors
- Do not use within 20 days of reserpine
- Strong CYP2D6 inhibitors (fluoxetine, paroxetine, quinidine) approximately double levels requiring reduction in dose. Weaker 2D6 inhibitors (duloxetine, amiodarone, or sertraline) may also increase levels

- Sedation increases with the use of CNS depressants, such as alcohol

Other Warnings/ Precautions
- May elevate prolactin levels
- May cause severe depression that may lead to suicide

Do Not Use
- Proven hypersensitivity, active depression or history of suicidal tendencies, or hepatic disease

SPECIAL POPULATIONS

Renal Impairment
- Patients with renal insufficiency may adjust poorly to lowered blood pressure

Hepatic Impairment
- Concentrations of drug and metabolites and elimination half-life are dramatically increased. Do not use

Cardiac Impairment
- May increase QTc interval. Avoid in patients with congenital long QT syndrome or in patients on QT-prolonging medications. Patients with recent myocardial infarction or unstable disease were excluded from clinical trials

Elderly
- No known effects

Children and Adolescents
- Not well studied but occasionally used for the treatment of generalized dystonias. Monitor for parkinsonism and hypotension. A trial of levodopa should be considered to rule out dopa-responsive dystonia

Pregnancy
- Category C. Use only if there is a clear need

Breast Feeding
- Unknown if excreted in breast milk. Use only if clearly needed

THE ART OF NEUROPHARMACOLOGY

Potential Advantages

- Useful for the treatment of hyperkinetic movement disorders, with fewer AEs than reserpine

Potential Disadvantages

- Not available in many countries. Drowsiness and parkinsonism limit titration. Multiple doses per day needed

Primary Target Symptoms

- Reduction in severity of chorea, dystonia, myoclonus, or tics

Pearls

- Most effective in the treatment of tardive dyskinesias, tardive dystonia, HD, and myoclonus
- Somewhat effective in idiopathic dystonia and GTS

- Dyskinesia related to Parkinson's disease should be treated with lowering levodopa medication doses and using extended-release forms, amantadine, or clozapine. Tetrabenazine may worsen orthostatic hypotension
- In refractory dystonia, tetrabenazine with trihexyphenidyl and pimozide may be effective
- For the treatment of chorea in HD, aripiprazole often has fewer AEs and is more likely to improve depression rather than worsen symptoms
- Parkinsonism is more common at higher doses (100 mg or greater)
- Although common, weight gain is less common than with neuroleptics in the treatment of GTS
- Compared to reserpine, has a shorter half-life and has fewer peripheral effects (lower incidence of GI AEs and hypotension)

Suggested Reading

Fernandez HH, Friedman JH. Classification and treatment of tardive syndromes. Neurologist 2003;9(1):16–27.

Kenney C, Hunter C, Jankovic J. Long-term tolerability of tetrabenazine in the treatment of hyperkinetic movement disorders. Mov Disord 2007;22(2):193–7.

Paleacu D, Giladi N, Moore O, Stern A, Honigman S, Badarny S. Tetrabenazine treatment in movement disorders. Clin Neuropharmacol 2004;27(5):230–3.

Setter SM, Neumiller JJ, Dobbins EK, Wood L, Clark J, DuVall CA, Santiago A. Treatment of chorea associated with Huntington's disease: focus on tetrabenazine. Consult Pharm 2009;24(7):524–37.

TIAGABINE

THERAPEUTICS

Brands
- Gabitril

Generic?
Yes

 Class
- Antiepileptic drug (AED)

Commonly Prescribed for
(FDA approved in bold)
- **Partial seizures in adults and children age 12 or older**
- Temporal lobe epilepsy (children and adults)
- Panic disorder

 How the Drug Works
- Enhances activity of GABA by binding to sites associated with GABA uptake into presynaptic neurons, allowing more GABA to be available to bind to receptors on postsynaptic cells

How Long Until It Works
- Seizures – should decrease by 2 weeks

If It Works
- Seizures – goal is the remission of seizures. Continue as long as effective and well-tolerated. Consider tapering and slowly stopping after 2 years without seizures

If It Doesn't Work
- Increase to highest tolerated dose
- Epilepsy: consider changing to another agent, adding a second agent or referral for epilepsy surgery evaluation

 Best Augmenting Combos for Partial Response or Treatment-Resistance
- Epilepsy: titration and combination regimen depends on whether the patient is on an enzyme-inducing drug or not

Tests
- No regular blood tests are recommended

ADVERSE EFFECTS (AEs)

How Drug Causes AEs
- CNS AEs are probably caused by excess GABA effect

Notable AEs
- Confusion, stuttering, muscle tremor, dizziness, sedation, paresthesias (usually doses > 8 mg/day), abdominal pain
- Less commonly, behavioral symptoms such as amnesia, extreme confusion, or seizures or seizure-like symptoms

 Life-Threatening or Dangerous AEs
- Can precipitate seizure in some patients (rare)
- Severe rash (rare) including Stevens-Johnson syndrome
- Falls producing accidental injury

Weight Gain
- Common

unusual / not unusual / **common** / problematic

Sedation
- Common

unusual / not unusual / **common** / problematic

What to Do About AEs
- Decreasing dose may improve CNS AEs, especially weakness and sedation
- Titrate more slowly

Best Augmenting Agents for AEs
- Initially dose at night to avoid sedation

DOSING AND USE

Usual Dosage Range
- Epilepsy: 16–56 mg/day

Dosage Forms
- Tablets: 2 mg, 4 mg, 12 mg, 16 mg

How to Dose
- For adults on enzyme-inducing AEDs (phenytoin, carbamazepine, primidone, phenobarbital), start at 4 mg. Increase dose by 4–8 mg in 1 week and continue to

increase by 4–8 mg/week as needed, to a maximum of 56 mg daily. At final doses give in divided doses 2–4 times daily
• In patients not on enzyme-inducing AEDs, give only half the dose and titrate more slowly

 Dosing Tips
• Food and specifically fats slow absorption rate but not the extent of absorption. Most patients take with food
• Titrate slowly in patients not on enzyme-inducing AEDs

Overdose
• Somnolence, weakness, agitation, confusion, depression, respiratory depression, and myoclonus have been reported. Rarely precipitates non-convulsive status epilepticus

Long-Term Use
• Safe for long-term use

Habit Forming
• No

How to Stop
• Taper slowly
• Abrupt withdrawal can lead to seizures in patients with epilepsy

Pharmacokinetics
• Elimination half-life is 2–5 hours in patients on inducing AEDs, but 7–9 hours in others. Most drug is metabolized by CYP-450 3A system. Bioavailability is about 90% and drug is 96% protein bound

 Drug Interactions
• Carbamazepine, phenytoin, phenobarbital, and primidone increase clearance of tiagabine by about 60%
• Use with other highly protein-bound drug may increase free levels and drug effect
• Valproate may slightly increase free tiagabine levels and tiagabine causes a slight decrease in valproate concentrations. Usually not clinically relevant

 Other Warnings/ Precautions
• CNS AEs increase when used with other CNS depressants

Do Not Use
• Hypersensitivity to drug

SPECIAL POPULATIONS

Renal Impairment
• No known effects

Hepatic Impairment
• Lower dose, as patients with moderate disease have reduced clearance by 60%

Cardiac Impairment
• No known effects

Elderly
• May need lower dose

 Children and Adolescents
• For children age 12–18 on enzyme-inducing AEDs (phenytoin, carbamazepine, primidone, phenobarbital), start at 4 mg. Increase dose to 8 mg in 1 week and continue to increase by 4–8 mg/week as needed, to a maximum of 32 mg daily. At final doses, give in divided doses 2–4 times daily
• In children not on enzyme-inducing AEDs, give only half the dose and titrate more slowly

 Pregnancy
• Risk category C. Multiple malformations in animals. Use only if benefits of using drug outweigh potential risk to fetus
• Supplementation with 0.4 mg of folic acid before and during pregnancy is recommended

Breast Feeding
• Some drug is found in mother's breast milk
• Generally recommendations are to discontinue drug or bottle feed

THE ART OF NEUROPHARMACOLOGY

Potential Advantages
- Useful for partial seizures, especially with coexisting panic disorder

Potential Disadvantages
- Depression and cognitive impairment. Does not treat generalized epilepsies

Primary Target Symptoms
- Seizure frequency and severity

Pearls
- Contraindicated in generalized epilepsy and may precipitate non-convulsive status epilepticus
- There are reports of patients with spike-wave discharges who experience exacerbations of EEG abnormalities which correlate with cognitive or neuropsychological reactions on tiagabine

Suggested Reading

Aikiä M, Jutila L, Salmenperä T, Mervaala E, Kälviäinen R. Comparison of the cognitive effects of tiagabine and carbamazepine as monotherapy in newly diagnosed adult patients with partial epilepsy: pooled analysis of two long-term, randomized, follow-up studies. Epilepsia 2006;47(7):1121–7.

Bauer J, Cooper-Mahkorn D. Tiagabine: efficacy and safety in partial seizures – current status. Neuropsychiatr Dis Treat 2008;4(4):731–6.

Koepp MJ, Edwards M, Collins J, Farrel F, Smith S. Status epilepticus and tiagabine therapy revisited. Epilepsia 2005;46(10):1625–32.

Sheehan DV, Sheehan KH, Raj BA, Janavs J. An open-label study of tiagabine in panic disorder. Psychopharmacol Bull 2007;40(3):32–40.

Zwanzger P, Baghai TC, Schüle C, Minov C, Padberg F, Möller HJ, Rupprecht R. Tiagabine improves panic and agoraphobia in panic disorder patients. J Clin Psychiatry 2001;62(8):656–7.

TIMOLOL

THERAPEUTICS

Brands
- Blocadren (oral), Betimol, Betim, Timoptic, Istalol (ocular solution)

Generic?
Yes

Class
- Antihypertensive, beta-blocker (non-selective)

Commonly Prescribed for
(FDA approved in bold)
- **Migraine prophylaxis**
- **Hypertension**
- **Myocardial infarction**
- **Chronic open angle glaucoma or ocular hypertension (ocular solution)**
- Congestive heart failure (stable)
- Angina pectoris due to coronary atherosclerosis
- Prevention of variceal bleeding

How the Drug Works
- Migraine: Proposed mechanisms include inhibition of adrenergic pathway, interaction with serotonin system and receptors, inhibition of nitric oxide production, and normalization of contingent negative variation. Prevention of cortical spreading depression may be the mechanism of action for all migraine preventives

How Long Until It Works
- Migraines – within 2 weeks, but can take up to 3 months on a stable dose to see full effect

If It Works
- In migraine, the goal is a 50% or greater decrease in migraine frequency or severity. Consider tapering or stopping if headaches remit for more than 6 months or if considering pregnancy

If It Doesn't Work
- Increase to highest tolerated dose
- Migraine: address other issues, such as medication-overuse, other coexisting medical disorders, such as anxiety, and consider changing to another drug or adding a second drug

Best Augmenting Combos for Partial Response or Treatment-Resistance
- Migraine: For some patients, low-dose polytherapy with 2 or more drugs may be better tolerated and more effective than high-dose monotherapy. May use in combination with AEDs, antidepressants, natural products, and non-pharmacologic treatments, such as biofeedback, to improve headache control

Tests
- None required

ADVERSE EFFECTS (AEs)

How Drug Causes AEs
- Antagonism of beta receptors

Notable AEs
- Bradycardia, hypotension, hyper- or hypoglycemia, weight gain
- Bronchospasm, cold/flu symptoms, sinusitis, pneumonias
- Dizziness, vertigo, fatigue/tiredness, depression, sleep disturbances
- Sexual dysfunction, decreased libido, dysuria, urinary retention, joint pain
- Exacerbation of symptoms in peripheral vascular disease and Raynaud's syndrome

Life-Threatening or Dangerous AEs
- In acute CHF, may further depress myocardial contractility
- Can blunt premonitory symptoms of hypoglycemia in diabetes and mask clinical signs of hyperthyroidism
- Non-selective beta-blockers, such as timolol, can inhibit bronchodilation, making them contraindicated in asthma, severe COPD
- Risk of excessive myocardial depression in general anesthesia

Weight Gain
- Not unusual

unusual — not unusual — common — problematic

Sedation
- Common

unusual — not unusual — common — problematic

What to Do About AEs

- Lower dose, take higher dose in the evening or switch to another drug

Best Augmenting Agents for AEs

- When patients have significant benefit from beta-blocker therapy but hypotension limits treatment, consider alpha-agonists (midodrine) or volume expanders (fludrocortisones) for symptomatic relief

DOSING AND USE

Usual Dosage Range

- 10–60 mg/day

Dosage Forms

- Tablets: 5, 10, 20 mg
- Ocular solution: 0.25 or 0.5%

How to Dose

- Migraine: Initial dose 10 mg twice daily in migraine. Can gradually increase weekly to usual effective dose: 20–60 mg/day

 Dosing Tips

- Patients on a stable dose of 20 mg/day can take the entire dose once daily, usually in the evening

Overdose

- Bradycardia, hypotension, low-output heart failure, shock, seizures, coma, hypoglycemia, apnea, cyanosis, respiratory depression, and bronchospasm. Epinephrine and dopamine are used to treat toxicity

Long-Term Use

- Safe for long-term use

Habit Forming

- No

How to Stop

- Do not abruptly discontinue. Gradually reduce dosage over 1–2 weeks. Stopping may exacerbate angina, and there are reports of tachyarrhythmias or myocardial infarction with rapid discontinuation in patients with cardiac disease

Pharmacokinetics

- Half-life 4 hours. Bioavailability is 75%. Hepatic metabolism. Metabolities are excreted by kidney. <10% protein binding. Lower lipid solubility than propranolol

 Drug Interactions

- Oral contraceptives, ciprofloxacin, and hydroxychloroquine can increase levels and/or effects of timolol and other beta-blockers
- Use with calcium channel blockers can be synergistic or additive, use with caution
- Barbiturates, penicillins, rifampin, calcium and aluminum salts, thyroid hormones, and cholestyramine can decrease effects of beta-blockers
- NSAIDs, sulfinpyrazone and salicylates inhibit prostaglandin synthesis and may inhibit the antihypertensive activity of beta-blockers
- Timolol can increase levels of lidocaine, resulting in toxicity
- Increased postural hypotension with prazosin and peripheral ischemia with ergot alkaloids
- Sudden discontinuation of clonidine while on beta-blockers or when stopping together can cause life-threatening increases in blood pressure

 Other Warnings/ Precautions

- Slight increases in blood urea, serum potassium, and uric acid, with decrease of HDL cholesterol and hematocrit. These alterations are not progressive or clinically significant
- Rare development of antinuclear antibodies (ANA)
- May worsen muscle weakness in myasthenia gravis

Do Not Use

- Sinus bradycardia, greater than first-degree heart block, cardiogenic shock
- Bronchial asthma, severe COPD
- Proven hypersensitivity to beta-blockers

Renal Impairment

- No significant changes in half-life or concentration with moderate failure, but marked hypotensive episodes have occurred in patients undergoing dialysis. Use with caution

Hepatic Impairment

- May need to reduce dose with significant hepatic disease

Cardiac Impairment

- Do not use in acute shock, MI, hypotension, and greater than first-degree heart block, but indicated in clinically stable patients post-MI to reduce risk of reinfarction. Metoprolol, another beta-blocker, is commonly used to reduce mortality and hospitalization for patients with stable CHF, in patients already receiving ACE inhibitors and diuretics

Elderly

- Use with caution. May increase risk of stroke

 Children and Adolescents

- Not studied in children. The pediatric dose is unknown

 Pregnancy

- Category C. Embryotoxic in animal studies only at doses much higher than maximum recommended human doses. May reduce perfusion of the placenta. Use if potential benefit outweighs risk to the fetus. Most beta-blockers are class C, except atenolol, which is D and acebutolol, pindolol and sotalol, which are B

Breast Feeding

- Not recommended. Timolol is found in breast milk

THE ART OF NEUROPHARMACOLOGY

Potential Advantages

- Proven effectiveness in migraine and fewer drug interactions than propranolol. Perhaps fewer CNS side effects

Potential Disadvantages

- Multiple potential AEs including bradycardia, hypotension, and fatigue. Less known efficacy for treating coexisting conditions, such as anxiety and tremor, compared with propranolol

Primary Target Symptoms

- Migraine frequency and severity

 Pearls

- Alternative beta-blockers for migraine: metoprolol 100–200 mg/day, propranolol 40–400 mg/day (FDA approved), atenolol 50–200 mg/day, nadolol 20–160 mg/day
- Beta-blockers that are partial agonists, with intrinsic sympathomimetic activity, are not effective in migraine prophylaxis. These include acebutolol, alprenolol, and pindolol
- Often used in combination with other drugs in migraine
- Not effective for cluster headache
- Beta-1 selective antagonists, such as metoprolol, may be an option for patients with asthma or severe COPD
- Recent studies have downgraded beta-blockers as a first-line treatment for hypertension compared with other classes due to lack of effectiveness, increased rate of stroke in elderly, and risk of provoking type II diabetes
- Often used in combination with other agents for hypertension, especially thiazide diuretics

Suggested Reading

Law MR, Morris JK, Wald NJ. Use of blood pressure lowering drugs in the prevention of cardiovascular disease: meta-analysis of 147 randomised trials in the context of expectations from prospective epidemiological studies. BMJ 2009;338:b1665.

Ramadan NM. Current trends in migraine prophylaxis. Headache 2007;47 (Suppl 1):S52–7.

Silberstein SD. Preventive migraine treatment. Neurol Clin 2009;27(2):429–43.

Taylor FR. Weight change associated with the use of migraine-preventive medications. Clin Ther 2008;30(6):1069–80.

TIZANIDINE

THERAPEUTICS

Brands
• Zanaflex, Sirdalud

Generic?
No

Class
• Skeletal muscle relaxant, centrally acting; alpha-2 agonist

Commonly Prescribed for
(FDA approved in bold)
• **Acute and intermittent management of increased muscle tone related to spasticity**
• Spasticity can result from neurological conditions, such as multiple sclerosis (MS), amyotrophic lateral sclerosis (ALS), primary lateral sclerosis, and spinal cord injury
• Migraine prophylaxis
• Neck pain/lower back pain
• Myofascial pain

How the Drug Works
• Alpha-2 adrenergic agonist (mostly at alpha-2A receptors) which also acts at imidazoline receptors. Reduces spasticity by increasing presynaptic inhibition of motor neurons

How Long Until It Works
• Pain – hours-weeks

If It Works
• Slowly titrate to most effective tolerated dose

If It Doesn't Work
• Increase to highest tolerated dose. If ineffective, gradually reduce dose and consider alternative medications

Best Augmenting Combos for Partial Response or Treatment-Resistance
• Botulinum toxin is effective, especially as an adjunct for focal spasticity, i.e., post-stroke or head injury affecting the upper limbs. For conditions with multiple areas of spasticity, i.e., cerebral palsy, this combination can be very useful
• May be used carefully in combination with baclofen, although additive sedation can be problematic

• Use other centrally acting muscle relaxants with caution due to potential additive CNS depressant effect

Tests
• Monitor liver and renal function at baseline and at 1, 2, and 3 months. Monitor hepatic enzymes at 6 months and periodically after that

ADVERSE EFFECTS (AEs)

How Drug Causes AEs
• Related to alpha-2 adrenergic agonist effect causing hypotension. Increased sedation may be due to actions at the imidazoline receptors

Notable AEs
• Dry mouth, weakness, and somnolence are most common. Dizziness, hypotension, and elevation of hepatic transaminases
• Hallucinations (usually visual) occur in about 3% of patients

Life-Threatening or Dangerous AEs
• Bradycardia and prolongation of QTc interval with higher doses. Tizanidine withdrawal can cause rebound hypertension

Weight Gain
• Not unusual

unusual not unusual common problematic

Sedation
• Common

unusual not unusual common problematic

What to Do About AEs
• Lower the dose and titrate more slowly

Best Augmenting Agents for AEs
• Most AEs cannot be improved by an augmenting agent. MS-related fatigue can respond to CNS stimulants such as modafinil but it is easier to temporarily lower the dose until tolerance develops

DOSING AND USE

Usual Dosage Range
- 6–24 mg/day in 3–4 divided doses, maximum 32 mg/day

Dosage Forms
- Tablets: 2, 4 mg
- Capsules: 2, 4, 6 mg

How to Dose
- Start with one 2 or 4 mg tablet daily. Increase by 2–4 mg every 3 days as tolerated to a goal of 24 mg/daily – either 8 mg 3 times a day or 6 mg 4 times a day – or until desired clinical effect is met. Some patients may increase to 32 mg/day if no AEs

 Dosing Tips
- Sedation peaks the first week. Slower titration may reduce AEs

Overdose
- One case of profound respiratory depression reported. Ensure adequate airway protection and intubate if needed. Gastric lavage and forced diuresis with furosemide and mannitol may be helpful

Long-Term Use
- Not well studied

Habit Forming
- No

How to Stop
- Taper slowly to avoid rebound tachycardia and hypertension (although much less problematic than clonidine)

Pharmacokinetics
- Bioavailability is 40%, with hepatic metabolism into inactive metabolites. 30% protein bound. Half-life is 2–2.5 hours and peak effect at 1–1.5 hours. The duration of effect is 3–6 hours. Food delays peak effect and half-life

 Drug Interactions
- Oral contraceptives decrease tizanidine clearance by about 50%
- Alcohol impairs tizanidine clearance and adds to depressant effect

- Tizanidine delays the effect of acetaminophen
- Use with other CNS depressants increases sedation

 Other Warnings/ Precautions
- Decreased spasticity can be problematic for some patients who require tone to maintain upright posture, balance, and ambulation
- In animal studies, dose-related corneal opacities and retinal degeneration occurred

Do Not Use
- Known hypersensitivity

SPECIAL POPULATIONS

Renal Impairment
- Clearance is reduced in patients with creatinine clearance less than 25 mL/min. Reduce dose

Hepatic Impairment
- Due to potential for elevation of hepatic transaminases, use with caution in any patient with significant hepatic disease

Cardiac Impairment
- No known effects

Elderly
- Drug metabolism is slower in elderly patients. Use with caution

 Children and Adolescents
- Not studied in children

 Pregnancy
- Category C. Use only if there is a clear need

Breast Feeding
- Unknown if excreted in breast milk but likely due to lipid solubility. Do not use

THE ART OF NEUROPHARMACOLOGY

Potential Advantages

- Effective treatment for spasticity with relatively benign AE profile. Effectiveness is similar to diazepam and oral baclofen with fewer AEs and less severe withdrawal

Potential Disadvantages

- Hypotension can be problematic in some and rebound hypertension from discontinuation may be confused for autonomic dysreflexia. Sedation often limits use

Primary Target Symptoms

- Spasticity, pain

Pearls

- Generally well-tolerated alternative to other muscle relaxants, such as oral baclofen, dantrolene, and diazepam
- Chemically similar to another alpha-2 adrenergic agonist, clonidine, but has only a fraction (1/10 to 1/50th) of the blood pressure lowering effect
- In migraine prophylaxis, may be helpful for some patients either as an acute pain medication or as a "bridge" treatment for daily pain. Some studies suggest usefulness as a longer-term prophylactic agent but AEs often outweigh benefit
- Effective for some patients with acute myofascial pain, back pain and neck pain

Suggested Reading

Freitag FG. Preventative treatment for migraine and tension-type headaches: do drugs having effects on muscle spasm and tone have a role? CNS Drugs 2003;17(6):373–81.

Kamen L, Henney HR 3rd, Runyan JD. A practical overview of tizanidine use for spasticity secondary to multiple sclerosis, stroke, and spinal cord injury. Curr Med Res Opin 2008;24(2):425–39.

Mathew NT. The prophylactic treatment of chronic daily headache. Headache 2006;46(10):1552–64.

Saulino M, Jacobs BW. The pharmacological management of spasticity. J Neurosci Nurs 2006;38(6):456–9.

Smith H, Elliott J. Alpha(2) receptors and agonists in pain management. Curr Opin Anaesthesiol 2001;14(5):513–18.

TOPIRAMATE

THERAPEUTICS

Brands
- Topamax, Epitomax, Topamac

Generic?
Yes

 Class
- Antiepileptic drug (AED)

Commonly Prescribed for
(FDA approved in bold)
- **Partial-onset seizures (adjunctive; adults and pediatric patients age 2–16)**
- **Primary generalized tonic-clonic seizures (adjunctive; adults and pediatric patients age 2–16)**
- **Migraine prophylaxis**
- Drop attacks associated with Lennox-Gastaut syndrome
- Obesity
- Bipolar disorder
- Binge-eating disorder/bulimia
- Cluster headache prophylaxis
- Idiopathic intracranial hypertension
- Alcohol dependence
- Essential tremor

 How the Drug Works
There are multiple mechanisms of action, and it is uncertain which of these give the drug its effectiveness
- Augmentation of the GABA-A receptor
- Sodium channel blocker
- Carbonic anhydrase inhibitor, isoenzymes II and IV
- Glutamate receptor (specifically the AMPA/kainate subtype) antagonist
- May work by inhibiting protein kinase activity
- Possible serotonin activity on 5-HT2$_C$ receptors

How Long Until It Works
- Seizures – may decrease by 2 weeks
- Migraines – may decrease in as little as 2 weeks, but can take up to 3 months on a stable dose to see full effect

If It Works
- Seizures – goal is the remission of seizures. Continue as long as effective and well-tolerated. Consider tapering slowly, stopping after 2 years without seizures, depending on the type of epilepsy
- Migraine – goal is a 50% or greater reduction in migraine frequency or severity. Consider tapering or stopping if headaches remit for more than 6 months or if considering pregnancy

If It Doesn't Work
- Increase to highest tolerated dose
- Epilepsy: consider changing to another agent, adding a second agent or referral for epilepsy surgery evaluation
- Migraine: address other issues, such as medication-overuse, other coexisting medical disorders, such as anxiety, and consider changing to another agent or adding a second agent

 Best Augmenting Combos for Partial Response or Treatment-Resistance
- For some patients with epilepsy or migraine, low-dose polytherapy with 2 or more drugs may be better tolerated and more effective than high-dose monotherapy
- Epilepsy: keep in mind drug interactions and their effect on levels
- Migraine: consider beta-blockers, antidepressants, natural products, other AEDs, and non-medication treatments such as biofeedback to improve headache control

Tests
- Mild to moderate decreases in bicarbonate can occur with topiramate, but are uncommon reasons for discontinuation. Routine screening for metabolic acidosis is not recommended

ADVERSE EFFECTS (AEs)

How Drug Causes AEs
- CNS AEs may be caused by sodium channel blockade or GABA-A receptor augmentation
- Carbonic anhydrase inhibition causes paresthesias, metabolic acidosis; may lead to kidney stones

Notable AEs
- Sedation, cognitive problems, especially word-finding difficulties, mood problems, paresthesias
- Anorexia. diarrhea, weight loss

- Pallinopsia – a visual disturbance that causes persistence of images (rare and frightening for the patient but benign)

 ### Life-Threatening or Dangerous AEs

- Metabolic acidosis
- Kidney stones (calcium phosphate)
- Narrow angle-closure glaucoma (rare)
- Fever, dehydration and lack of sweating (more common in children)

Weight Gain

- Unusual

Sedation

- Common

What to Do About AEs

- AEs often decrease or remit after a longer time on a stable dose
- Paresthesias may respond to high potassium diets or potassium tablets
- Cognitive AEs tend to improve with small decreases in dose
- For patients with kidney stones, check the type of stone. Topiramate usually causes calcium phosphate stones

Best Augmenting Agents for AEs

- Paresthesias related to topiramate may improve with high potassium diet or tablets
- Other AEs are more likely to improve by lowering dose

DOSING AND USE

Usual Dosage Range

- Epilepsy: 200 – 400 mg/day in adults, with maximum 1600 mg/day. 5–9 mg/kg/day in pediatric patients. Given as 2 divided doses
- Migraine: 25–200 mg/day. Patients can take qhs to increase compliance. Can use higher doses as tolerated

Dosage Forms

- 15 mg sprinkle capsule. 25 mg, 50 mg, 100 mg, 200 mg

How to Dose

- Adults: increase by 50 mg/week for epilepsy or as tolerated, and by 25 mg/week for migraine until goal dose
- Pediatrics – see children and adolescents

 ### Dosing Tips

- Adverse events increase with dose increases
- Weight loss is often dose related, but patients on lower doses (50 mg) still lose weight
- Slow titration minimizes sedation and other AEs
- Some patients need higher doses for migraine or cluster headache prophylaxis

Overdose

- Convulsions, drowsiness, sleep disturbance, blurred vision, diplopia, stupor, hypotension, abdominal pain, agitation, dizziness, lethargy, depression, and metabolic acidosis. No reported deaths except with poly-drug overdoses

Long-Term Use

- Safe for long-term use

Habit Forming

- No

How to Stop

- Taper slowly
- Abrupt withdrawal can lead to seizures in patients with epilepsy. Tremor is also common
- Headaches may return within days to months of stopping, but patients often continue to do well for 6 or more months after stopping

Pharmacokinetics

- Renally excreted. Peak levels at 2 hr and half-life 21 hours

 ### Drug Interactions

- Phenytoin, carbamazepine, valproic acid, and pioglitazone can increase topiramate clearance and decrease topiramate levels
- Lamotrigine and hydrochlorothiazide may increase topiramate levels
- Topiramate may increase levels of amitriptyline

- Topiramate can decrease levels of lithium, digoxin, and valproic acid
- Carbonic anhydrase inhibitors such as acetazolamide increase the risk of kidney stones
- Topiramate can interact with CNS depressants and alcohol with neuropsychiatric and cognitive consequences
- Higher-dose topiramate (> 200 mg) can decrease plasma concentrations of estrogens and progestins in patients taking oral contraceptives. Use a higher dose of estrogen or consider alternative methods of contraception

 Other Warnings/ Precautions

- Patients taking a ketogenic diet for seizures are more likely to experience severe metabolic acidosis on topiramate

Do Not Use

- Patients with a proven allergy to topiramate

 Pregnancy

- Risk category C. Teratogenic in animal studies but no studies in humans
- Associated with hypospadias in male infants
- Risks of stopping medication must outweigh risk to fetus for patients with epilepsy. Seizures and potential status epilepticus place the woman and fetus at risk and can cause reduced oxygen and blood supply to the womb
- Patients with migraine should generally stop topiramate before considering pregnancy. Migraine usually improves in the last 2 trimesters
- Supplementation with 0.4 mg of folic acid before and during pregnancy is recommended

Breast Feeding

- Some drug is found in mother's breast milk
- Generally recommendations are to discontinue drug or bottle feed
- If topiramate is used, then need to monitor infant for sedation, poor feeding or irritability

SPECIAL POPULATIONS

Renal Impairment

- Topiramate is renally excreted and removed by hemodialysis. Lower dose and give an extra dose after dialysis sessions

Hepatic Impairment

- May be decreased in patients with significant liver disease

Cardiac Impairment

- No known effects

Elderly

- Elderly patients may be more susceptible to AEs

 Children and Adolescents

- Approved for treatment of children over age 2 for epilepsy management
- Starting dose 1–3 mg/kg/day at night, increasing every 1–2 weeks by 1–3 mg/kg/day until goal dose of 5–9 mg/kg/day in 2 divided doses
- Paresthesias and cognitive AEs are less common in children

THE ART OF NEUROPHARMACOLOGY

Potential Advantages

- Effectively treats both migraine and epilepsy. Usually causes weight loss, unlike many other medications for epilepsy and migraine

Potential Disadvantages

- Cognitive AEs. Weight loss in thin patients can be troublesome. Kidney stones and metabolic acidosis

Primary Target Symptoms

- Seizure frequency and severity
- Migraine frequency and severity

 Pearls

- For epilepsy, higher doses may be needed. AEs are more common when using in combination with other drugs that can produce CNS depression
- Broad-spectrum AED effective against almost all seizure types (maybe even infantile spasms)

- For migraine, the individual dose may vary widely. Some patients benefit from doses as low as 25 mg/day but others may require much higher doses than the 100 mg/day approved for migraine prophylaxis
- Topiramate may be effective in treating idiopathic intracranial hypertension (pseudotumor cerebrii) and is often easier to tolerate with more weight loss than acetazolamide

- Topiramate is not a first-line medication for cluster headache
- Topiramate is used for treatment of manic symptoms in bipolar disorder, but its efficacy was not established in clinical trials
- Topiramate is useful for essential tremor, although often higher doses are needed to see an effect

Suggested Reading

Celebisoy N, Gökçay F, Sirin H, Akyürekli O. Treatment of idiopathic intracranial hypertension: topiramate vs acetazolamide, an open-label study. Acta Neurol Scand 2007;116(5):322–7.

Connor GS, Edwards K, Tarsy D. Topiramate in essential tremor: findings from double-blind, placebo-controlled, crossover trials. Clin Neuropharmacol 2008;31(2):97–103.

Guerrini R, Parmeggiani L. Topiramate and its clinical applications in epilepsy. Expert Opin Pharmacother 2006;7(6):811–23.

Silberstein SD. Preventive migraine treatment. Neurol Clin 2009;27(2):429–43.

Silberstein SD, Lipton RB, Dodick DW, Freitag FG, Ramadan N, Mathew N, Brandes JL, Bigal M, Saper J, Ascher S, Jordan DM, Greenberg SJ, Hulihan J; Topiramate Chronic Migraine Study Group. Efficacy and safety of topiramate for the treatment of chronic migraine: a randomized, double-blind, placebo-controlled trial. Headache 2007;47(2):170–80.

Taylor FR. Weight change associated with the use of migraine-preventive medications. Clin Ther 2008;30(6):1069–80.

van Passel L, Arif H, Hirsch LJ. Topiramate for the treatment of epilepsy and other nervous system disorders. Expert Rev Neurother 2006;6(1):19–31.

TRIENTINE HYDROCHLORIDE

Brands
• Syprine

Generic?
Yes

 Class
• Chelating agent

Commonly Prescribed for
(FDA approved in bold)
• **Wilson's disease (WD) in patients intolerant of penicillamine**

 How the Drug Works
• In WD copper accumulates in body tissues (especially the liver and CNS), causing neurological/psychiatric problems and/or liver failure. Trientine binds to (chelates) copper, allowing it to be excreted in the urine

How Long Until It Works
• 6 months or more

If It Works
• Continue treatment, if tolerated. Most patients remain on drug for the rest of their life but if serum copper returns to normal (< 10 µg/dL) consider changing to elemental zinc or zinc sulfate. Monitor for recurrence of symptoms or changes in urinary copper excretion

If It Doesn't Work
• Increase to as much as 2000 mg daily for poor clinical response or if free serum copper is above 20 mcg/dL. For liver failure or truly refractory patients, liver transplantation is curative

 Best Augmenting Combos for Partial Response or Treatment-Resistance
• Change to penicillamine if ineffective. A diet low in copper-containing foods, such as nuts, chocolate, liver, and dried fruit, is recommended

Tests
• Adequately treated patients should have free serum copper below 10 mcg/dL. Monitor 24-hour urinary copper excretion every 6–12 months (should be between 0.5–1 mg)

How Drug Causes AEs
• Unknown

Notable AEs
• Heartburn, iron deficiency anemia, anorexia, cramps, muscle pain, and epigastric pain have been reported. Rarely muscle spasm or dystonia have occurred. The relationship of these symptoms to trientine is unclear

 Life-Threatening or Dangerous AEs
• Myasthenia gravis and systemic lupus erythematosus have been reported

Weight Gain
• Unusual

Sedation
• Unusual

What to Do About AEs
• Discontinue only for serious AEs

Best Augmenting Agents for AEs
• Most cannot be improved with the use of an augmenting agent

Usual Dosage Range
• 1000 mg – 2000 mg/day

Dosage Forms
• Tablets: 250 mg

How to Dose
• Start at 750 – 1250 mg/day in 2–4 divided doses. Increase to as much as 2 g daily in divided doses as needed

Dosing Tips
- Give at least 1 hour before or 2 hours after meals to ensure absorption

Overdose
- Symptoms unknown

Long-Term Use
- Safe for long-term use

Habit Forming
- No

How to Stop
- No need to taper

Pharmacokinetics
- Not available

 Drug Interactions
- Mineral supplements block the absorption of trientine. Do not give within 2 hours of iron supplements

 Other Warnings/ Precautions
- Capsule contents can cause contact dermatitis

Do Not Use
- Known hypersensitivity

SPECIAL POPULATIONS

Renal Impairment
- Use with caution

Hepatic Impairment
- Usually improves hepatic disease in WD, even if severe

Cardiac Impairment
- No known effects

Elderly
- Use with caution

 Children and Adolescents
- WD can occur in children, usually ages 5 or older. In children 12 or younger, start at 500–750 mg/day in 2–4 divided doses. Increase to maximum of 1500 mg/day. Dose children over 12 as adults

 Pregnancy
- Category C. Use only if needed

Breast Feeding
- Unknown if excreted in breast milk

THE ART OF NEUROPHARMACOLOGY

Potential Advantages
- Compared to penicillamine, fewer AEs and easier to dose. Small head-to-head studies show effectiveness is similar

Potential Disadvantages
- Penicillamine has been used for a longer period of time with more evidence of effectiveness

Primary Target Symptoms
- Monitor serum and urinary copper to determine effectiveness. Treatment should improve neurological symptoms, including parkinsonism, dystonia, ataxia, depression, and psychosis

 Pearls
- The high incidence of paradoxical worsening and multiple AEs seen with penicillamine have led many to suggest that trientine should be the first-line agent in WD
- Not indicated for rheumatoid arthritis or cystinuria
- Other agents with known effects in WD include tetrathiomolybdate and intramuscular dimercaprol
- In asymptomatic individuals diagnosed by abnormal test results or family screening, it is uncertain if zinc, trientine or penicillamine is most appropriate initial treatment

Suggested Reading

Brewer GJ. Novel therapeutic approaches to the treatment of Wilson's disease. Expert Opin Pharmacother 2006;7(3):317–24.

Brewer GJ. The risks of free copper in the body and the development of useful anticopper drugs. Curr Opin Clin Nutr Metab Care 2008;11(6):727–32.

Das SK, Ray K. Wilson's disease: an update. Nat Clin Pract Neurol 2006;2(9):482–93.

Wiggelinkhuizen M, Tilanus ME, Bollen CW, Houwen RH. Systematic review: clinical efficacy of chelator agents and zinc in the initial treatment of Wilson disease. Aliment Pharmacol Ther 2009;29(9):947–58.

TRIHEXYPHENIDYL

THERAPEUTICS

Brands
- Artane

Generic?
Yes

Class
- Antiparkinson agent, anticholinergic

Commonly Prescribed for
(FDA approved in bold)
- **Extrapyramidal disorders**
- **Parkinsonism**
- Idiopathic generalized dystonia
- Focal dystonias
- Dopa-responsive dystonia

How the Drug Works
- In PD, there is a relative excess of cholinergic input. Trihexyphenidyl is a synthetic anticholinergic with relatively greater CNS activity than most other anticholinergics
- May also inhibit the reuptake and storage of dopamine at dopamine neurons and transporters, prolonging dopamine action

How Long Until It Works
- PD/extrapyramidal disorders – minutes-hours

If It Works
- PD – do not abruptly discontinue or change doses of other PD treatments. Usually most effective in combination with other medications

If It Doesn't Work
- PD – Generally trihexyphenidyl is an adjunctive medication for common PD symptoms, such as tremor, rigidity, and drooling. Other cardinal PD symptoms, such as bradykinesia and gait difficulties, are most likely to improve with other PD treatments, such as levodopa, dopamine agonists, amantadine, or MAO-B inhibitors
- Extrapyramidal disorders – increase to highest tolerated dose. Long-standing disorders are less likely to respond to treatment

Best Augmenting Combos for Partial Response or Treatment-Resistance
- For bradykinesia or gait disturbances causing significant functional disturbance, levodopa is most effective. For idiopathic PD patients, especially younger patients with normal cognition and milder disability, dopamine agonists are also a good first choice. Amantadine and MAO-B inhibitors may also be useful
- Depression is common in PD and may respond to low-dose SSRIs

Tests
- None

ADVERSE EFFECTS (AEs)

How Drug Causes AEs
- Prevents the action of acetylcholine on muscarinic receptors

Notable AEs
- Dry mouth, tachycardia, palpitations, hypotension, disorientation, confusion, hallucinations, constipation, nausea/vomiting, dilation of colon, rash, blurred vision, diplopia, urinary retention, elevated temperature, decreased sweating, erectile dysfunction

Life-Threatening or Dangerous AEs
- May precipitate narrow-angle glaucoma. Risk of heat stroke, especially in elderly patients. Can precipitate tachycardia, cardiac arrhythmias and hypotension in susceptible patients. May cause urinary retention in patients with prostate hypertrophy

Weight Gain
- Unusual

unusual · not unusual · common · problematic

Sedation
- Common

unusual · not unusual · common · problematic

What to Do About AEs

- Confusion, hallucinations – if possible stop trihexyphenidyl and any other anticholinergics
- Sedation – can take entire dose at night or lower dose
- Dry mouth – chewing gum or water can help
- Urinary retention: if drug cannot be discontinued, obtain urological evaluation

Best Augmenting Agents for AEs

- Most AEs cannot be improved with the use of an augmenting agent

DOSING AND USE

Usual Dosage Range

- PD – 6–15 mg/daily
- Extrapyramidal reactions: 5–15 mg daily

Dosage Forms

- Tablets: 2, 5 mg
- Elixir: 2 mg/5 mL

How to Dose

- PD: start at 1 mg the first few days. Then increase in 2 mg increments every 3–5 days as tolerated or until clinical effect reached. Divide total dose and give 3 times daily, usually with meals. Patients on very high doses may elect to take 4 doses daily: with meals and at bedtime. Usual dose is 6–10 mg in idiopathic PD but higher on average (12–15 mg) in post-encephalitic PD
- Drug-induced extrapyramidal disorders: wait a few hours to assess effect and increase dose empirically as tolerated. The total daily dose varies from patient to patient. To achieve more rapid relief, temporarily lower dose of the offending agent (phenothiazine, thioxanthene, or butyrophenone) when starting

 Dosing Tips

- Taking with meals may reduce AEs

Overdose

- Complications may include circulatory collapse, cardiac arrest, respiratory depression or arrest, CNS depression or stimulation, psychosis, shock, coma, seizures, ataxia, combativeness, anhidrosis and hyperthermia, fever, dysphagia, decreased bowel sounds, and sluggish pupils. Induce emesis, use gastric lavage or activated charcoal. Oxygen or intubation may be needed for respiratory depression. Catheterize for urinary retention. Treat hyperthermia appropriately with cooling devices, local miotics for mydriasis/cycloplegia. Use physostigmine to reverse cardiac effects and use fluids and vasopressors if needed

Long-Term Use

- Safe for long-term use. Effectiveness may decrease over time (years) in PD and AEs, such as sedation and cognitive impairment, can worsen

Habit Forming

- No

How to Stop

- No need to taper

Pharmacokinetics

- Half-life is 6–10 hours, but the time to peak effect is at 1–1.3 hours. Mostly urinary excretion. Bioavailability is about 100% but metabolism not well understood

 Drug Interactions

- Use with amantadine may increase AEs
- Trihexyphenidyl and all other anticholinergics may increase serum levels and effects of digoxin
- Can lower concentration of haloperidol and other phenothiazines, causing worsening of schizophrenia symptoms. Phenothiazines tend to increase anticholinergic AEs with concurrent use
- Can decrease gastric motility, resulting in increased gastric deactivation of levodopa and reduction in efficacy

 Other Warnings/ Precautions

- Use with caution in hot weather – may increase susceptibility to heat stroke
- Anticholinergics have additive effects when used with drugs of abuse, such as cannabinoids, barbiturates, opioids, and alcohol

Do Not Use

• Known hypersensitivity to the drug, glaucoma (especially angle-closure type), pyloric or duodenal obstruction, stenosing peptic ulcers, prostate hypertrophy or bladder neck obstructions, achalasia, or megacolon

SPECIAL POPULATIONS

Renal Impairment

• Use with caution but no known effects

Hepatic Impairment

• Use with caution but no known effects

Cardiac Impairment

• Use with caution in patients with known arrhythmias, especially tachycardia

Elderly

• Use with caution. More susceptible to AEs

Children and Adolescents

• Do not use in children aged 3 or less. Generalized dystonias may respond to anticholinergic treatment; young patients usually tolerate the medication better than the elderly

Pregnancy

• Category C. Use only if benefit of medication outweighs risks

Breast Feeding

• Concentration in breast milk unknown. May inhibit lactation. Use only if benefits outweigh risk

THE ART OF NEUROPHARMACOLOGY

Potential Advantages

• Useful adjunctive agent for some PD patients, especially post-encephalitic and younger patients with bothersome tremor. First-line agent for generalized dystonias and well tolerated in the younger age groups

Potential Disadvantages

• Multiple dose-dependent AEs associated with muscarinic effects limit use. Not effective in most idiopathic PD patients. Patients with long-standing extrapyramidal disorders may not respond to treatment

Primary Target Symptoms

• Tremor, akinesia, rigidity, drooling, dystonia

 Pearls

• Useful adjunct in younger PD patients with tremor
• Useful in the treatment of post-encephalitic PD
• Sedation limits use, especially in older patients. Patients with mental impairment do poorly
• Post-encephalitic PD patients usually tolerate higher doses better than idiopathic PD patients
• Generalized dystonias are more likely to benefit from anticholinergic therapy than focal dystonias
• Dystonias related to cerebral palsy, head injuries, and stroke may improve with trihexyphenidyl, especially in younger, cognitively normal patients
• Schizophrenic patients may abuse trihexyphenidyl and other anticholinergic medications to relieve negative symptoms, for a stimulant effect or to improve symptoms of drug-induced parkinsonism

Suggested Reading

Brocks DR. Anticholinergic drugs used in Parkinson's disease: an overlooked class of drugs from a pharmacokinetic perspective. J Pharm Pharm Sci 1999;2(2):39–46.

Colosimo C, Gori MC, Inghilleri M. Post-encephalitic tremor and delayed-onset parkinsonism. Parkinsonism Relat Disord 1999;5(3):123–4.

Costa J, Espírito-Santo C, Borges A, Ferreira JJ, Coelho M, Sampaio C. Botulinum toxin type A versus anticholinergics for cervical dystonia. Cochrane Database Syst Rev 2005;(1): CD004312.

Sanger TD, Bastian A, Brunstrom J, Damiano D, Delgado M, Dure L, Gaebler-Spira D, Hoon A, Mink JW, Sherman-Levine S, Welty LJ; Child Motor Study Group. Prospective open-label clinical trial of trihexyphenidyl in children with secondary dystonia due to cerebral palsy. J Child Neurol 2007;22(5):530–7.

Zemishlany Z, Aizenberg D, Weiner Z, Weizman A. Trihexyphenidyl (Artane) abuse in schizophrenic patients. Int Clin Psychopharmacol 1996;11(3): 199–202.

VALPROIC ACID AND DERIVATIVES (DPX)

Brands
- Depakote, Depakote ER, Depakene, Depacon, Episenta, Epilim, Epival, Divalproex, Dicorate, Disorate, Divaa, Divalpro, Soval DX, Trend XR, Valna, Stavzor

Generic?
Yes, except for ER formulation

 ## Class
- Antiepileptic drug (AED)

Commonly Prescribed for
(FDA approved in bold)
- **Complex partial seizures (monotherapy and adjunctive)**
- **Simple and complex absence seizures (monotherapy and adjunctive)**
- **Adjunctive therapy for multiple seizure types, including absence seizures**
- **Migraine prophylaxis**
- **Acute mania in bipolar disorder**
- Cluster headache
- Generalized tonic-clonic seizures, including juvenile myoclonic epilepsy
- Infantile spasms (West syndrome)
- Lennox-Gastaut syndrome
- Status epilepticus
- Post-hypoxic myoclonus
- Landau-Kleffner syndrome (acquired epileptic aphasia)
- Spinal muscular atrophy
- Acute migraine or status migrainosus
- Bipolar depression
- Schizophrenia/psychosis

 ## How the Drug Works
Unknown but there are multiple mechanisms of action
- Activates glutamic acid decarboxylase to increase gamma-aminobutyric acid (GABA) production
- Inhibits GABA transaminase and the catabolism of GABA
- Sodium channel antagonist
- T-type calcium currents in thalamus
- May suppress NMDA excitatory neurotransmission

How Long Until It Works
- Seizures – 2 weeks
- Migraines – effective within a few weeks but can take up to 3 months to see full effect
- Mania – usually effective in days

If It Works
- Seizures – goal is the remission of seizures. Continue as long as effective and well-tolerated. Consider slowly tapering and stopping after 2 years seizure-free, depending on the type of epilepsy
- Migraine – goal is a 50% or greater reduction in migraine frequency or severity. Consider tapering or stopping if headaches remit for more than 6 months or if patient considering pregnancy

If It Doesn't Work
- Increase to highest tolerated dose. Check a drug level if compliance an issue
- Epilepsy: consider changing to another agent, adding a second agent or referral for epilepsy surgery evaluation. When adding a second agent keep in mind the drug interactions
- Migraine: address other issues, such as medication-overuse, other coexisting medical disorders, such as anxiety, and consider changing to or adding a second agent

 ## Best Augmenting Combos for Partial Response or Treatment-Resistance
- Epilepsy: drug interactions complicate multi-drug therapy, especially the older AEDs. Most of the newer drugs, such as gabapentin, topiramate, oxcarbazepine, and zonisamide, are easier to use with DPX
- Migraine: consider beta-blockers, antidepressants, natural products, other antiepileptics, and non-medication treatments, such as biofeedback, to improve headache control

Tests
- Obtain liver function testing and platelet counts before starting, optional to monitor regularly for the first few months and once or twice a year after that. Test urgently if any symptoms of liver disease or new bleeding or easy bruising
- Monitor for weight gain and signs of metabolic syndrome (weight gain, hyperlipidemia, elevated fasting glucose)

- Hyperammonemia may occur, even with normal liver function tests. Often asymptomatic. Check a level for any clinically significant symptoms

ADVERSE EFFECTS (AEs)

How Drug Causes AEs

- CNS AEs may be caused by sodium or calcium channel effects or GABA effects
- DPX-associated hyperammonemia can cause delirium, tremor
- DPX-associated hepatic toxicity can cause nausea, anorexia, or jaundice

Notable AEs

- Sedation, tremor, dizziness, diplopia, blurred vision, cognitive problems
- Nausea, vomiting, abdominal pain, diarrhea, anorexia, constipation
- Weight gain, peripheral edema, bronchitis, pharyngitis, alopecia, carnitine depletion

Life-Threatening or Dangerous AEs

- Hepatotoxicity and liver disease, especially in children under 2 on multiple anti-epilepsy medications. More commonly patients have mild-moderate elevations of serum liver enzymes that are asymptomatic. Patients usually recover
- Rare pancreatitis can occur months to years after starting DPX. Most patients recover but can be fatal
- Thrombocytopenia
- Polycystic ovarian syndrome, including obesity, elevated androgen concentrations, anovulation, and hirsutism
- Significant weight gain and development of insulin resistance/metabolic syndrome (controversial)

Weight Gain

- Problematic

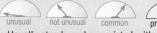

- Usually steady and associated with carbohydrate craving

Sedation

- Common

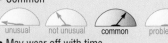

- May wear off with time

What to Do About AEs

- May be decreased with extended-release formulation
- Decrease dose
- Small elevations in liver enzymes or increased ammonia are common. If there are no symptoms, then the decision to decrease or maintain dose depends on the patient and the severity of the condition treated
- Change to another drug

Best Augmenting Agents for AEs

- Propranolol for tremor
- Weight gain may improve with augmentation or transition to Zonegran or topiramate
- Zinc and selenium can help alopecia

DOSING AND USE

Usual Dosage Range

- Epilepsy: 10–60 mg/kg/day, may need to increase in some patients
- Migraine: 1000 mg/day, some need a higher dose
- Cluster: 500–2000 mg/day
- Acute mania: Usually 1000 mg/day or more

Dosage Forms

- As valproic acid: 250 mg (Depakene) or 250 mg /5 mL syrup
- As divalproex sodium compound: 125 mg sprinkles or delayed release 125 mg, 250 mg, 500 mg, Depakote ER: 250 mg, 500 mg
- Valproate sodium solution for injection: 100 mg/mL in 5 mL vials

How to Dose

- Epilepsy: Start at 10–15 mg/kg/day and increase to goal dose
- Migraine: Start 250–500 qhs
- As valproic acid: tid; as delayed release divalproex sodium: bid. Depakote ER can be taken once daily

Dosing Tips

- Easier to rapidly increase dose than many other AEDs; IV Depacon available for emergency use to treat seizures, status migrainosis and mania
- When converting to Depakote ER, plasma levels are generally 10–20% lower than immediate release for a given dose
- Oral loading with 20–30 mg/kg per day is an alternative to IV loading
- Depakote ER has less GI AEs; avoids peak levels
- For most conditions levels 50–100 µg/mL are effective, but in some cases higher levels are needed, i.e., cluster headache and mania

Overdose

- Stupor and coma, increased intracranial pressure. Fever. Respiratory insufficiency and supraventricular tachycardia. Supportive care and gastric lavage. Can be fatal

Long-Term Use

- Regular platelet counts and liver function testing. Optional unless patient symptomatic

Habit Forming

- No

How to Stop

- Taper slowly and keep drug interactions in mind
- Abrupt withdrawal can lead to seizures in patients with epilepsy
- Headaches may return within days to months of stopping

Pharmacokinetics

- Mainly hepatic metabolism. Metabolized in part by CYP450 system. Plasma half-life is 9–16 hours. 100% bioavailability and 93% protein bound

Drug Interactions

- DPX causes interactions by displacing other medications from plasma proteins and inhibiting hepatic metabolism. Drugs that affect the expression of hepatic enzymes such as glucuronosyltransferases can alter DPX clearance

- Increases levels of carbamazepine, lamotrigine, phenobarbital, and ethosuximide
- Increases free levels of phenytoin (which can cause toxicity even if serum levels are in a normal therapeutic range)
- DPX increases levels of warfarin, amitriptyline, nortriptyline, zidovudine, valium, cimetadine, chlorpromazine, erythromycin, and nimodipine
- Phenytoin, phenobarbital, primidone, cholestyramine, rifampin, and carbamazepine (hepatic inducers) can lower DPX levels
- Addition of salicylates, erythromycin, felbamate, and chlorpromazine can increase DPX levels

Other Warnings/ Precautions

- CNS AEs increase when taken with other CNS depressants or with most acute or chronic illnesses
- Hepatotoxicity: nausea, vomiting, jaundice, edema
- Pancreatitis: abdominal pain, anorexia, nausea
- Teratogenic effects: neural tube defects
- Urea cycle disorders: unexplained delirium in children, mental retardation, vomiting, lethargy and hyperammonemia

Do Not Use

- Patients with a proven allergy to DPX. Also contraindicated in patients with thrombocytopenia, liver disease, urea cycle disorders, and pancreatitis

SPECIAL POPULATIONS

Renal Impairment

- No known effects. Highly protein bound, easier to use in patients on dialysis than most other AEDs

Hepatic Impairment

- Do not use

Cardiac Impairment

- No known effects

Elderly

- Use a lower dose and watch for AEs and nutritional intake

 Children and Adolescents

- Approved for use in children and often used in generalized seizures, such as absence and juvenile myoclonic epilepsy
- May help treat infantile spasms related to tuberous sclerosis, especially if ACTH is ineffective or cannot be used
- For infants with new-onset unexplained seizures, metabolic diseases are not rare. Consider using an alternative agent until ruled out

 Pregnancy

- Risk category D. Increased risk of neural tube defects, cardiac defects, craniofacial abnormalities, and hepatic failure
- Women who continue taking DPX during pregnancy should be considered high-risk and take folate
- If a patient continues taking during pregnancy, consider vitamin K during the last 6 weeks of pregnancy to reduce risk of bleeding
- Patients taking DPX for conditions other than epilepsy should generally stop DPX before considering pregnancy. Migraine usually improves in the last 2 trimesters

Breast Feeding

- Relatively low (3%) in breast milk and safer than most other AEDs
- Monitor infant for sedation, poor feeding or irritability

THE ART OF NEUROPHARMACOLOGY

Potential Advantages

- Highly effective for multiple types of epilepsy due to broad spectrum of action. Treats generalized seizures as well as partial and is approved as monotherapy. Effective for both migraine and cluster headache. Useful for patients with more than one, condition, such as migraine and epilepsy or mania

Potential Disadvantages

- Weight gain. Tremor. Risk of polycystic ovarian syndrome and teratogenicity

make difficult to use in women of childbearing age. Protein binding and enzyme induction cause drug interactions. Liver disease and hepatotoxicity in children under 2

Primary Target Symptoms

- Seizure frequency and severity
- Headache frequency and severity

 Pearls

- Drug of choice for patients with generalized epilepsies, however may not be as effective as carbamazepine for focal seizures
- Useful in status epilepticus for patients with contraindications to phenytoin. Loading dose 20–30 mg/kg. Less respiratory depression than other AEDs
- Highly effective for migraine and cluster prophylaxis. For cluster, DPX is more likely to be effective at the upper end of the therapeutic range
- May be useful as an acute headache treatment in the emergency room or infusion setting as IV Depacon. (300–1000 mg as rapid infusion.) For use as a preventive drug after discharge, you can load the medication (15 mg/kg) and then administer 5 mg/kg every 8–12 hours. IV Depacon for acute headache is especially useful for patients who cannot tolerate or have contraindications to other medications
- As a headache prophylactic agent for patients in the emergency room, consider giving an intravenous treatment followed by an initial dose of 1000 mg/day
- For migraine patients on DPX with tremor and suboptimal headache control, propranolol may improve headaches and treat tremor
- DPX may have neuroprotective properties, such as inhibition of apoptosis and slowing of neurofibrillary tangle formation, suggesting usefulness for treatment of neurodegenerative diseases. However, studies for treatment of Alzheimer's dementia and associated psychosis have been largely negative, with poor tolerability in this population
- Preliminary studies suggest utility in treating spinal muscular atrophy, especially in young children

Suggested Reading

Apostol G, Cady RK, Laforet GA, Robieson WZ, Olson E, Abi-Saab WM, Saltarelli M. Divalproex extended-release in adolescent migraine prophylaxis: results of a randomized, double-blind, placebo-controlled study. Headache 2008;48(7):1012–25.

Cohen AS, Matharu MS, Goadsby PJ. Trigeminal autonomic cephalalgias: current and future treatments. Headache 2007;47(6):969–80.

Limdi NA, Knowlton RK, Cofield SS, Ver Hoef LW, Paige AL, Dutta S, Faught E. Safety of rapid intravenous loading of valproate. Epilepsia 2007;48(3):478–83.

Mackay MT, Weiss SK, Adams-Webber T, Ashwal S, Stephens D, Ballaban-Gill K, Baram TZ, Duchowny M, Hirtz D, Pellock JM, Shields WD, Shinnar S, Wyllie E, Snead OC 3rd; American Academy of Neurology; Child Neurology Society. Practice parameter: medical treatment of infantile spasms: report of the American Academy of Neurology and the Child Neurology Society. Neurology 2004;62(10):1668–81.

Posner EB, Mohamed K, Marson AG. Ethosuximide, sodium valproate or lamotrigine for absence seizures in children and adolescents. Cochrane Database Syst Rev 2005;(4): CD003032.

Rauchenzauner M, Haberlandt E, Scholl-Bürgi S, Ernst B, Hoppichler F, Karall D, Ebenbichler CF, Rostasy K, Luef G. Adiponectin and visfatin concentrations in children treated with valproic acid. Epilepsia 2008;49(2):353–7.

Silberstein SD. Preventive migraine treatment. Neurol Clin 2009;27(2):429–43.

Swoboda KJ, Scott CB, Reyna SP, Prior TW, LaSalle B, Sorenson SL, Wood J, Acsadi G, Crawford TO, Kissel JT, Krosschell KJ, D'Anjou G, Bromberg MB, Schroth MK, Chan GM, Elsheikh B, Simard LR. Phase II open label study of valproic acid in spinal muscular atrophy. PLoS One 2009;4(5):e5268.

Trinka E. The use of valproate and new antiepileptic drugs in status epilepticus. Epilepsia 2007;48 (Suppl 8): 49–51.

Brands
- Effexor, Effexor XR, Effexor XL, Efectin, Efexor, Trevilor, Venla

Generic?
Yes (except XR form)

Class
- Serotonin and norepinephrine reuptake inhibitor (SNRI), antidepressant

Commonly Prescribed for
(FDA approved in bold)
- **Depression**
- **Generalized anxiety disorder**
- **Panic disorder**
- **Social phobia**
- Migraine or tension-type headache prophylaxis
- Diabetic neuropathy
- Other painful peripheral neuropathies
- Cancer pain (neuropathic)
- Depression secondary to stroke
- Stress urinary incontinence
- Fibromyalgia
- Binge-eating disorder
- Insomnia
- Post-traumatic stress disorder
- ADHD
- Perimenopausal/menopausal hot flashes

How the Drug Works
- Blocks serotonin and norepinephrine reuptake pumps, increasing their levels within hours, but antidepressant effects take weeks. Effect is more likely related to adaptive changes in serotonin and norepinephrine receptor systems over time
- Weakly blocks dopamine reuptake pump (dopamine transporter)

How Long Until It Works
- Migraines – effective in as little as 2 weeks, but can take up to 10 weeks on a stable dose to see full effect
- Tension-type headache prophylaxis – effective in 4–8 weeks
- Neuropathic pain – usually some effect within 4 weeks

- Diabetic neuropathy – may have significant improvement with high doses within 6 weeks
- Depression – 2 weeks but up to 2 months for full effect

If It Works
- Migraine/tension-type headache – goal is a 50% or greater reduction in headache frequency or severity. Consider tapering or stopping if headaches remit for more than 6 months or if considering pregnancy
- Neuropathic pain – the goal is to reduce pain intensity and symptoms, but usually does not produce remission. Continue to use and monitor for AEs
- Diabetic neuropathy – the goal is to reduce pain intensity and reduce use of analgesics, but usually does not produce remission. Continue to use and maintain strict glycemic control and diabetic management
- Depression – continue to use and monitor for AEs. May continue for 1 yr following first depression episode or indefinitely if >1 episode of depression

If It Doesn't Work
- Increase to highest tolerated dose
- Migraine and tension-type headache: address other issues, such as medication-overuse, other coexisting medical disorders, such as anxiety, and consider changing to another agent or adding a second agent
- Neuropathic pain: either change to another agent or add a second agent

Best Augmenting Combos for Partial Response or Treatment-Resistance
- Headache: For some patients, low-dose polytherapy with 2 or more drugs may be better tolerated and more effective than high-dose monotherapy. May use in combination with AEDs, antihypertensives, natural products, and non-medication treatments, such as biofeedback, to improve headache control
- Neuropathic pain: AEDs, such as gabapentin, pregabalin, carbamazepine and capsaicin, mexiletine are agents used for neuropathic pain. Opioids are appropriate for long-term use in some cases but require careful monitoring

Tests
- Check blood pressure at baseline and when increasing dose

Usual Dosage Range
- 37.5–375 mg/day

Dosage Forms
- Tablet: 25 mg, 37.5 mg, 50 mg, 75 mg, 100 mg
- Extended release: 37.5 mg, 75 mg, 150 mg

How to Dose
- Initial dose 37.5–75 mg taken daily. Increase by 75 mg in 1 week. Titrate as tolerated to effective dose, typically 150–375 mg for pain syndromes. Dose once daily as extended release or divided into 2–3 doses as immediate release

 Dosing Tips
- Higher doses are typically used for pain. Extended-release formulation allows for once-a-day dosing and may be better tolerated

Overdose
- Signs and symptoms may include cardiac arrhythmias, usually tachycardia, ECG changes (prolonged QTc interval or bundle branch block), sedation, seizures, bowel perforation, serotonin syndrome, fever, rhabdomyolysis, hyponatremia, blood pressure abnormalities, extrapyramidal effects, headache, nervousness, tremor; death can occur

Long-Term Use
- Safe for long-term use with monitoring of blood pressure

Habit Forming
- No

How to Stop
- Taper slowly (no more than 50% reduction every 3–4 days until discontinuation) to avoid withdrawal. Pain often worsens shortly after decreasing dose

Pharmacokinetics
- Metabolized via the CYP2D6 isoenzyme. Venlafaxine is a weak inhibitor of this isoenzyme. O-desmethylvenlafaxine is the only major active metabolite of venlafaxine.

ADVERSE EFFECTS (AEs)

How Drug Causes AEs
- By increasing serotonin and norepinephrine on non-therapeutic responsive receptors throughout the body. Most AEs are dose- and time-dependent

Notable AEs
- Constipation, dry mouth, sweating, blurry vision, loss of appetite, nausea, weight loss or gain, hypertension, headache, asthenia, dizziness, tremor, dream disorder, insomnia, somnolence, abnormal ejaculation, impotence, orgasm disorder, sweating, itching, sedation, nervousness, restlessness

 Life-Threatening or Dangerous AEs
- Serotonin syndrome
- Rare hepatitis
- Rare activation of mania or suicidal ideation
- Rare worsening of coexisting seizure disorders

Weight Gain
- Not unusual

unusual   not unusual   common   problematic

Sedation
- Not unusual

unusual   not unusual   common   problematic
- May cause insomnia in some patients

What to Do About AEs
- For minor AEs, lower dose, titrate more slowly, or switch to another agent
- For serious AEs, lower dose and consider stopping, taper to avoid withdrawal

Best Augmenting Agents for AEs
- Try magnesium for constipation

Half-life 5 h venlafaxine and 11hrs for active metabolite O-desmethylvenlafaxine

Drug Interactions

- CYP2D6 inhibitors (paroxetine, fluoxetine, bupropion), cimetidine, and valproic acid and CYP3A4 inhibitors (clarithromycin, ketoconazole, itraconazole) may increase drug concentration
- The release of serotonin by platelets is important for maintaining hemostasis. Combined use of SSRIs or SNRI's (such as venlafaxine) and NSAIDs, and/or drugs that effect anticoagulation have been associated with an increased risk of bleeding
- CYP2D6 and 1A2 enzyme inducers, including rifampin, nicotine, phenobarbital, can lower levels
- May decrease effects of antihypertensive medications, such as metoprolol
- May decrease clearance and increase effect of antipsychotics (haloperidol, clozapine.)
- May increase the risk of seizure with tramadol
- May cause serotonin syndrome when used within 14 days of MAO inhibitors
- May increase risk of cardiotoxicity and arrhythmia when used with tricyclic antidepressants

⚠ Other Warnings/ Precautions

- May increase risk of seizure
- Patients should be observed closely for clinical worsening, suicidality, and changes in behavior in known or unknown bipolar disorder

Do Not Use

- Proven hypersensitivity to drug
- Concurrently with MAOI; allow at least 14 days between discontinuation of an MAOI and initiation of venlafaxine or at least 7–14 days between discontinuation of venlafaxine and initiation of an MAOI
- In patient with uncontrolled narrow angle-closure glaucoma

Renal Impairment

- Use with caution. Decrease usual dose by 25–50%

Hepatic Impairment

- Use with caution. Decrease usual dose by 50%

Cardiac Impairment

- Use with caution. Dose-dependent effect on blood pressure

Elderly

- No adjustments necessary

Children and Adolescents

- Safety and efficacy not established. Use with caution. Observe closely for clinical worsening, suicidality, and changes in behavior, in known or unknown bipolar disorder. Parents should be informed and advised of the risks

Pregnancy

- Category C. Generally not recommended for the treatment of headaches or neuropathic pain during pregnancy. Neonates exposed to venlafaxine or other SNRIs or SSRIs late in the third trimester have developed complications necessitating extended hospitalizations, respiratory support, and tube feeding. Respiratory distress, cyanosis, apnea, seizures, temperature instability, feeding difficulty, vomiting, hypoglycemia, hypotonia, hyperreflexia, tremor, jitteriness, irritability, and constant crying consistent with a toxic effect of the drug or drug discontinuation syndrome have been reported

Breast Feeding

- Some drug is found in breast milk and use while breast feeding is not recommended

Potential Advantages

- Very effective in the treatment of multiple pain disorders. Effective for treatment of comorbid depression and anxiety in chronic pain. Less sedation than tertiary amine tricyclic antidepressants (TCAs) (e.g., amitriptyline)

Potential Disadvantages
- May cause or worsen hypertension. Usually higher doses are need for pain disorders than for depression

Primary Target Symptoms
- Reduction in headache frequency, duration and/or intensity
- Reduction in neuropathic pain

Pearls
- Effect on norepinephrine receptors relative to serotonin is greater at higher doses (150 mg or above). This may explain why higher doses are needed in pain disorders than depression and anxiety
- In patients with migraine or tension-type headache, best responders were those on dosages of 150 mg (XR formulation) or

more, and safety and efficacy has been reported at those doses
- May treat chronic pain with effects similar to TCAs with no antihistamine, fewer anticholinergic AEs (e.g., sedation, orthostatic hypotension, etc.)
- Efficacy as well as AEs are usually dose-dependent
- XR formulations allows for once-daily dosing, improves tolerability, and reduces certain AEs (e.g., nausea)
- If high blood pressure is not a major concern, may work well with metoprolol in migraine prophylaxis, as venlafaxine lowers the antihypertensive effect of metoprolol
- Venlafaxine can often precipitate mania in patients with bipolar disorder. Use with caution
- For post-stroke depression, may be superior to SSRIs and may even increase survival
- May be useful as an adjunct for patients with pain and coexisting ADHD

Suggested Reading

Ozyalcin SN, Talu GK, Kiziltan E, Yucel B, Ertas M, Disci R. The efficacy and safety of venlafaxine in the prophylaxis of migraine. Headache 2005; 45(2):144–52.

Saarto T, Wiffen PJ. Antidepressants for neuropathic pain. Cochrane Database Syst Rev 2007;(4):CD005454.

Wellington K, Perry CM. Venlafaxine extended-release: a review of its use in the management of major depression. CNS Drugs 2001;15(8):643–69.

Zissis NP, Harmoussi S, Vlaikidis N, Mitsikostas D, Thomaidis T, Georgiadis G, Karageorgiou K. A randomized, double-blind, placebo-controlled study of venlafaxine XR in out-patients with tension-type headache. Cephalalgia 2007; 27(4):315–24.

VERAPAMIL

THERAPEUTICS

Brands
- Calan, Cordilox, Securon, Verapress, Vertab, Univer, Covera-HS, Verelan, Isoptin SR

Generic?
Yes

 Class
- Antihypertensive, calcium channel blocker

Commonly Prescribed for
(FDA approved in bold)
- **Angina (vasospastic or effort associated)**
- **Essential hypertension**
- **Paroxysmal supraventricular tachycardia, atrial fibrillation/flutter (IV formulation)**
- Migraine prophylaxis
- Cluster headache prophylaxis
- Peyronie's disease, plantar fibromatosis, Dupuytren's disease (gel)

 How the Drug Works
- Migraine/cluster: Proposed prior mechanisms included inhibition of smooth muscle contraction preventing arterial spasm and hypoxia, prevention of vasoconstriction or platelet aggregation, and alterations of serotonin release and uptake. Prevention of cortical spreading depression may be the mechanism of action for all migraine preventives
- Voltage-gated L-calcium channels mediate calcium influx and are important in regulating neurotransmitter and hormone release

How Long Until It Works
- Migraines – may decrease in as little as 2 weeks, but can take up to 3 months on a stable dose to see full effect
- Cluster – usually effective in weeks

If It Works
- Migraine – goal is a 50% or greater reduction in migraine frequency or severity. Consider tapering or stopping if headaches remit for more than 6 months or if considering pregnancy
- Cluster – reduction in the severity or frequency of attacks

If It Doesn't Work
- Increase to highest tolerated dose

- Migraine/cluster: address other issues, such as medication-overuse, other coexisting medical disorders, such as anxiety, and consider changing to another agent or adding a second agent

 Best Augmenting Combos for Partial Response or Treatment-Resistance
- Migraine: For some patients with migraine, low-dose polytherapy with 2 or more drugs may be better tolerated and more effective than high-dose monotherapy. May use in combination with AEDs, antidepressants, natural products, and non-medication treatments, such as biofeedback, to improve headache control
- Cluster: At the start of the cycle can use a steroid slam and taper. Valproic acid, lithium, topiramate, and methysergide are effective for many cluster patients

Tests
- At higher doses, monitor ECG for PR interval

ADVERSE EFFECTS (AEs)

How Drug Causes AEs
- Direct effects of calcium receptor antagonism, slowing of AV conduction

Notable AEs
- Bradycardia, hypotension, weakness, headache
- Constipation, nausea, myalgia
- Allergic rhinitis, ankle edema, gingival hyperplasia
- First degree AV block
- Upper respiratory infection, flu-like syndrome

 Life-Threatening or Dangerous AEs
- Pulmonary edema, worsening of CHF in patients with moderate to severe cardiac function
- Rarely produces second or third degree AV block
- Rare hypertrophic cardiomyopathy
- Can worsen muscle transmission and cause weakness in patients with muscular dystrophies

Weight Gain
- Unusual

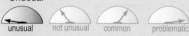

Sedation
- Unusual

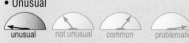

What to Do About AEs
- For common AEs, lower dose, change to extended-release formulation, or switch to another agent. For serious AEs, do not use

Best Augmenting Agents for AEs
- Constipation can be treated by usual agents, such as magnesium

---

DOSING AND USE

Usual Dosage Range
- 120–480 mg/day

Dosage Forms
- Tablets: 40, 80, 120 mg. Extended release 120, 180, 240 mg
- Extended-release capsules: 100, 180, 240, 300, 360 mg
- Injection: 2.5 mg/mL
- Gel: 15% transdermal

How to Dose
- Migraine: Initial dose 40–120 mg/day and effective usually at 120–360 mg/day for most patients. Gradually increase over days to weeks to usual effective dose. Immediate release dose TID. Sustained or extended release BID or once daily
- Cluster: Start at 120–240 mg daily and increase by 40–120 mg/week until attacks are suppressed or a daily dose of 960 mg/day. May use as much as 1200 mg/day with ECG monitoring

 Dosing Tips
- Doses above 360 mg had no additional antihypertensive effect in clinical trials
- Can titrate with immediate release then change to longer acting once at a stable dose

Overdose
- Bradycardia, hypotension, with the possibility of low-output heart failure and shock. Treat with lavage, charcoal, cathartics. For hypotension, use dopamine, IV calcium, beta-agonists, or norepinephrine. For AV block, atropine is also helpful. For rapid ventricular rate due to anterograde conduction, use D.C. cardioversion or IV lidocaine

Long-Term Use
- Safe for long-term use

Habit Forming
- No

How to Stop
- Decrease 2 weeks after cessation of cluster attacks. Less risk of rebound tachycardia than beta-blockers

Pharmacokinetics
- Metabolized by CYP450 system, especially CYP3A4. Half-life 2.8–7.4 h with 1 dose but increased with repetitive dosing. SR about 12 h. Tmax 1–2 h, 11 h extended release, 7–9 h sustained release. Oral bioavailability 20–35%. 90% protein binding

 Drug Interactions
- Verapamil can alter hepatic function, increasing plasma concentrations and effect of anesthetics, digoxin, statins, ethanol, buspirone, imipramine, prazosin, sirolimus, tacrolimus, carbamazepine, theophyllines, some benzodiazepines, and muscle relaxants
- Verapamil can lower lithium levels but increase toxicity
- Phenytoin, rifampin, and calcium salts decrease concentration of verapamil
- Potent CYP3A4 inhibitors such as ketoconazole increase levels
- H2 antagonists (cimetidine, ranitidine) increase verapamil levels
- Use with beta-blockers can be synergistic or additive, use with caution

 Other Warnings/ Precautions
- Increased intracranial pressure with verapamil IV in patients with supratentorial tumors
- Elevated liver enzymes have occurred

Do Not Use

- Sick sinus syndrome, greater than first-degree heart block
- Severe CHF, cardiogenic shock, severe left ventricular dysfunction
- Hypotension less than 90 mm Hg systolic
- Proven hypersensitivity to verapamil or other calcium channel blockers
- Do not give IV verapamil in close proximity to IV beta-blockers

 Pregnancy

- Category C (all calcium channel blockers). Use only if potential benefit outweighs risk to the fetus

Breast Feeding

- Not recommended. Verapamil is found in breast milk

SPECIAL POPULATIONS

Renal Impairment

- About 70% of verapamil metabolites are secreted by the kidney. Monitor for PR interval prolongation and side effects. Use with caution

Hepatic Impairment

- Verapamil is highly metabolized by the liver. Give about 30% of usual dose to patients with severe dysfunction

Cardiac Impairment

- Do not use in acute shock, severe CHF, hypotension, and greater than first-degree heart block as above

Elderly

- Use with caution and start with lower doses

 Children and Adolescents

- Little is known about efficacy or safety. Use with caution if at all

THE ART OF NEUROPHARMACOLOGY

Potential Advantages

- Proven effectiveness in cluster headache and better tolerated than most other preventive options, but may need a very high dose

Potential Disadvantages

- Not a first-line agent in migraine (limited evidence of efficacy). Multiple potential drug interactions

Primary Target Symptoms

- Headache frequency and severity

 Pearls

- Relatively little evidence for effectiveness in migraine, but first-line agent for cluster headache
- For patients with cycles of cluster headache, taper off starting 2 weeks after last attack
- May help patients with migraine with atypical or prolonged aura (i.e., hemiplegic migraine)

There is no evidence that verapamil is more effective in the treatment of hypertension beyond 360 mg/day

Suggested Reading

Cohen AS, Matharu MS, Goadsby PJ. Trigeminal autonomic cephalalgias: current and future treatments. Headache 2007;47(6): 969–80.

Cohen AS, Matharu MS, Goadsby PJ. Electrocardiographic abnormalities in patients with cluster headache on verapamil therapy. Neurology 2007;69(7):668–75.

Law MR, Morris JK, Wald NJ. Use of blood pressure lowering drugs in the prevention of cardiovascular disease: meta-analysis of 147 randomised trials in the context of expectations from prospective epidemiological studies. BMJ 2009;338:b1665.

Silberstein SD. Preventive migraine treatment. Neurol Clin 2009;27(2):429–43.

VIGABATRIN

THERAPEUTICS

Brands
- Sabril

Generic?
No

 Class
- Antiepileptic drug (AED)

Commonly Prescribed for
(FDA approved in bold)
- **Infantile spasms in children (ages 1 month-2 years)**
- Adjunctive for treatment-resistant epilepsy
- Complex partial seizures
- Cocaine or methamphetamine dependence

 How the Drug Works
- Inhibits catabolism of GABA by inhibiting gamma-aminobutyric acid transaminase (GABA-T). This increases synaptic levels of GABA. Does not act directly on GABA receptors. May decrease levels of excitatory neurotransmitters (glutamate, aspartate, glutamine) in the brain

How Long Until It Works
- Seizures –by 2 weeks

If It Works
- Seizures – goal is the remission of seizures. Continue as long as effective and well-tolerated

If It Doesn't Work
- Increase to highest tolerated dose
- Epilepsy: consider changing to another agent, adding a second agent or referral for epilepsy surgery evaluation

 Best Augmenting Combos for Partial Response or Treatment-Resistance
- Often used in combination with other AEDs. Lack of significant drug interactions make it easier to use than many other AEDs

Tests
- No regular blood tests are recommended

ADVERSE EFFECTS (AEs)

How Drug Causes AEs
- CNS AEs are probably caused by changes in GABA levels

Notable AEs
- Somnolence, fatigue, weight gain, headache, dizziness, anxiety, depression, ataxia, hyperactivity (children), psychosis (adults)

 Life-Threatening or Dangerous AEs
- Retinal atrophy and visual field defects in about 1/3 of patients, peaking at 1 year but occurring as soon as a few weeks. Visual field loss may be irreversible

Weight Gain
- Not unusual

Sedation
- Not unusual

What to Do About AEs
- Decrease dose
- Vision loss may require stopping drug

Best Augmenting Agents for AEs
- Most AEs cannot be improved by an augmenting agent

DOSING AND USE

Usual Dosage Range
- Epilepsy: 2–4 g/day

Dosage Forms
- Tablets: 500 mg

How to Dose
- In adults, start at 1 or 2 g/day. Increase or decrease by 500 mg depending on clinical response and tolerability. Usual most effective dose is 2–4 g/day in once- or twice-daily doses

Dosing Tips
- Food slows rate but not extent of absorption

Overdose
- Vertigo and tremor have been reported

Long-Term Use
- Safe

Habit Forming
- No

How to Stop
- Taper slowly over 2 weeks or more
- Abrupt withdrawal can lead to seizures in patients with epilepsy

Pharmacokinetics
- Most drug is excreted unchanged in urine. No hepatic metabolism. Bioavailability is 80–90%. Peak levels at 2 hours. Half-life is 5–8 hours in young adults but 12–13 hours in the elderly

 Drug Interactions
- Vigabatrin lowers phenytoin levels by 20% but there are no other significant interactions with other AEDs

Do Not Use
- Patients with a proven allergy to vigabatrin

SPECIAL POPULATIONS

Renal Impairment
- May require lowering of dose if creatinine clearance is less than 60 mL/min

Hepatic Impairment
- No known effects

Cardiac Impairment
- No known effects

Elderly
- May need lower dose

 Children and Adolescents
- Start at 40 mg/kg/day. Increase to 80–100 mg/kg/day depending on clinical response. Alternatively, start at 500 mg and increase by 500 mg per week to optimal dose. Children over 50 kg will use the adult dose

 Pregnancy
- Risk category C. Use only if risks of stopping drug outweigh potential risk to fetus
- Supplementation with 0.4 mg of folic acid before and during pregnancy is recommended

Breast Feeding
- Generally recommendations are to discontinue drug or bottle feed
- Monitor infant for sedation, poor feeding or irritability

THE ART OF NEUROPHARMACOLOGY

Potential Advantages
- Effective in infantile spasm and low drug interactions

Potential Disadvantages
- Vision loss. May not be effective for many types of epilepsy

Primary Target Symptoms
- Seizure frequency and severity

 Pearls
- Usually used in combination with other AEDs in refractory epilepsy
- The effect of the drug is related to the resynthesis of GABA-T enzyme molecules rather than vigabatrin plasma levels
- Patients with symptomatic infantile spasms, i.e., related to tuberous sclerosis, may improve more rapidly. Infantile spasms usually remit by age 5, but are often replaced by other types of seizures
- Visual field deficits can be monitored by formal visual field testing. Consider checking electroretinography for monitoring vision loss in infants and children that cannot perform perimetry

Suggested Reading

Curatolo P, Bombardieri R, Cerminara C. Current management for epilepsy in tuberous sclerosis complex. Curr Opin Neurol. 2006;19(2):119–23.

Fechtner RD, Khouri AS, Figueroa E, Ramirez M, Federico M, Dewey SL, Brodie JD. Short-term treatment of cocaine and/or methamphetamine abuse with vigabatrin: ocular safety pilot results. Arch Ophthalmol 2006;124(9):1257–62.

Gaily E, Jonsson H, Lappi M. Visual fields at school-age in children treated with vigabatrin in infancy. Epilepsia 2009;50(2):206–16.

Parisi P, Bombardieri R, Curatolo P. Current role of vigabatrin in infantile spasms. Eur J Paediatr Neurol 2007;11(6):331–6.

WARFARIN

THERAPEUTICS

Brands
- Coumadin, Jantoven, Carfin, Marevan, Panwarfin, Warx

Generic?
Yes

Class
- Anticoagulant

Commonly Prescribed for
(FDA approved in bold)
- **Prophylaxis or treatment of thromboembolic complications associated with atrial fibrillation or cardiac valve replacement, and to prevent embolism after myocardial infarction (MI)**
- **Venous thrombosis/pulmonary embolism**

How the Drug Works
- Interferes with the synthesis of vitamin K-dependent clotting factors II, VII, IX, and X and anticoagulant proteins C and S. This decreases risk of thromboembolism

How Long Until It Works
- Anticoagulant effect is delayed for up to 7 days. Heparin is preferred for rapid anticoagulation

If It Works
- Continue to use with appropriate monitoring

If It Doesn't Work
- Patients can still have stroke despite treatment. Warfarin is only superior to antiplatelet agents for cardiogenic stroke, i.e., related to atrial fibrillation or ventricular thrombus
- Control all stroke risk factors, such as smoking, hyperlipidemia, and hypertension
- For acute events, admit patients for treatment and diagnostic testing. Check international normalized ratio (INR) to determine drug effectiveness

Best Augmenting Combos for Partial Response or Treatment-Resistance
- The combination of aspirin and warfarin in patients with mechanical heart valves appears beneficial despite increased risk of bleeding. Aspirin combined with warfarin did not appear to reduce risk of stroke, systemic embolism, or myocardial infarction in patients with atrial fibrillation in the SPORTIF trials

Tests
- Monitor prothrombin time (PT) and INR to determine effectiveness

ADVERSE EFFECTS (AEs)

How Drug Causes AEs
- Anticoagulation increases bleeding risk

Notable AEs
- Abdominal pain/cramping, elevated liver enzymes/jaundice, hypotension, weakness, paresthesias, diarrhea, nausea, pruritus and alopecia

Life-Threatening or Dangerous AEs
- Bleeding complications, especially with elevated INRs. Hemorrhage in organs or tissues can cause death
- Necrosis associated with local thrombosis can occur within days of starting treatment
- Patients with venous thrombosis and heparin-induced thrombocytopenia have a risk of limb ischemia, necrosis, and gangrene when stopping heparin and starting warfarin
- May increase risk of cholesterol plaque emboli, typically 3–10 weeks after starting therapy
- "Purple toes syndrome" is a dark, mottled, often purple discoloration on the sides and plantar surface of toes; may be reversible or may lead to necrosis or gangrene

Weight Gain
- Unusual

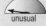
unusual not unusual common problematic

Sedation
- Unusual

unusual not unusual common problematic

WARFARIN (continued)

What to Do About AEs
- Stop or lower dose or give vitamin K based on INR and presence of bleeding. For systemic atheroemboli/microemboli, stop drug

Best Augmenting Agents for AEs
- Most AEs cannot be improved by an augmenting agent

DOSING AND USE

Usual Dosage Range
- 2–10 mg daily

Dosage Forms
- Tablets: 1, 2, 2.5, 3, 4, 5, 6, 7.5 and 10 mg
- Injection: 5.4 mg (2 mg/mL)

How to Dose
Give once daily, usually starting at 2 to 5 mg/day. Start at lower dose in patients with genetic variations in CYP2C9 or VKORC1 enzymes, the elderly or debilitated and those with potentially greater than expected PT/INR response to warfarin. Adjust dose based on PT/INR determinations. Loading doses of warfarin do not offer more protection against thrombi formation and may increase bleeding risk

Intravenous warfarin dosing is the same as oral. Use in patients without the ability to take oral drugs
- Goal INR is 2–3 for most conditions, including acute MI, atrial fibrillation, pulmonary embolism, venous thrombosis, valvular heart disease, and tissue heart valves
- Goal INR is 2.5–3.5 for patients with mechanical heart valves and for prevention of recurrent MI
- Continue heparin therapy for 4–5 days after starting warfarin until the desired therapeutic response has been reached based on INR. Then stop heparin. Patients with supratherapeutic INR:
- < 5: lower or omit a dose
- ≥ 5 but < 9: if no significant bleeding, omit next few doses, increase monitoring frequency and resume warfarin at a lower dose once INR is therapeutic. When there is significant bleeding, omit dose and give ≤ 5 mg of vitamin K. If there is still significant bleeding and INR has not normalized, give an additional 1–4 mg vitamin K

- ≥ 9: If no significant bleeding, hold warfarin and give 5–10 mg vitamin K orally
- For any serious or life-threatening bleeding, hold warfarin, give vitamin K 10 mg intravenously, and supplement with plasma or prothrombin complex concentrate

 Dosing Tips
- Food decreases rate of absorption. If a dose is missed, do not double the next dose
- Asian patients may also require lower initiation and maintenance doses

Overdose
- Bleeding complications, such as blood in stools or urine, excessive menstrual bleeding, petechiae, or oozing from superficial injuries. Check INR and treat by holding warfarin therapy and giving vitamin K if indicated

Long-Term Use
- Safe for long-term use

Habit Forming
- No

How to Stop
- No need to taper, but patients will be at increased risk of thromboembolic complications soon after

Pharmacokinetics
- Extensive metabolism by CYP450 isoenzymes into inactive metabolites, which are excreted in urine and bile. Half-life ranges from 20–60 hours (mean 40). Drug 99% protein bound

 Drug Interactions
- Increased anticoagulant effect due to inhibition of hepatic metabolism: proton pump inhibitors, statins, allopurinol, azole antifungals, quinidine, quinine, sulfonamides
- Increased anticoagulant effect due to reduced clearance: macrolide antibiotics (azithromycin, erythromycin)
- Increased anticoagulant effect due to displacement from binding sites: loop diuretics (furosemide), valproate, nalidixic acid

- Increased anticoagulant effect due to interference with vitamin K: aminoglycosides, tetracyclines, vitamin E
- Increased anticoagulant effect due to effects on platelet function or GI irritant effects: NSAIDs, penicillins, salicylates, diflunisal
- Increased anticoagulant effect due to unclear reasons: SSRIs, cox-2 inhibitors, cephalosporins, beta-blockers, heparin, isonazid, influenza vaccine, quinolines (ciprofloxacin), ropinirole, tamoxifen, thyroid hormones, tramadol, zafirlukast, methylphenidate
- Decreased anticoagulant effect due to hepatic induction: barbiturates, nafcillin, carbamazepine, rifamycins
- Decreased anticoagulant effect due to decreased absorption or increased elimination: spironolactone, thiazide diuretics, azathioprine
- Decreased anticoagulant effect due to unclear reasons: clozapine, haloperidol, estrogens, griseofulvin, protease inhibitors, trazodone, ribavirin, isoretinoin, cyclosporine, chlordiazepoxide, oral contraceptives
- May increase or decrease anticoagulant effect: alcohol, corticosteroids, phenytoin, pravastatin, chloral hydrate, ranitidine, propylthiouracil
- Many herbal medications can reportedly increase (ginkgo, dong quai, garlic, among others) or decrease (coenzyme q10 and St. John's wort) the effect of warfarin
- Vitamin-K-rich vegetables such as broccoli, spinach, seaweed, and turnips decrease warfarin effects

 Other Warnings/ Precautions

- Use warfarin with great caution in patients at risk for trauma, infections of intestinal flora, indwelling catheters, known or suspected protein C or S deficiency, moderate-severe renal insufficiency, exposed raw surfaces, or severe hypertension

Do Not Use

- Hypersensitivity to the drug; pregnancy; recent or impending surgery or procedure such as lumbar puncture or lumbar anesthesia; bleeding tendencies with active ulceration or overt bleeding of GI, GU or respiratory tracts; malignant hypertension; eclampsia or preeclampsia; aortic dissection; cerebral aneurysm; bacterial endocarditis; CNS hemorrhage; and unsupervised patients with senility, substance abuse, or psychosis

SPECIAL POPULATIONS

Renal Impairment

- Patients with renal dysfunction are more likely to experience bleeding complications, perhaps due to increase in the unbound fraction of the drug. Use with caution

Hepatic Impairment

- Use with much caution. Patients with moderate-severe disease have an increased risk of bleeding complications due to decreased metabolism and decreased synthesis of clotting factors

Cardiac Impairment

- No known effects

Elderly

- Lower initiation and maintenance doses needed

 Children and Adolescents

- Not well-studied in children but appears effective for prevention of thromboembolic complications. May require more frequent monitoring

 Pregnancy

- Category X. Associated with multiple serious birth malformations, including CNS and spontaneous abortions. Do not use. Heparin is preferred in pregnant patients who require anticoagulation

Breast Feeding

- Not detected in limited studies in breast milk, but may increase bleeding time. Monitor bleeding time closely and perform coagulation tests in infants at risk

THE ART OF NEUROPHARMACOLOGY

Potential Advantages

- Drug of choice for ischemic stroke in patients with mechanical heart valves, cardiac thrombus, or atrial fibrillation

Potential Disadvantages

- Not as useful for non-cardiac ischemic stroke. Serious bleeding risks and drug interactions require frequent monitoring

Primary Target Symptoms

- Prevention of the neurological complications that result from ischemic stroke

 Pearls

- There is no evidence to suggest that warfarin is superior to antiplatelet medications for secondary stroke prevention unless there is a clear cardiac source (i.e., atrial fibrillation or cardiac thrombus). It is also not superior for preventing stroke due to patent foramen ovale

- The WARSS trial compared warfarin to aspirin for the prevention of ischemic stroke. Warfarin was not more effective than aspirin, but the use of lower goal INR (1.4–2.8) could have affected results
- The WASID trial compared warfarin to high-dose aspirin for the secondary prevention of stroke due to intracranial stenosis. Warfarin was associated with greater AEs but not improved efficacy
- Goal INR may be increased in patients with recurrent embolism (to 3 or 3.5) despite therapeutic INR, but INR of 4 or greater does not appear more effective and is associated with more bleeding AEs
- Multiple drug interactions due mostly to hepatic metabolism, often unpredictable, require frequent monitoring with the addition or change of any medication – even those only for short-term use (e.g., antibiotics)
- CYP2C9 and VKORC1 genotypes may help predict dose variability, but routine testing before starting warfarin is not recommended

 Suggested Reading

ESPRIT. Oral anticoagulation in patients after cerebral ischemia of arterial origin and risk of intracranial hemorrhage. Stroke 2003;34(6): e45–6.

Ferder N, Eby CS, Deych E, Harris JK, Ridker PM, Milligan P, Goldhaber SZ, King CR, Giri T, McLeod HL, Glynn RJ, Gage BF. Ability of VKORC1 and CYP2C9 to predict therapeutic warfarin dose during the initial weeks of therapy. J Thromb Haemost 2010;8(1):95–100.

Flaker GC, Gruber M, Connolly SJ, Goldman S, Chaparro S, Vahanian A, Halinen MO, Horrow J, Halperin JL; SPORTIF Investigators. Risks and benefits of combining aspirin with anticoagulant therapy in patients with atrial fibrillation: an exploratory analysis of stroke prevention using an oral thrombin inhibitor in atrial fibrillation (SPORTIF) trials. Am Heart J 2006;152 (5):967–73.

Hylek EM, Frison L, Henault LE, Cupples A. Disparate stroke rates on warfarin among contemporary cohorts with atrial fibrillation: potential insights into risk from a comparative analysis of SPORTIF III versus SPORTIF V. Stroke 2008;39(11):3009–14.

Redman AR, Allen LC. Warfarin versus aspirin in the secondary prevention of stroke: the WARSS study. Curr Atheroscler Rep 2002;4(4):319–25.

ZOLMITRIPTAN

THERAPEUTICS

Brands
• Zomig, Zomig MLT

Generic?
No

 Class
• Triptan

Commonly Prescribed for
(FDA approved in bold)
• **Migraine**
• Cluster headache (nasal spray)

 How the Drug Works
• Selective 5-HT1 receptor agonist, working predominantly at the B and D receptor subtypes. Effectiveness may be due to blocking the transmission of pain signals from the trigeminal nerve to the trigeminal nucleus caudalis and preventing the release of inflammatory neuropeptides rather than just causing vasoconstriction

How Long Until It Works
• 1 hour or less

If It Works
• Continue to take as needed. Patients taking acute treatment more than 2 days/week are at risk for medication-overuse headache, especially if they have migraine

If It Doesn't Work
• Treat early in the attack – triptans are less likely to work after the development of cutaneous allodynia, a marker of central sensitization
• For patients with partial response or reoccurrence, add an NSAID
• Change to another agent

 Best Augmenting Combos for Partial Response or Treatment-Resistance
• NSAIDs or neuroleptics are often used to augment response

Tests
• None required

ADVERSE EFFECTS (AEs)

How Drug Causes AEs
• Direct effect on serotonin receptors

Notable AEs
• Paresthesias, dizziness, sensation of pressure (chest or jaw), palpitation somnolence, nausea

 Life-Threatening or Dangerous AEs
• Rare cardiac events including acute MI, cardiac arrhythmias, and coronary artery vasospasm have been reported with zolmitriptan

Weight Gain
• Unusual

unusual | not unusual | common | problematic

Sedation
• Unusual

unusual | not unusual | common | problematic

What to Do About AEs
• In most cases, only reassurance is needed. Lower dose, change to another triptan or use an alternative headache treatment

Best Augmenting Agents for AEs
• Treatment of nausea with antiemetics is acceptable. Other AEs improve with time

DOSING AND USE

Usual Dosage Range
• 2.5–5 mg, maximum 10 mg/day

Dosage Forms
• Tablets: 2.5 and 5 mg
• Orally disintegrating tablets: 2.5 mg
• Nasal spray: 5 mg

How to Dose
• Tablets: 1 pill (either 2.5 or 5 mg) at the onset of an attack and repeat in 2 hours for a partial response or if headache returns. Maximum 10 mg/day. Limit 10 days per month
• Nasal spray: Give 1 spray and repeat in 2 hours if needed. Maximum 10 mg/day

Dosing Tips

- Treat early in the attack. Side effects are greater with 5 mg dose

Overdose

- May cause hypertension, cardiovascular symptoms. Other possible symptoms include seizure, tremor, extremity erythema, cyanosis or ataxia. For patients with angina, perform ECG and monitor for ischemia for at least 15 hours

Long-Term Use

- Monitor for cardiac risk factors with continued use

Habit Forming

- No

How to Stop

- No need to taper. Patients who overuse triptans often experience withdrawal headaches lasting up to several days

Pharmacokinetics

- Half-life 2.5 hours tablet and 3 for disintegrating tablets and nasal spray. Tmax 1.5–3 hours, longer with nasal spray. Bioavailability is 40%. Metabolism mostly by CYP1A2 isoenzyme but MAO-A is important for further metabolism of the metabolites. 25% protein binding

 Drug Interactions

- MAO inhibitors may make it difficult for drug to be metabolized
- Theoretical interactions with SSRI/SNRI. It is unclear that triptans pose any risk for the development of serotonin syndrome in clinical practice
- Concurrent propranolol use increases peak concentrations – use the 5 mg dose
- Use with sibutramine, a weight loss drug, may cause a serotonin syndrome including weakness, irritability, myoclonus and confusion

⚠ **Other Warnings/ Precautions**

- For phenylketonurics: Orally disintegrating tablets contain phenylalanine

Do Not Use

- Within 2 weeks of MAO inhibitors, or 24 hours of ergot-containing medications such as dihydroergotamine
- Patients with proven hypersensitivity to sumatriptan, known cardiovascular disease, uncontrolled hypertension, or Prinzmetal's angina
- Rizatriptan was not studied in patients with hemiplegic and basilar migraine
- May worsen symptoms in ischemic bowel disease

SPECIAL POPULATIONS

Renal Impairment

- Concentration increases in those with severe renal impairment (creatinine clearance less than 25 mL/min). May be at increased cardiovascular risk

Hepatic Impairment

- Drug metabolism significantly decreased with hepatic disease. Use lower doses and do not use with severe hepatic impairment

Cardiac Impairment

- Do not use in patients with known cardiovascular or peripheral vascular disease

Elderly

- May be at increased cardiovascular risk

 Children and Adolescents

- Safety and efficacy has not been established. Triptan trials in children were negative, due to higher placebo response

 Pregnancy

- Category C. Use only if potential benefit outweighs risk to the fetus. Migraine often improves in pregnancy, and other acute agents (opioids, neuroleptics, prednisone) have more proven safety

Breast Feeding

- Zolmitriptan is found in breast milk. Use with caution

THE ART OF NEUROPHARMACOLOGY

Potential Advantages

- Effectiveness equal to other triptans. Available as melt formulation and nasal spray
- Better taste than sumatriptan nasal spray. Less risk of abuse than opioids or barbiturate-containing treatments

Potential Disadvantages

- Cost, potential for medication-overuse headache. Relatively greater rate of CNS AEs than other triptans

Primary Target Symptoms

- Headache pain, nausea, photo- and phonophobia

 Pearls

- Early treatment of migraine is most effective
- Compared to other triptans, it has one of the highest 2-hour pain-free responses

- May not be effective when taking during aura, before headache begins
- In patients with "status migrainosus" (migraine lasting more than 72 hours) neuroleptics and DHE are more effective
- Triptans were not originally studied for use in the treatment of basilar or hemiplegic migraine
- Patients taking triptans more than 10 days/month are at increased risk of medication-overuse headache which is less responsive to treatment
- Chest and throat tightness are usually benign and may be related to esophageal spasm rather than cardiac ischemia. These symptoms occur more commonly in patients without cardiac risk factors
- Recent studies suggest zolmitriptan nasal spray is useful for acute cluster headache

 Suggested Reading

Dodick D, Lipton RB, Martin V, Papademetriou V, Rosamond W, MaassenVanDenBrink A, Loutfi H, Welch KM, Goadsby PJ, Hahn S, Hutchinson S, Matchar D, Silberstein S, Smith TR, Purdy RA, Saiers J; Triptan Cardiovascular Safety Expert Panel. Consensus statement: cardiovascular safety profile of triptans (5-HT agonists) in the acute treatment of migraine. Headache 2004; 44(5):414–25.

Ferrari MD, Roon KI, Lipton RB, Goadsby PJ. Oral triptans (serotonin 5-HT(1B/1D) agonists) in acute migraine treatment: a meta-analysis of 53 trials. Lancet 2001;358(9294):1668–75.

Gladstone JP, Gawel M. Newer formulations of the triptans: advances in migraine management. Drugs 2003;63(21):2285–305.

Lewis DW, Winner P, Hershey AD, Wasiewski WW; Adolescent Migraine Steering Committee. Efficacy of zolmitriptan nasal spray in adolescent migraine. Pediatrics 2007;120(2):390–6.

Rapoport AM, Mathew NT, Silberstein SD, Dodick D, Tepper SJ, Sheftell FD, Bigal ME. Zolmitriptan nasal spray in the acute treatment of cluster headache: a double-blind study. Neurology 2007;69(9):821–6.

ZONISAMIDE

THERAPEUTICS

Brands
• Zonegran

Generic?
Not in US

Class
• Antiepileptic drug (AED), structurally a sulfonamide

Commonly Prescribed for
(FDA approved in bold)
• **Partial-onset seizures (adjunctive in adults)**
• Partial-onset seizures (adjunctive in pediatric patients)
• Primary generalized tonic-clonic seizures (adjunctive; adults and pediatric patients age 2–16)
• Myoclonic epilepsy, Lennox-Gastaut syndrome
• Infantile spasms (West syndrome)
• Migraine prophylaxis
• Obesity
• Bipolar disorder
• Binge-eating disorder/bulimia
• Neuropathic pain
• Parkinson's disease

How the Drug Works
Unknown but there are multiple mechanisms of action that may be important
• Sodium channel antagonist
• Modulates T-type calcium channels
• Binds to GABA receptors
• Weak carbonic anhydrase inhibitor
• MAO-B inhibition
• May help facilitate dopamine and serotonin neurotransmission

How Long Until It Works
• Seizures – by 2–3 weeks
• Migraines – can take up to 3 months on a stable dose to see full effect

If It Works
• Seizures – goal is the remission of seizures. Continue as long as effective and well-tolerated. Consider tapering and slowly stopping after 2 years seizure-free, depending on the type of epilepsy

• Migraine – goal is a 50% or greater reduction in migraine frequency or severity. Consider tapering or stopping if headaches remit for more than 6 months or if patient considering pregnancy

If It Doesn't Work
• Increase to highest tolerated dose
• Epilepsy: consider changing to another agent, adding a second agent or referral for epilepsy surgery evaluation
• Migraine: address other issues such as medication-overuse, other coexisting medical disorders, such as anxiety, and consider changing to another agent or adding a second agent

Best Augmenting Combos for Partial Response or Treatment-Resistance
• For some patients with epilepsy or migraine, low-dose polytherapy with 2 or more drugs may be better tolerated and more effective than high-dose monotherapy
• Epilepsy: keep in mind drug interactions and their effect on levels
• Migraine: consider beta-blockers, antidepressants, natural products, other AEDs, and non-medication treatments, such as biofeedback, to improve headache control

Tests
• Mild to moderate decreases in bicarbonate can occur with zonisamide, but are uncommon reasons for discontinuation. Routine screening for metabolic acidosis is not recommended

ADVERSE EFFECTS (AEs)

How Drug Causes AEs
• CNS AEs may be caused by sodium or calcium channel effects or GABA effects
• Carbonic anhydrase inhibition causes metabolic acidosis and may lead to kidney stones

Notable AEs
• Sedation, depression, irritability, fatigue, ataxia
• Anorexia, abdominal pain, nausea
• Kidney stones

Life-Threatening or Dangerous AEs
- Metabolic acidosis
- Increased BUN and creatinine (non-progressive)
- Kidney stones (calcium or urate)
- Blood dyscrasias (aplastic anemia or agranulocytosis)
- Rare serious allergic rash (Stevens-Johnson syndrome)
- Fever, dehydration and oligohidrosis (more common in children)

Weight Gain
- Unusual

Sedation
- Common

What to Do About AEs
- May decrease or remit after a longer time on a stable dose
- Paresthesias may respond to high potassium diets or potassium tablets
- A small decrease in dose may improve AEs

Best Augmenting Agents for AEs
- Paresthesias may improve with high potassium diet or tablets
- Other AEs are more likely to improve by lowering dose

DOSING AND USE

Usual Dosage Range
- Epilepsy: 100–600 mg/day in adults. Most patients do best at 400 mg or less. One/day dosing is fine
- Migraine: 100–600 mg/day. Most studies use 400 mg
- Parkinson's disease – used as low-dose adjunctive medication, typically 25–100 mg/day

Dosage Forms
- 25 mg, 50 mg, 100 mg

How to Dose
- In adults, start at low dose (100 mg/day for epilepsy, or 50 mg/day for migraine). After 1 week, increase to 200 mg/day. Wait at least 2 weeks before increasing to 300 mg and for each new increase
- For children, start at 2–4 mg/kg/day, dosed once or twice daily and increase by 2 mg/kg/day every 1–2 weeks until at maintenance dose of 4–8 mg/kg/day. Maximum pediatric dose 12 mg/kg/day

 Dosing Tips
- AEs increase with dose increases but can be delayed due to the long half-life of the drug
- Weight loss is often dose related
- Slow titration can help minimize sedation and other AEs

Overdose
- Nystagmus, drowsiness, slurred speech, blurred vision, diplopia, stupor, hypotension, and bradycardia, respiratory depression, and metabolic acidosis. No reported deaths except with poly-drug overdoses

Long-Term Use
- Safe for long-term use

Habit Forming
- No

How to Stop
- Taper slowly
- Abrupt withdrawal can lead to seizures in patients with epilepsy. Tremor is also common
- Headaches may return within days to months of stopping

Pharmacokinetics
- Majority is renally excreted. Metabolized in part by CYP450 3A4 system. Plasma half-life is 63 hours

 Drug Interactions
- Any drug that affects hepatic CYP3A4 can affect zonisamide levels
- CYP3A4 inhibitors such as nefazodone, fluoxetine, fluvoxamine, ketoconazole,

clarithromycin, and many antivirals increase zonisamide levels
- CYP3A4 inducers such as phenytoin, phenobarbital, primidone, and especially carbamazepine decrease zonisamide levels
- May interact with carbonic anhydrase inhibitors, increasing risk of kidney stones

Other Warnings/ Precautions

- CNS AEs increase when taken with other CNS depressants
- Patients taking a ketogenic diet for seizures are more likely to experience severe metabolic acidosis on zonisamide
- Can be associated with severe rash – new-onset rash may be sign of hypersensitivity syndrome
- Any unusual bleeding or bruising, fever, or mouth sores should raise concern for rare blood dyscrasias that can occur with zonisamide

Do Not Use

- Proven allergy to zonisamide. Because zonisamide contains a sulfa moiety, it may cause allergy in patients with proven sulfa allergy

Renal Impairment

- Zonisamide is primarily renally excreted and patients with severe renal disease may require a slower titration

Hepatic Impairment

- Clearance may be decreased in patients with severe liver disease

Cardiac Impairment

- No known effects

Elderly

- May be more susceptible to CNS AEs

Children and Adolescents

- Approved for children aged 16 and up; little data about its use in younger patients but is used off-label for epilepsy and migraine

- May help treat infantile spasms related to tuberous sclerosis, especially if ACTH is ineffective or cannot be used

Pregnancy

- Risk category C. Teratogenic in animal studies but no studies in humans
- Risks of stopping medication must outweigh risk to fetus for patients with epilepsy. Seizures and potential status epilepticus place the woman and fetus at risk and can cause reduced oxygen and blood supply to the womb
- Supplementation with 0.4 mg of folic acid before and during pregnancy is recommended
- Patients taking for conditions other than epilepsy should generally stop zonisamide before considering pregnancy. Migraine usually improves in the last 2 trimesters

Breast Feeding

- Some drug is found in mother's breast milk
- Generally recommendations are to discontinue drug or bottle feed
- Monitor infant for sedation, poor feeding or irritability

Potential Advantages

- Highly effective for epilepsy, useful for migraine. Usually causes weight loss, unlike many other medications. Ability to use once daily due to long half-life can increase compliance

Potential Disadvantages

- Weight loss in thin patients can be troublesome. Kidney stones. Fatigue and other CNS AEs

Primary Target Symptoms

- Seizure frequency and severity
- Migraine frequency and severity

Pearls

- For epilepsy, higher doses may be needed. AEs are more common when using in combination with other drugs that can produce CNS symptoms
- For migraine, Zonegran may be better tolerated but is less effective than topiramate

- Recent studies suggest low-dose zonisamide (25 mg) can effectively treat motor symptoms in Parkinson's disease and decrease "off" time, perhaps by facilitation of monoamine transmission
- Zonisamide is used for treatment of essential tremor, but in clinical trials was only of modest benefit

- Early studies suggest utility in the treatment of neuropathic pain, such as diabetic neuropathy
- No proven effectiveness in bipolar disorder, and not a first-line treatment
- Occasionally used to offset weight gain seen with psychotropic agents or to treat binge-eating disorder

Suggested Reading

Ashkenazi A, Benlifer A, Korenblit J, Silberstein SD. Zonisamide for migraine prophylaxis in refractory patients. Cephalalgia 2006;26(10):1199–202.

Bigal ME, Krymchantowski AV, Rapoport AM. Prophylactic migraine therapy: emerging treatment options. Curr Pain Headache Rep 2004;8(3):178–84.

Jain KK. An assessment of zonisamide as an antiepileptic drug. Expert Opin Pharmacother 2000;1(6):1245–60.

Leppik IE. Zonisamide: chemistry, mechanism of action, and pharmacokinetics. Seizure. 2004;13 (Suppl 1):S5–9; discussion S10.

Yang LP, Perry CM. Zonisamide: in Parkinson's disease. CNS Drugs 2009;23(8):703–11.

List of abbreviations

5-HT	serotonin
ACE	angiotensin-converting enzyme
ADHD	attention deficit hyperactivity disorder
ALT	alanine aminotransferase
ANA	antinuclear antibodies
bid	twice a day
BMI	body mass index
CNS	central nervous system
CYP450	cytochrome P450
dL	deciliter
DLB	dementia with Lewy bodies
EEG	electroencephalogram
FDA	Food and Drug Administration
GAD	generalized anxiety disorder
GI	gastrointestinal
HDL	high-density lipoprotein
HMG CoA	beta-hydroxy-beta-methylglutaryl coenzyme A
IM	intramuscular
IV	intravenous
lb	pound
MAO	monoamine oxidase
MAO-B	monoamine oxidase B
MDD	major depressive disorder
mg	milligram
mL	milliliter
mm Hg	millimeters of mercury
NMDA	N-methyl-D-aspartate
qhs	once a day at bedtime
SNRI	dual serotonin and norepinephrine reuptake inhibitor
SSRI	selective serotonin reuptake inhibitor
TCA	tricyclic antidepressant

Index by drug name

Abobotulinumtoxin A (botulinum toxin type A) 40
acetazolamide 1
acetylsalicylic acid *see* aspirin
Activase (alteplase) 8
Adartrel (ropinirole) 315
Aggrenox (dipyridamole and aspirin) 103
Alertec (modafinil) 224
Alka-Seltzer (aspirin) 24
Alkabel (phenobarbital) 251
Allegron (nortriptyline) 240
Almogran (almotriptan) 5
almotriptan 5
alteplase 8
Alupram (diazepam) 96
amantadine 11
Amerge (naratriptan) 231
Amethopterin (methotrexate) 205
Amifampridine (3,4-diaminopyridine) 93
amitriptyline 14
Amrix (cyclobenzaprine) 78
Antegren (natalizumab) 234
Antivert (meclizine) 194
Apo-Cyclobenzaprine (cyclobenzaprine) 78
Apo-go (apomorphine) 18
Apokyn (apomorphine) 18
apomorphine 18
Arbil (carbamazepine) 51
Aricept (donepezil) 107
Aricept Evess (donepezil) 107
Ariclaim (duloxetine) 113
armodafinil 21
Artane (trihexyphenidyl) 349
Ascriptin (aspirin) 24
Aspergum (aspirin) 24
aspirin 24
aspirin and dipyridamole 103
Asprimox (aspirin) 24
Atamet (carbidopa/levodopa) 55
Atensine (diazepam) 96
Aventyl (nortriptyline) 240
Avonex (interferon-beta) 173
Axert (almotriptan) 5
Azamun (azathioprine) 28
Azasan (azathioprine) 28
azathioprine 28
Azilect (rasagiline) 296
AZM (acetazolamide) 1
Azomid (acetazolamide) 1

baclofen 32
Banzel (rufinamide) 319
Bayer Aspirin (aspirin) 24

benztropine 36
Betaseron (interferon-beta) 173
Betim (timolol) 335
Betimol (timolol) 335
Blocadren (timolol) 335
Bonine (meclizine) 194
Botox (botulinum toxin type A) 40
botulinum toxin type A 40
botulinum toxin type B 45
bromocriptine 48
Buccastem (prochlorperazine) 279
Bufferin (aspirin) 24

Calan (verapamil) 362
Camcolit (lithium) 187
Caramet (carbidopa/levodopa) 55
Carbagen (carbamazepine) 51
carbamazepine 51
Carbatrol (carbamazepine) 51
carbidopa/levodopa 55
Carbolith (lithium) 187
Carfin (warfarin) 369
Carimune (immune globulin intravenous) 165
Carisoma (carisoprodol) 59
carisoprodol 59
Catapres (clonidine) 69
CellCept (mycophenolate mofetil) 228
chlorpromazine 62
Cicloral (cyclosporine) 84
ciclosporin *see* cyclosporine
CinnoVex (interferon-beta) 173
clonazepam 65
clonidine 69
clopidogrel 72
Clopine (clozapine) 75
Clorpres (clonidine) 69
clozapine 75
Clozaril (clozapine) 75
Co-careldopa (carbidopa/levodopa) 55
Cogentin (benztropine) 36
Compazine (prochlorperazine) 279
Comptan (entacapone) 123
Copaxone (glatiramer acetate) 149
Copolymer 1 (glatiramer acetate) 149
Cordilox (verapamil) 362
Cordrol (prednisone) 266
Coumadin (warfarin) 369
Covera-HS (verapamil) 362
Cuprimine (penicillamine) 248
cyclobenzaprine 78
cyclophosphamide 81
cyclosporine 84

Cymbalta (duloxetine) 113
cyproheptadine 87
Cypromar (cyproheptadine) 87
Cytoxan (cyclophosphamide) 81

Dantamacrin (dantrolene) 90
Dantrium (dantrolene) 90
Dantrolen (dantrolene) 90
dantrolene 90
Dazamide (acetazolamide) 1
Deltasone (prednisone) 266
Denzapine (clozapine) 75
Depacon (valproic acid) 353
Depakene (valproic acid) 353
Depakote (valproic acid) 353
Depakote ER (valproic acid) 353
Depen (penicillamine) 248
Deseril (methysergide) 212
DHE-45 (dihydroergotamine) 100
Dialar (diazepam) 96
3,4-diaminopyridine 93
Diamox (acetazolamide) 1
Diastat (diazepam) 96
Diazemuls (diazepam) 96
diazepam 96
Dicorate (valproic acid) 353
Dihydergot (dihydroergotamine) 100
dihydroergotamine (DHE) 100
Dilantin (phenytoin) 255
dipyridamole and aspirin 103
Disorate (valproic acid) 353
Divaa (valproic acid) 353
Divalpro (valproic acid) 353
Divalproex (valproic acid) 353
Dixarit (clonidine) 69
donepezil 107
Dozic (haloperidol) 158
droperidol 110
duloxetine 113
Duraclon (clonidine) 69
Dysport (botulinum toxin type A) 40

Ebixa (memantine) 197
Ecotrin (aspirin) 24
edrophonium 117
Efectin (venlafaxine) 358
Efexor (venlafaxine) 358
Effexor (venlafaxine) 358
Effexor XL (venlafaxine) 358
Effexor XR (venlafaxine) 358
Elatrol (amitriptyline) 14
Elavil (amitriptyline) 14
Eldepryl (selegiline) 322
eletriptan 120
Emeside (ethosuximide) 126
Empirin (aspirin) 24

Emsam (selegiline) 322
Emthexate (methotrexate) 205
Endep (amitriptyline) 14
Endoxan (cyclophosphamide) 81
Enlon (edrophonium) 117
Enlon-Plus (edrophonium) 117
entacapone 123
Epanutin (phenytoin) 255
Epilim (valproic acid) 353
Epimaz (carbamazepine) 51
Episenta (valproic acid) 353
Epitomax (topiramate) 342
Epival (valproic acid) 353
Equetro (carbamazepine) 51
Eskalith (lithium) 187
ethosuximide 126
Evacalm (diazepam) 96
Exelon (rivastigmine) 309
Extavia (interferon-beta) 173

felbamate 129
Felbatol (felbamate) 129
Fexmid (cyclobenzaprine) 78
Flebogamma (immune globulin intravenous) 165
Flexeril (cyclobenzaprine) 78
flunarizine 132
Fluox (fluoxetine) 135
fluoxetine 135
Formula Q (quinine sulfate) 293
Frova (frovatriptan) 139
frovatriptan 139

gabapentin 142
Gabarone (gabapentin) 142
Gabitril (tiagabine) 332
galantamine 146
Gammagard (immune globulin intravenous) 165
Gamunex (immune globulin intravenous) 165
Gengraf (cyclosporine) 84
glatiramer acetate 149
guanfacine 152
guanidine hydrochloride 155

Haldol (haloperidol) 158
Halfprin (aspirin) 24
haloperidol 158
Harmonyl (reserpine) 300
Heartline (aspirin) 24
Hep-lock (heparin) 161
heparin 161
Hepflush (heparin) 161

Imigran (sumatriptan) 326
Imitrex (sumatriptan) 326
immune globulin intravenous (IGIV) 165
Imuran (azathioprine) 28

Imurel (azathioprine) 28
Inapsine (droperidol) 110
Inderal (propranolol) 282
Inderal-LA (propranolol) 282
Indochron E-R (indomethacin) 169
Indocid (indomethacin) 169
Indocin (indomethacin) 169
Indocin-SR (indomethacin) 169
indomethacin 169
InnoPran XL (propranolol) 282
Inovelon (rufinamide) 319
interferon-beta 173
Intuniv (guanfacine) 152
Isoptin SR (verapamil) 362
Istalol (timolol) 335
Iveegam (immune globulin
    intravenous) 165

Jantoven (warfarin) 369

Keppra (levetiracetam) 184
Keppra XR (levetiracetam) 184
Kernstro (baclofen) 32
Ketipinor (quetiapine) 289
Klonopin (clonazepam) 65
Kopodex (levetiracetam) 184

lacosamide 177
Lamictal (lamotrigine) 180
Lamictin (lamotrigine) 180
lamotrigine 180
Laradopa (levodopa) 55
Largactil (chlorpromazine) 62
Laroxyl (amitriptyline) 14
Ledertrexate (methotrexate) 205
Legatrim (quinine sulfate) 293
Leponex (clozapine) 75
levetiracetam 184
levodopa see carbidopa/levodopa
Lioresal (baclofen) 32
Litarex (lithium) 187
Lithicarb (lithium) 187
lithium 187
Lithotab (lithium) 187
Lodosyn (carbidopa) 55
Luminal (phenobarbital) 251
Lyrica (pregabalin) 272

MabThera (rituximab) 306
Magnaprin (aspirin) 24
mannitol 191
Marevan (warfarin) 369
Maxalt (rizatriptan) 312
Maxolon (metoclopramide) 215
Maxtrex (methotrexate) 205
Mazepine (carbamazepine) 51

meclizine 194
memantine 197
Memorit (donepezil) 107
Mestinon (pyridostigmine) 286
Mestinon Timespan (pyridostigmine) 286
metaxalone 200
Methergine (methylergonovine) 209
methocarbamol 202
methotrexate 205
methylergonovine 209
methysergide 212
Meticorten (prednisone) 266
metoclopramide 215
Metoject (methotrexate) 205
Mexate (methotrexate) 205
mexiletine 218
Mexitil (mexiletine) 218
Migard (frovatriptan) 139
Migranal (dihydroergotamine) 100
Mirapex (pramipexole) 262
Mirapexin (pramipexole) 262
mitoxantrone 221
modafinil 224
Modiodal (modafinil) 224
MTX (methotrexate) 205
mycophenolate mofetil 228
Myfortic (mycophenolate mofetil) 228
Myobloc (botulinum toxin type B) 45
Mysoline (primidone) 275

Namenda (memantine) 197
naproxen
Naramig (naratriptan) 231
naratriptan 231
natalizumab 234
Neoral (cyclosporine) 84
Neosar (cyclophosphamide) 81
Neupentin (gabapentin) 142
Neurobloc (botulinum toxin type B) 45
Neuronox (botulinum toxin type A) 40
Neurontin (gabapentin) 142
Neurostil (gabapentin) 142
nimodipine 237
Nimotop (nimodipine) 237
Nitoman (tetrabenazine) 329
Norpress (nortriptyline) 240
Nortrilen (nortriptyline) 240
nortriptyline 240
Novantrone (mitoxantrone) 221
Novo-Carbamaz (carbamazepine) 51
Novo-Zolamide (acetazolamide) 1
Nuvigil (armodafinil) 21

Octagam (immune globulin intravenous) 165
Onabotulinumtoxin A (botulinum toxin type A) 32
Orasone (prednisone) 266

Osmitrol (mannitol) 191
oxcarbazepine 244

Pamelor (nortriptyline) 240
Panasol (prednisone) 266
Panglobulin (immune globulin intravenous) 165
Panwarfin (warfarin) 369
Parcopa (carbidopa/levodopa) 55
Parlodel (bromocriptine) 48
penicillamine 248
Periactin (cyproheptadine) 87
Periavit (cyproheptadine) 87
phenobarbital 251
Phenytek (phenytoin) 255
phenytoin 255
pizotifen 259
Plavix (clopidogrel) 72
Polygam (immune globulin intravenous) 165
pramipexole 262
Prednicot (prednisone) 266
prednisone 266
pregabalin 272
Priadel (lithium) 187
primidone 275
Privigen (immune globulin intravenous) 165
prochlorperazine 279
Procytox (cyclophosphamide) 81
Prometax (rivastigmine) 309
propranolol 282
Provigil (modafinil) 224
Prozac (fluoxetine) 135
pyridostigmine 286
Pyrohep (cyproheptadine) 87

Qualaquin (quinine sulfate) 293
quetiapine 289
Quilonum (lithium) 187
quinine sulfate 293

rasagiline 296
Razadyne (galantamine) 146
Rebif (interferon-beta) 173
Redomex (amitriptyline) 14
Reglan (metoclopramide) 215
Regonal (pyridostigmine) 286
Relert (eletriptan) 120
Relpax (eletriptan) 120
Reminyl (galantamine) 146
Requip (ropinirole) 315
reserpine 300
Reversol (edrophonium) 117
Revimmune (cyclophosphamide) 81
Rheumatrex (methotrexate) 205
Rilutek (riluzole) 303
riluzole 303
Rimabotulinum toxin B (botulinum toxin type B) 45

Rimapam (diazepam) 96
Rituxan (rituximab) 306
rituximab 306
rivastigmine 309
Rivotril (clonazepam) 65
rizatriptan 312
Robaxin (methocarbamol) 202
ropinirole 315
rufinamide 319

Sabril (vigabatrin) 366
Sandimmune (cyclosporine) 84
Sanoma (carisoprodol) 59
Sanomigran (pizotifen) 259
Sansert (methysergide) 212
Sarafem (fluoxetine) 135
Saroten (amitriptyline) 14
Securon (verapamil) 362
selegiline 322
Sensoval (nortriptyline) 240
Serenace (haloperidol) 158
Serocryptin (bromocriptine) 48
Seroquel (quetiapine) 289
Seroquel XR (quetiapine) 289
Sibelium (flunarizine) 132
Sinemet (carbidopa/levodopa) 55
Sirdalud (tizanidine) 339
Skelaxin (metaxalone) 200
Solis (diazepam) 96
Soma (carisoprodol) 59
Soval DX (valproic acid) 353
Stalevo (entacapone) 123
Stavzor (valproic acid) 353
Stemetil (prochlorperazine) 279
Sterapred (prednisone) 266
Stesolid (diazepam) 96
sumatriptan 326
sumatriptan/naproxen 326
Symbyax (fluoxetine) 135
Symmetrel (amantadine) 11
Syprine (trientine hydrochloride) 346

Taloxa (felbamate) 129
Tegretol (carbamazepine) 51
Tegretol XR (carbamazepine) 51
Tenex (guanfacine) 152
Tensilon (edrophonium) 117
Tensium (diazepam) 96
Teril (carbamazepine) 51
tetrabenazine 329
Thorazine (chlorpromazine) 62
tiagabine 332
timolol 335
Timonil (carbamazepine) 51
Timoptic (timolol) 335
tizanidine 339

Topamac (topiramate) 342
Topamax (topiramate) 342
topiramate 342
Trend XR (valproic acid) 353
Trepiline (amitriptyline) 14
Trevilor (venlafaxine) 358
Trexall (methotrexate) 205
Treximet (sumatriptan) 326
trientine hydrochloride 346
trihexyphenidyl 349
Trileptal (oxcarbazepine) 244
Triptafen (amitriptyline) 14
Triptyl (amitriptyline) 14
Tryptanol (amitriptyline) 14
Tryptizol (amitriptyline) 14
Tysabri (natalizumab) 234

Univer (verapamil) 362
Uprima (apomorphine) 18

Valclair (diazepam) 96
Valium (diazepam) 96
Valna (valproic acid) 353
valproic acid and derivatives (DPX) 353
Venla (venlafaxine) 358
venlafaxine 358
verapamil 362

Verapress (verapamil) 362
Verelan (verapamil) 362
Vertab (verapamil) 362
vigabatrin 366
Vimpat (lacosamide) 177
Vistabel (botulinum toxin type A) 40

warfarin 369
Warx (warfarin) 369

Xenazine (tetrabenazine) 329
Xeomin (botulinum toxin type A) 40
Xeristar (duloxetine) 113

Yentreve (duloxetine) 113

Zanaflex (tizanidine) 339
Zaponex (clozapine) 75
Zarontin (ethosuximide) 126
Zeegap (pregabalin) 272
Zelapar (selegiline) 322
zolmitriptan 373
Zomig MLT (zolmitriptan) 373
Zomig (zolmitriptan) 373
Zonegran (zonisamide) 376
zonisamide 376
ZORprin (aspirin) 24

Index by use

Drug names in **bold** are FDA approved

Achalasia
  botulinum toxin type A 40
Acromegaly
  bromocriptine 48
Acute coronary syndrome
  clopidogrel 72
Acute demyelinating encephalomyelitis
    (ADEM)
  immune globulin intravenous (IGIV) 165
  prednisone 266
Adrenoleukodystrophy
  immune globulin intravenous (IGIV) 165
Agoraphobia
  clonazepam 65
Akathisia
  propranolol 282
Alcohol dependence *see* Alcoholism
Alcohol withdrawal
  carbamazepine 51
  clonidine 69
  diazepam 96
  gabapentin 142
  guanfacine 152
  oxcarbazepine 244
  phenobarbital 251
  pregabalin 272
Alcoholism
  baclofen
  quetiapine 289
  topiramate 342
Allergic conditions
  prednisone 266
Allodynia
  gabapentin 142
Alternating hemiplegia of childhood
  flunarizine 132
Alzheimer's dementia (AD)
  donepezil 107
  galantamine 146
  immune globulin intravenous (IGIV) 165
  memantine 197
  rasagiline 296
  rivastigmine 309
  selegiline 322
Amyotrophic lateral sclerosis (ALS)
  immune globulin intravenous (IGIV) 165
  riluzole 303
Anemia
  cyclosporine 84
  prednisone 266
Anesthesia
  clonidine 69

Angina
  aspirin 24
  heparin 161
  propranolol 282
  timolol 335
  verapamil 362
Angioplasty
  aspirin 24
Ankylosing spondylitis
  indomethacin 169
Anxiety
  amitriptyline 14
  chlorpromazine 62
  diazepam 96
  nortriptyline 240
  phenobarbital 251
  pizotifen 259
  prochlorperazine 279
  quetiapine 289
  selegiline 322
  see also Generalized anxiety disorder (GAD)
Arthritic disorders
  amitriptyline 14
  aspirin 24
  indomethacin 169
  prednisone 266
  see also Osteoarthritis; Rheumatoid arthritis
Asthma
  prednisone 266
Atrial fibrillation
  clonidine 69
  heparin 161
  verapamil 362
  warfarin 369
Attention deficit hyperactivity disorder (ADHD)
  amantadine 11
  clonidine 69
  donepezil 107
  guanfacine 152
  memantine 197
  modafinil 224
  nortriptyline 240
  venlafaxine 358
Autism
  donepezil 107
  quetiapine 289

Back pain
  amitriptyline 14
  cyclobenzaprine 78
  nortriptyline 240
  tizanidine 339

Behavioral problems
  haloperidol 158
Bipolar depression
  fluoxetine 135
  lamotrigine 180
  lithium 187
  valproic acid 353
Bipolar disorder
  carbamazepine 51
  clozapine 75
  gabapentin 142
  haloperidol 158
  lamotrigine 180
  lithium 187
  oxcarbazepine 244
  pregabalin 272
  quetiapine 289
  topiramate 342
  valproic acid 353
  zonisamide 376
  see also Mania
Blepharospasm
  botulinum toxin type A 40
  botulinum toxin type B 45
Bone marrow transplantation
  cyclophosphamide 81
Breast cancer
  cyclophosphamide 81
  methotrexate 205
  mitoxantrone 221
Bulimia nervosa/binge eating
  amitriptyline 14
  fluoxetine 135
  memantine 197
  nortriptyline 240
  topiramate 342
  venlafaxine 358
  zonisamide 376
Burkitt's disease
  cyclophosphamide 81
Burning mouth syndrome
  clonazepam 65
Bursitis
  indomethacin 169
  prednisone 266

Carcinoid syndrome
  methysergide 212
Cardiac arrhythmias
  mexiletine 218
  phenytoin 255
  propranolol 282
  verapamil 362
Carotid endarterectomy
  aspirin 24
Central pontine myelinolysis

immune globulin intravenous (IGIV) 165
Central venous access device, restoration of function
  alteplase 8
Cerebral edema
  prednisone 266
Cerebral palsy
  botulinum toxin type A 40
  botulinum toxin type B 45
Cervical dystonia (CD)
  botulinum toxin type A 40
  botulinum toxin type B 45
Chorea
  baclofen 32
  reserpine 300
  tetrabenazine 300
Chronic inflammatory demyelinating
    polyneuropathy (CIDP)
  immune globulin intravenous (IGIV) 165
  prednisone 266
  rituximab 306
Chronic obstructive pulmonary disease
  prednisone 266
Churg-Strauss syndrome
  immune globulin intravenous (IGIV) 165
  mycophenolate mofetil 228
Clinically isolated syndromes (CIS)
  glatiramer acetate 149
  interferon-beta 173
Clotting prevention
  heparin 161
Coagulopathies
  heparin 161
Cognitive impairment
  donepezil 107
Congestive heart failure
  propranolol 282
  timolol 335
Coronary artery bypass graft (CABG)
  aspirin 24
Cosmesis
  botulinum toxin type A 40
Crohn's disease
  methotrexate 205
  natalizumab 234
  prednisone 266
Curare antagonism
  edrophonium 117
Cystinuria
  penicillamine 248

Deep vein thrombosis (DVT)
  heparin 161
  see also Thromboembolism
Dementia *see* Alzheimer's dementia (AD); Dementia
  with Lewy bodies (DLB); HIV dementia;
  Vascular dementia

Dementia with Lewy bodies (DLB)
  clozapine 75
  donepezil 107
  galantamine 146
  memantine 197
  quetiapine 289
  rivastigmine 309
Depression
  amitriptyline 14
  duloxetine 113
  fluoxetine 135
  lithium 187
  modafinil 224
  nortriptyline 240
  quetiapine
  selegiline 322
  venlafaxine 358
Dermatomyositis (DM)
  azathioprine 28
  cyclophosphamide 81
  immune globulin intravenous
    (IGIV) 165
  methotrexate 205
  prednisone 266
  rituximab 306
Detrusor sphincter dyssynergia
  botulinum toxin type A 40
Diabetic amyotrophy
  immune globulin intravenous (IGIV) 165
Diabetic gastroparesis
  metoclopramide 215
Diabetic neuropathy
  amitriptyline 14
  botulinum toxin type A 40
  duloxetine 113
  nortriptyline 240
  pregabalin 272
  venlafaxine 358
Diarrhea
  methysergide 212
Diuresis
  mannitol 191
Drug dependence
  vigabatrin 366
Drug withdrawal
  diazepam 96
  gabapentin 142
  phenobarbital 251
  pregabalin 272
Duchenne muscular dystrophy (DMD)
  prednisone 266
Dupuytren's disease
  verapamil 362
Dyskinesias
  reserpine 300
  tetrabenazine 329

Dystonias
  benztropine 36
  botulinum toxin type A 40
  botulinum toxin type B 45
  carbidopa/levodopa 55
  diazepam 96
  reserpine 300
  tetrabenazine 329
  trihexyphenidyl 349

Edema
  acetazolamide 1
  prednisone 266
Epidermoid cancer
  methotrexate 205
Epilepsy
  acetazolamide 1
  carbamazepine 51
  clonazepam 65
  ethosuximide 126
  flunarizine 132
  immune globulin intravenous
    (IGIV) 165
  lamotrigine 180
  levetiracetam 184
  oxcarbazepine 244
  tiagabine 332
  valproic acid 353
  vigabatrin 366
  zonisamide 376
  see also Seizures
Episodic ataxias
  acetazolamide 1
Essential tremor
  primidone 275
  propranolol 282
  topiramate 342
Extrapyramidal disorders
  amantadine 11
  benztropine 36
  trihexyphenidyl 349

Fatigue
  modafinil 224
  see also Sleepiness, excessive
Fever
  aspirin 24
Fibromyalgia
  amitriptyline 14
  cyclobenzaprine 78
  duloxetine 113
  gabapentin 142
  nortriptyline 240
  pramipexole 262
  pregabalin 272
  venlafaxine 358

Gastroesophageal reflux
  metoclopramide 215
Generalized anxiety disorder (GAD)
  clonazepam 65
  duloxetine 113
  fluoxetine 135
  gabapentin 142
  pregabalin 272
  propranolol 282
  venlafaxine 358
  see also Anxiety
Gestational choriocarcinoma
  methotrexate 205
Gilles de la Tourette syndrome (GTS)
  clonidine 69
  guanfacine 152
  haloperidol 158
  metoclopramide 215
  reserpine 300
  tetrabenazine 329
Glabellar lines
  botulinum toxin type A 40
  botulinum toxin type B 45
Glaucoma
  acetazolamide 1
  timolol 335
Glossopharyngeal neuralgia
  carbamazepine 51
  phenytoin 255
Graves ophthalmopathy
  prednisone 266
Growth delay
  clonidine 69
Guillain Barre syndrome (GBS)
  immune globulin intravenous (IGIV) 165

Headache
  amitriptyline 14
  aspirin 24
  botulinum toxin type A 40
  botulinum toxin type B 45
  cyproheptadine 87
  dihydroergotamine (DHE) 100
  duloxetine 113
  fluoxetine 135
  haloperidol 158
  indomethacin 169
  levetiracetam 184
  lithium 187
  methylergonovine 209
  methysergide 212
  mexiletine 218
  nortriptyline 240
  pizotifen 259
  prednisone 266
  sumatriptan 326

topiramate 342
valproic acid 353
venlafaxine 358
verapamil 362
zolmitriptan 373
see also Migraine
Heart failure
  acetazolamide 1
Heat stroke
  dantrolene 90
Hemiballism
  reserpine 300
  tetrabenazine 329
Hemicrania
  indomethacin 169
Hemifacial spasm
  botulinum toxin type A 40
  botulinum toxin type B 45
Hiccups
  chlorpromazine 62
HIV
  immune globulin intravenous (IGIV) 165
HIV dementia
  donepezil 107
  memantine 197
Hodgkin's disease
  cyclophosphamide 81
Hot flashes
  fluoxetine 135
  venlafaxine 358
Human T-cell lymphotrophic virus-1 (HTLV-1)
    infection
  immune globulin intravenous (IGIV) 165
Huntington's disease
  baclofen 32
  reserpine 300
  tetrabenazine 329
Hyperactivity
  chlorpromazine 62
  haloperidol 158
Hyperalgesia
  gabapentin 142
Hyperhidrosis
  botulinim toxin type B 45
  botulinum toxin type A 40
  clonidine 69
Hyperprolactinemia
  bromocriptine 48
Hypersensitivity reactions
  cyproheptadine 87
  prednisone 266
Hypertension
  clonidine 69
  guanfacine 152
  nimodipine 237
  propranolol 282

reserpine 300
tetrabenazine 329
timolol 335
verapamil 362
Hyperthyroidism
propranolol 282
Hypertrophic subaortic stenosis
propranolol 282

Idiopathic thrombocytopenic purpura
immune globulin intravenous (IGIV) 165
prednisone 266
Immunodeficiency
immune globulin intravenous (IGIV) 165
Incontinence
botulinum toxin type A 40
duloxetine 113
venlafaxine 358
Infantile spasms
felbamate 129
valproic acid 353
vigabatrin 366
zonisamide 376
Inflammatory myopathies
azathioprine 28
immune globulin intravenous (IGIV) 165
methotrexate 205
prednisone 266
Influenza-A
amantadine 11
Insomnia
amitriptyline 14
carisoprodol 59
clonazepam 65
clonidine 69
diazepam 96
gabapentin 142
nortriptyline 240
quetiapine 289
venlafaxine 358
Intracranial hypertension
acetazolamide 1
mannitol 191
prednisone 266
topiramate 342
Intraoccular pressure reduction
mannitol 191
timolol 335
Irritable bowel syndrome
diazepam 96

Junctional epidermolysis bullosa
phenytoin 255

Kawasaki syndrome
immune globulin intravenous (IGIV) 165

Lambert-Eaton myasthenic syndrome (LEMS)
3,4-diaminopyridine 93
guanidine hydrochloride 155
Landau-Kleffner syndrome
valproic acid 353
Leg cramps
quinine sulfate 293
Lennox-Gastaut syndrome
carbamazepine 51
clonazepam 65
felbamate 129
immune globulin intravenous (IGIV) 165
lamotrigine 180
rufinamide 319
topiramate 342
valproic acid 353
zonisamide 376
Leukemia
cyclosporine 84
immune globulin intravenous (IGIV) 165
mitoxantrone 221
prednisone 266
rituximab 306
Long QT syndrome
primidone 275
Lung cancer
methotrexate 205
Lupus nephritis
mycophenolate mofetil 228
Lymphoma
cyclophosphamide 81
methotrexate 205
mitoxantrone 221
prednisone 266
rituximab 306

Major depressive disorder (MDD) *see* Depression
Malaria
quinine sulfate 293
Malignancies
cyclophosphamide 81
methotrexate 205
Malignant hyperthermia (MT)
dantrolene 90
Mania
chlorpromazine 62
clonazepam 65
diazepam 96
levetiracetam 184
lithium 187
pregabalin 272
prochlorperazine 279
valproic acid 353
see also Bipolar disorder
Marfan syndrome
acetazolamide 1

Menopausal symptoms
  clonidine 69
  venlafaxine 358
Menstrual pain
  aspirin 24
Migraine
  acetazolamide 1
  almotriptan 5
  amitriptyline 14
  baclofen 32
  chlorpromazine 62
  cyproheptadine 87
  dihydroergotamine (DHE) 100
  droperidol 110
  duloxetine 113
  eletriptan 120
  flunarizine 132
  fluoxetine 135
  frovatriptan 139
  gabapentin 142
  indomethacin 169
  lamotrigine 180
  memantine 197
  methylergonovine 209
  methysergide 212
  metoclopramide 215
  naratriptan 231
  nortriptyline 240
  phenytoin 255
  pizotifen 259
  prednisone 266
  pregabalin 272
  prochlorperazine 279
  propranolol 282
  rizatriptan 312
  selegiline 322
  sumatriptan 326
  timolol 335
  tizanidine 339
  topiramate 342
  valproic acid 353
  venlafaxine 358
  verapamil 362
  zolmitriptan 373
  zonisamide 376
Motion sickness
  meclizine 194
Mountain sickness
  acetazolamide 1
Multiple sclerosis (MS)
  amantadine 11
  azathioprine 28
  baclofen 32
  cyclophosphamide 81
  3,4-diaminopyridine 93
  glatiramer acetate 149

  immune globulin intravenous (IGIV) 165
  interferon-beta 173
  methotrexate 205
  mitoxantrone 221
  modafinil 224
  natalizumab 234
  prednisone 266
  rituximab 306
Muscle relaxant reversal
  pyridostigmine 286
Muscle relaxation
  diazepam 96
Muscle spasm
  carisoprodol 59
  cyclobenzaprine 78
  methocarbamol 202
Myasthenia gravis (MG)
  azathioprine 28
  cyclophosphamide 81
  cyclosporine 84
  3,4-diaminopyridine 93
  edrophonium 117
  guanidine hydrochloride 155
  immune globulin intravenous (IGIV) 165
  mycophenolate mofetil 228
  prednisone 266
  pyridostigmine 286
  rituximab 306
Mycosis fungoides
  cyclophosphamide 81
Myocardial infarction (MI)
  alteplase 8
  aspirin 24
  clopidogrel 72
  heparin 161
  propranolol 282
  timolol 335
  warfarin 369
Myoclonus
  reserpine 300
  rituximab 306
  tetrabenazine 329
  valproic acid 353
  see also Epilepsy; Seizures
Myotonia
  mexiletine 218
  phenytoin 255
  quinine sulfate 293

Narcolepsy
  armodafinil 21
  modafinil 224
Nausea and vomiting
  chlorpromazine 62
  diazepam 96
  droperidol 110

haloperidol 158
metoclopramide 215
prochlorperazine 279
Neck pain
amitriptyline 14
cyclobenzaprine 78
nortriptyline 240
tizanidine 339
Nephrotic syndrome
cyclophosphamide 81
prednisone 266
Neuroblastoma
cyclophosphamide 81
Neuroleptic malignant syndrome
dantrolene 90
Neuromyelitis optica
azathioprine 28
rituximab 306
Neuropathies
amitryiptyline 14
botulinum toxin type A 40
cyclophosphamide 81
duloxetine 113
fluoxetine 135
guanfacine 152
immune globulin intravenous (IGIV) 165
lacosamide 177
levetiracetam 184
memantine 197
mexiletine 218
nortriptyline 240
oxcarbazepine 244
pregabalin 272
rituximab 306
venlafaxine 358
zonisamide 376
Nightmares
cyproheptadine 87
Nocturnal enuresis
amitriptyline 14
Non-Hodgkin lymphoma
methotrexate 205
mitoxantrone 221
rituximab 306
Nystagmus
baclofen 32
botulinum toxin type A 40

Obesity
topiramate 342
zonisamide 376
Obsessive compulsive disorder
fluoxetine 135
quetiapine 289
Obstructive sleep apnea (OSA)/hypopnea
syndrome

armodafinil 21
modafinil 224
Opioid detoxification
clonidine 69
guanfacine 152
Optic neuritis
immune globulin intravenous (IGIV) 165
prednisone 266
Organ transplantation
azathioprine 28
cyclosporine 84
immune globulin intravenous (IGIV) 165
mycophenolate mofetil 228
Oscillopsia
botulinum toxin type A 40
Osteoarthritis
aspirin 24
indomethacin 169
Ovarian adenocarcinoma
cyclophosphamide 81

Pain relief
amitriptyline 14
aspirin 24
baclofen 32
botulinum toxin type A 40
botulinum toxin type B 45
carbamazepine 51
carisoprodol 59
clonidine 69
cyclobenzaprine 78
dantrolene 90
duloxetine 113
fluoxetine 135
gabapentin 142
guanfacine 152
indomethacin 169
lacosamide 177
memantine 197
metaxalone 200
methocarbamol 202
mexiletine 218
nortriptyline 240
oxcarbazepine 244
pregabalin 272
tizanidine 339
venlafaxine 358
zonisamide 376
see also Headache
Panic disorder
clonazepam 65
diazepam 96
fluoxetine 135
pregabalin 272
tiagabine 332
venlafaxine 358

Paraneoplastic syndromes
  immune globulin intravenous (IGIV) 165
Parkinsonian dysarthria
  clonazepam 65
Parkinsonian tremor
  propranolol 282
Parkinsonism
  amantadine 11
  benztropine 36
  entacapone 123
  trihexyphenidyl 349
Parkinson's disease (PD)
  amantadine 11
  apomorphine 18
  bromocriptine 48
  carbidopa/levodopa 55
  clozapine 75
  entacapone 123
  pramipexole 262
  quetiapine 289
  rasagiline 296
  rivastigmine 309
  ropinirole 315
  selegiline 322
  zonisamide 376
Periodic leg movements disorder (PLMD)
  clonazepam 65
Peripheral arterial disease
  clopidogrel 72
Peyronie's disease
  verapamil 362
Phantom limb pain
  amitriptyline 14
  nortriptyline 240
Pheochromocytoma
  propranolol 282
Plantar fibromatosis
  verapamil 362
Pleurisy
  aspirin 24
Polyarteritis nodosa
  cyclophosphamide 81
Polymyositis (PM)
  azathioprine 28
  cyclophosphamide 81
  immune globulin intravenous (IGIV) 165
  methotrexate 205
  prednisone 266
Porphyria
  chlorpromazine 62
Post-herpetic neuralgia
  amitriptyline 14
  gabapentin 142
  nortriptyline 240
  pregabalin 272
Post-traumatic stress disorder

cyproheptadine 87
fluoxetine 135
guanfacine 152
propranolol 282
venlafaxine 358
Preeclampsia
  diazepam 96
  phenytoin 255
Premature labor prevention
  indomethacin 169
Premenstrual dysphoric disorder
  fluoxetine 135
Preoperative medication
  diazepam 96
Prostate cancer
  mitoxantrone 221
Pseudobulbar affect
  amitriptyline 14
Psoriasis
  cyclosporine 84
  methotrexate 205
  mycophenolate mofetil 228
Psychosis
  carbamazepine 51
  chlorpromazine 62
  clozapine 75
  haloperidol 158
  lamotrigine 180
  primidone 275
  quetiapine 289
  reserpine 300
  tetrabenazine 329
  valproic acid 353
Pulmonary embolism (PE)
  alteplase 8
  heparin 161
  warfarin 369

Raynaud phenomenon
  fluoxetine 135
Restless legs syndrome (RLS)
  carbamazepine 51
  carbidopa/levodopa 55
  clonazepam 65
  clonidine 69
  pramipexole 262
  ropinirole 315
Revascularization procedures
  aspirin 24
Reversible cerebral vasoconstrictive syndromes
  nimodipine 237
Rheumatoid arthritis
  aspirin 24
  azathioprine 28
  cyclophosphamide 81
  cyclosporine 84

indomethacin 169
methotrexate 205
penicillamine 248
prednisone 266
rituximab 306

Sarcoidosis
  rituximab 306
Schizoaffective disorder
  clozapine 75
Schizophrenia
  carbamazepine 51
  chlorpromazine 62
  clonazepam 65
  clozapine 75
  haloperidol 158
  lamotrigine 180
  prochlorperazine 279
  quetiapine 289
  valproic acid 353
Sedation
  phenobarbital 251
Seizures
  carbamazepine 51
  clonazepam 65
  diazepam 96
  felbamate 129
  gabapentin 142
  lacosamide 177
  lamotrigine 180
  levetiracetam 184
  oxcarbazepine 244
  phenobarbital 251
  phenytoin 255
  pregabalin 272
  primidone 275
  rufinamide 319
  tiagabine 332
  topiramate 342
  valproic acid 353
  vigabatrin 366
  zonisamide 376
  see also Epilepsy
Serotonin syndrome
  pizotifen 259
Sexual dysfunction
  amantadine 11
Sialorrhea
  botulinum toxin type A 40
  botulinum toxin type B 45
Sleep apnea
  acetazolamide 1
  armodafinil 21
Sleepiness, excessive
  armodafinil 21
  modafinil 224

Small bowel intubation
  metoclopramide 215
Smoking cessation
  nortriptyline 240
Social phobia
  pizotifen 259
  venlafaxine 358
Spasmodic dysphonia
  botulinum toxin type A 40
  botulinum toxin type B 45
Spasmodic torticollis
  botulinum toxin type A 40
  botulinum toxin type B 45
Spasticity
  baclofen 32
  botulinum toxin type A 40
  botulinum toxin type B 45
  dantrolene 90
  diazepam 96
  metaxalone 200
  tizanidine 339
Spinal cord diseases
  baclofen 32
Spinal muscular atrophy
  valproic acid 353
Spondyloarthropathies
  aspirin 24
Status epilepticus
  diazepam 96
  levetiracetam 184
  phenobarbital 251
  phenytoin 255
  valproic acid 353
Stiff person syndrome
  diazepam 96
  immune globulin intravenous
    (IGIV) 165
Strabismus
  botulinum toxin type A 40
  botulinum toxin type B 45
Stroke
  alteplase 8
  aspirin 24
  clopidogrel 72
  dipyridamole and aspirin 103
  heparin 161
Subarachnoid hemorrhage (SAH)
  flunarizine 132
  nimodipine 237
Suicidal behaviour
  clozapine 75
SUNCT
  lamotrigine 180
Systemic lupus erythematosus (SLE)
  aspirin 24
  cyclophosphamide 81

Systemic lupus (cont.)
  methotrexate 205
  prednisone 266

Tardive dyskinesias
  baclofen 32
Temporal arteritis (TA)
  prednisone 266
Temporomandibular joint dysfunction
  botulinum toxin type A 40
Tendinitis
  indomethacin 169
Tension-type headache
  amitriptyline 14
  cyproheptadine 87
  duloxetine 113
  indomethacin 169
  nortriptyline 240
Tetanus
  chlorpromazine 62
  diazepam 96
Tetralogy of Fallot
  propranolol 282
Thrombocytopenic purpura
  rituximab 306
  see also Idiopathic thrombocytopenic
    purpura
Thromboembolism
  dipyridamole and aspirin 103
  heparin 161
  warfarin 369
Tics
  botulinum toxin type A 40
  carbamazepine 51
  clonidine 69
  guanfacine 152
  haloperidol 158
  metoclopramide 215
  reserpine 300
  tetrabenazine 329
Tinnitus
  flunarizine 132
Toothache
  aspirin 24
Tourette's syndrome
  baclofen 32
  flunarizine 132
  quetiapine 289
Toxemia of pregnancy
  aspirin 24
Transient ischemic attack (TIA)
  aspirin 24
  dipyridamole and aspirin 103
Traumatic brain injury
  amantadine 11

nimodipine 237
Trigeminal neuralgia
  baclofen 32
  carbamazepine 51
  lamotrigine 180
  oxcarbazepine 244
  phenytoin 255
Tuberculous meningitis
  prednisone 266

Ulcerative colitis
  clonidine 69
  cyclosporine 84
  methotrexate 205
  prednisone 266
Urologic irrigation
  mannitol 191
Uterine contractions/bleeding after
    delivery
  methylergonovine 209
Uveitis
  mycophenolate mofetil 228

Variceal bleeding prevention
  propranolol 282
  timolol 335
Vascular dementia
  donepezil 107
  galantamine 146
  memantine 197
  rivastigmine 309
Vasculitis
  cyclophosphamide 81
  methotrexate 205
Vasospasm
  flunarizine 132
  nimodipine 237
Venous thrombosis
  warfarin 369
Vertigo
  diazepam 96
  flunarizine 132
  meclizine 194
  prochlorperazine 279
Vomiting see Nausea and vomiting

Waldenstrom macroglobulinemia
  rituximab 306
Wegener's granulomatosis
  cyclophosphamide 81
  immune globulin intravenous
    (IGIV) 165
  methotrexate 205
West syndrome
  felbamate 129

immune globulin intravenous (IGIV) 165
valproic acid 353
vigabatrin 366
zonisamide 376
Wilson's disease

penicillamine 248
trientine hydrochloride 346
Writer's cramp
  botulinum toxin type A 40
  botulinum toxin type B 45

Index by class

Alpha-2 agonists
  clonidine
  guanfacine
  tizanidine
Antiadrenergics
  clonidine 69
  guanfacine 152
  reserpine 300
  tetrabenazine 329
Antiarrhythmics
  mexiletine 218
Anticholinergics
  benztropine
  trihexyphenidyl
Anticoagulants
  heparin 161
  warfarin 369
Anticonvulsants *see* Antiepileptic
  drugs (AED)
Antidepressants
  amitriptyline 14
  duloxetine 113
  fluoxetine 135
  notriptyline 240
  venlafaxine 358
Antidopaminergics
  tetrabenazine 329
Antiemetics
  chlorpromazine 62
  droperidol 110
  meclizine 194
  metoclopramide 215
  prochlorperazine 279
Antiepileptic drugs (AED)
  acetazolamide 1
  carbamazepine 51
  clonazepam 65
  diazepam 96
  ethosuximide 126
  gabapentin 142
  lacosamide 177
  lamogrigine 180
  levetiracetam 184
  oxcarbazepine 244
  phenobarbital 251
  phenytoin 255
  pregabalin 272
  primidone 275
  rufinamide 319
  tiagabine 332
  topiramate 342
  valproic acid 353

  vigabatrin 366
  zonisamide 376
Antihistamines
  cyproheptadine 87
  flunarizine 132
  meclizine
  pizotifen 259
Antihypertensives
  flunarizine 132
  propranolol 282
  timolol 335
  verapamil 362
Anti-inflammatory agents
  aspirin 24
  indomethacin 169
Antimalarials
  quinine sulfate 293
Antineoplastic agents
  mitoxantrone 221
Antiparkinson agents
  amantadine 11
  apomorphine
  benztropine 36
  bromocriptine
  carbidopa/levodopa 55
  entacapone 123
  pramipexole
  ropinirole
  trihexyphenidyl 349
Antiplatelet agents
  aspirin 24
  clopidogrel 72
  dipyridamole and aspirin 103
Antipsychotics
  chlorpromazine 62
  clozapine 75
  droperidol
  haloperidol 158
  metoclopramide
  prochlorperazine 279
  quetiapine 289

Barbiturates
  phenobarbital 251
Benzodiazepines
  clonazepam 65
  diazepam 96
Beta-blockers
  propranolol 282
  timolol 335

Calcium channel blockers
  flunarizine 132

Calcium channel (cont.)
  nimodipine 237
  verapamil 362
Carbonic anhydrase inhibitors
  acetazolamide 1
Chelating agents
  penicillamine
  trientine hydrochloride 346
Cholinergic agonists
  3,4-diaminopyridine 93
  guanidine hydrochloride 155
Cholinesterase inhibitors
  donepezil 107
  edrophonium 117
  galantamine 146
  pyridostigmine 286
  rivastigmine 309
Cystine-depleting agents
  penicillamine 248

Diuretics
  mannitol 191
Dopamine agonists
  apomorphine 18
  bromocriptine 48
  pramipexole 262
  ropinirole 315

Ergots
  bromocriptine 48
  dihydroergotamine (DHE) 100
  methylergonovine 209
  methysergide 212

Folic acid antagonists
  methotrexate 205

GI stimulants
  metoclopramide 215
Glucocorticoids
  prednisone 266

Immune globulins
  immune globulin intravenous
    (IGIV) 165
Immunomodulators
  azathioprine
  cyclophosphamide
  cyclosporine
  glatiramer acetate
  immune globulin intravenous (IGIV)
  interferon-beta 173
  methotrexate
  mitoxantrone
  mycophenolate mofetil
  natalizumab

prednisone
rituximab
Immunosuppressants
  azathioprine 28
  cyclophosphamide 81
  cyclosporine 84
  glatiramer acetate 149
  mycophenolate mofetil 228
  natalizumab 234
  rituximab 306

Migraine preventatives
  methylergonovine 209
  methysergide 212
Monamine oxidase type B
    (MAO-B)
  inhibitors
  rasagiline 296
  selegiline 322
Monoclonal antibodies
  rituximab 306
Mood stabilizers
  lithium 187
Muscle relaxants
  baclofen 32
  carisoprodol 59
  cyclobenzaprine 78
  dantrolene 90
  metaxalone 200
  methocarbamol 202
  tizanidine 339

Neuromuscular drugs
  dantrolene
  3,4-diaminopyridine
  guanidine hydrochloride
  quinine sulfate 293
  riluzole 303
Neurotoxins
  botulinum toxin type A 40
  botulinum toxin type B 45
NMDA receptor antagonists
  memantine 197
Non-steroidal anti-inflammatory drugs
    (NSAIDs)
  aspirin 24
  indomethacin 169

Osmotic diuretics
  mannitol

Potassium channel blockers
  3,4-diaminopyridine 93
Psychostimulants
  armodafinil
  modafinil

Selective serotonin reuptake inhibitors
(SSRI)
fluoxetine 135
Serotonin and norepinephrine reuptake inhibitors
(SNRI)
duloxetine 113
venlafaxine 358
Skeletal muscle relaxants *see* Muscle relaxants
Sulfonamides
zonisamide 376
Synaptic vesicle blockers
reserpine
tetrabenazine

Thrombolytic agents
alteplase agents
Tissue plasminogen activators (TPA)
alteplase 8

Tricyclic antidepressants (TCA)
amitriptyline 14
nortriptyline 240
Triptans
almotriptan 5
eletriptan 120
frovatriptan 139
naratriptan 231
rizatriptan 312
sumatriptan 326
zolmitriptan 373

Vestibular suppressants
meclizine 194

Wake-promoting agents
armodafinil 21
modafinil 224